COMPENDIUM OF THE EPILEPSIES

COMPENDIUM OF THE EPILEPSIES

By

ERNST NIEDERMEYER, M.D.

Electroencephalographer-in-Charge
The Johns Hopkins Hospital
Associate Professor
Department of Neurological Surgery
Department of Neurology
The Johns Hopkins University School of Medicine
Baltimore, Maryland

THOMAS BOOKS SYMBOL OF LEADERSHIP

CHARLES C THOMAS · PUBLISHER

Springfield · Illinois · U.S.A.

Published and Distributed Throughout the World by
CHARLES C THOMAS • PUBLISHER
BANNERSTONE HOUSE
301-327 East Lawrence Avenue, Springfield, Illinois, U.S.A.

ISBN 0-398-02878-8
Library of Congress Catalog Card Number: 73-6563

With THOMAS BOOKS *careful attention is given to all details of manufacturing and design. It is the Publisher's desire to present books that are satisfactory as to their physical qualities and artistic possibilities and appropriate for their particular use.* THOMAS BOOKS *will be true to those laws of quality that assure a good name and good will.*

Printed in the United States of America
N-1

Library of Congress Cataloging in Publication Data

Niedermeyer, Ernst, 1920-
Compendium of the epilepsies.

Bibliography: p.
1. Epilepsy. I. Title. [DNLM: 1. Epilepsy. WL 385 N666c 1973]
RC372.N53 616.8'53 73-6563
ISBN 0-398-02878-8

To my wife

ANNIE

PREFACE

THIS CONDENSED TEXTBOOK of Epileptology attempts to unfold a pluralistic picture of the epileptic manifestations and conditions. The phenomena are determined by biochemical and neurophysiological events and these facets of the seizure disorder must be understood in the light of modern advances of the basic sciences. What makes these epileptic events possible, however, is a wide variety of disease processes and dysfunctions; their knowledge is of utmost significance in clinical diagnosis and therapy. Both the basic science and the clinical viewpoint must be encompassed in a textbook-like presentation of the epilepsies.

This book has been written *for the clinician* and, for this reason, greater emphasis has been placed on the clinical segment. One is inclined to add that the clinical aspects of the epilepsies are less troubled by scientific controversies than the data provided by the basic sciences but this statement could be unwise and proven false in future years. The aim of this book is to provide clinicians of various specialties, general practitioners and medical students with helpful information about diagnosis and treatment of epileptic disorders. This goal, of course, cannot be reached without giving at least a very short outline of the abnormal physiology; its brevity, however, does not indicate a diminished emphasis on this area.

Much of the author's daily work is devoted to clinical electroencephalography but it has been his intention not to overstress this important diagnostic segment. Nevertheless, the reader will find a fairly large number of electroencephalographic tracings among the illustrations. The reason for the use of these text figures lies in the fact that some crucial characteristics of epileptic conditions are convincingly documented in the EEG whereas the pictorial demonstration of clinical seizures is limited by their rapid fluctuations and requires the use of cinematographic technique.

The large dimension of the therapeutic chapter indicates the importance of a sound active approach which, unfortunately, has its limitations, too. Human suffering always comprises interactions between patient and society and this is particularly true for the sufferer from seizures. The last two chapters of this book should convey the message that the treatment of epileptic seizures is not confined to writing prescriptions and must include an appraisal of the patient's personality and his human interrelations.

This book contains no historical introduction. The completeness of Owsei Temkin's "The falling sickness" (2nd ed., 1972) and the awesome achievements of this investigator discourage the amateur medico-historian from writing a poor surrogate.

ERNST NIEDERMEYER

INTRODUCTION

EPILEPTIC MANIFESTATIONS ARE abnormal reactions of the brain caused by a large number of diseases. These reactions either involve the brain in an almost global manner or the disturbance is confined to certain cerebral regions. The basic disorder may be located within the brain or the failure of other organs may give rise to secondary encephalopathies. In all these epileptic conditions, the role of genetic factors and individual predisposition to seizures may play a certain part. Epileptic phenomena cut across vast areas of the entire domain of medicine and, for this reason, the physician should be familiar with various facets of seizure disorders.

There has been a cloud of fear, superstition and prejudice around the epilepsies which, for many centuries, even pervaded the medical profession. Modern neurophysiology and clinical observation have lifted these shrouds of ignorance although basic processes in the generation of seizures and especially the role of genetic factors are still very poorly understood. Unfortunately, in spite of a growing bulk of sober knowledge, sufferers from rather mild epileptic seizure disorders are still bearers of a stigma which society has attached to them. The medical profession has not made all of the necessary efforts to help dispelling the last fragments of prejudice in order to make the occasional occurrence of seizures a socially acceptable event and to teach the public that one is dealing with a cerebral reaction, which theoretically could befall anyone.

Great epileptologists of the past few decades have aimed at a deeper comprehension of the epileptic conditions and propagated new insights to their confreres. We find in these ranks the late William G. Lennox, the philanthropic clinician, and Frederic A. Gibbs, the father of epileptological electroencephalography which technique has opened the eyes for the understanding of the basic electrophysiology in epileptic processes. The combined neurosurgical and neurophysiological approach to the seizure disorders by Wilder Penfield in Montreal and A. Earl Walker in Baltimore has shed further light on the epilepsies. Outside the North American continent, the astute clinical and electroencephalographic observations of Henri Gastaut in France have led clinical epileptology to further progress. The work of these great leaders and the contributions made by a host of investigators in the basic sciences (especially Herbert H. Jasper, Fréderic Brémer, Richard Jung, Sir John Eccles and Giuseppe Moruzzi) have built the platform on which present and future work can be done.

ERNST NIEDERMEYER

ACKNOWLEDGMENTS

THIS BOOK IS THE product of more than 20 years of intensive work with epileptic patients in clinics, on neurological wards and in the EEG laboratory. It started in the University Hospital Innsbruck (Austria) and was continued from 1960 to 1965 (with almost exclusive emphasis on electroencephalography) at the Medical Center of the University of Iowa in Iowa City. Most of this work, however, was conceived and carried out at the Johns Hopkins Hospital (EEG laboratory, Neurology Outpatient Clinic). The unusually stimulating atmosphere of this Medical Center has been perhaps the most productive catalyst for this work. A warm and close collaboration with my colleagues of the Departments of Neurology, Pediatrics and Internal Medicine has proved to be extremely fruitful; this is also true for the adjacent John F. Kennedy Institute for Habilitation of the Mentally and Physically Handicapped Child. Many severe cases of seizure disorder were referred by the Division of Neurological Surgery and a sizeable number of these patients were studied with implanted depth EEG electrodes. The surgical therapy was usually performed with the aid of electrocorticographic recordings. I am particularly grateful for the opportunity of using electroencephalographic techniques in this type of neurosurgical team work.

If one name has to be singled out among those who helped me to develop a fairly global picture of Epileptology, it would be that of Dr. A. Earl Walker, Professor emeritus of Neurological Surgery at the Johns Hopkins University School of Medicine. When I associate his name with "depth," this word does not solely pertain to the anatomical third dimension explored by special electrodes (which technique he introduced to me); it rather means depth of insight. His constant struggle for a universal comprehension of the neurological sciences (reaching far beyond his neurosurgical specialty) has taught me unforgettable lessons

In this context, I express my special gratitude for the kind permission to use his beautiful pictorial demonstration of temporal lobectomy.

Dr. Lee Neidengard's kind assistance was instrumental in many respects.

My co-workers in the EEG laboratory have been extremely helpful in this work; Mrs. Anna Maria Zobniw, R. EEG T.; Mrs. Marie Faircloth, R. EEG T.; Mrs. Rose Burnite, R. EEG T., and Mrs. Carrie Lou Gerdom deserve particular praise . The secretarial help of Mrs. Kathy Rogers, Mrs. Mary Dembeck and Miss Joann Devanko is also gratefully acknowledged. Most of the pictorial work and the graphs have been carried out by Miss Barbara Grossmann.

This book has been financially supported by a grant from the Hoffmann-LaRoche Inc., Nutley, New Jersey. When I extend my special thanks to this company and especially to Dr. Harrison M. Langrall and his understanding attitude, I can gratefully add that not the slightest strings were ever attached to this support and that everything could be written in full scientific freedom. Earlier work for this book had been supported by a research grant of the National Institute of Health (M. 556, 084).

E. N.

CONTENTS

COMPENDIUM OF THE EPILEPSIES

Chapter 1

BASIC CONSIDERATIONS OF EPILEPTIC MECHANISMS

1) Introductory remarks

THE SEARCH FOR THE origin of epileptic activity has led to a thorough study of various cerebral structures and their modifying role in the type of clinical seizure manifestations. More recent neurophysiological techniques have yielded some insight into the electrophysiology of single neurons and their behavior during epileptic activity. There is good evidence that the recorded seizure discharge is nothing but an epiphenomenon of a primary biochemical disturbance.

Clinical neurologists have witnessed the shift of emphasis from the outward clinical sign to associated alterations of cerebral structures in all areas of Neurology. The focus of interest has shifted further from cerebral macromorphology to microstructures and thence into the world of ultramicromorphology and molecular biology. Many investigators feel that the future of Neurology depends chiefly on the discovery of the *primum movens* at the molecular level. This fascinating development during the past two decades has also been fostered by giant strides made in the basic sciences of clinical genetics.

Epileptology as a subspecialty of the neurological sciences went through analogous stages. This domain became naturally overwhelmed by electrophysiological insights when the EEG (more precisely: the macroelectroencephalogram) provided the epileptologists with impressive correlates of various seizure manifestations. Then the microelectrodes of the neurophysiologists were reaching for the single neuron where the behavior of the neurocellular membrane indicated a crucial link between biochemical and electrophysiological processes. More recently, the focus of attention has been moving from the *sparks* (the bioelectrical phenomena) to the *soup* of biochemical activities.

2) *Neurobiochemistry*

A multitude of chemical disturbances have been thought to be related to epileptic processes and it is therefore necessary to divide the chemical changes from different angles of view. The following classification appears to be justified:

a) Disease-specific chemical changes creating a predisposition to seizures
b) Chemical changes occurring in focal lesions (trauma, tumor, infection etc.)
c) Facilitation and precipitation of seizures due to chemical changes
d) Chemical changes occurring during epileptic seizures
e) Chemical changes related to the termination of seizures

Metaphorically speaking, one could distinguish the spark of an igniting mechanism (and the conditions which provide the ground for such an ignition system) from the fuel needed for the occurrence and maintenance of the discharge.

As to the *disease-specific chemical changes,* a long list of hereditary *inborn errors of metabolism* is growing longer from year to year and many of these diseases lead to early or delayed brain damage with epileptic seizures. This will be discussed more extensively in the chapter dealing with the etiologies of seizures. One could speculate that the so-called idiopathic epilepsy (also called "centrencephalic") and discussed later under the heading of "Common Generalized Epilepsy" may be caused by a hitherto unknown biochemical disturbance.

Very little is known about the *chemical basis of epileptic activity generated within an epileptogenic focus.* According to Tower (1960), accumulation of free acetylcholine leads to seizure activity and a chronic defect in acetylcholine metabolism is felt to play an important part. Thus, excessive free acetylcholine would give rise to depolarization of the soma-dendritic membrane and resulting post-synaptic potentials would produce epileptic discharges.

Concerning the *facilitation and precipitation of seizures,* the excitability of the membrane stands in the foreground. The just mentioned action of a transmitter substance such as acetylcholine would render the membrane hyperexcitable; increased influx of sodium and depletion of intracellular potassium would also enhance the excitability of the membrane (Fig. 1). Tower (1960) also considered the *failure of transmitter substances with inhibitory action* such as gamma-aminobutyric acid (GABA) as a possibly important factor in the generation of seizure activity. An *intrinsic instability of the membrane* has been thought to be a basic disturbance in epileptic processes (Matsumoto and Ajmone Marsan, 1964). This could be due to a) abnormal increase

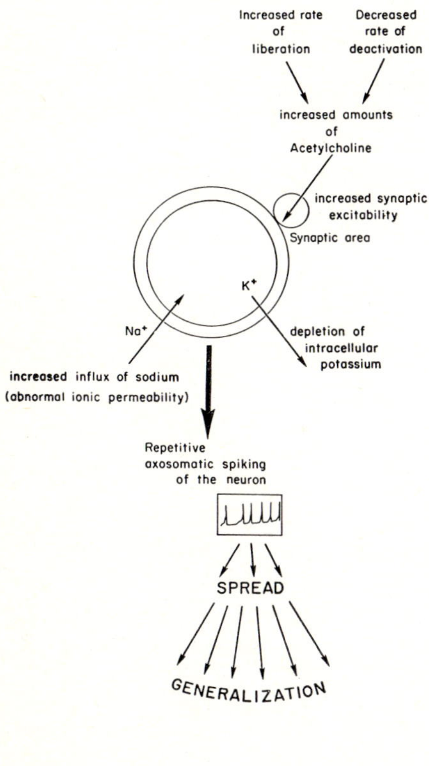

FIGURE 1. The genesis of cellular epileptic activity (modified after Tower 1960). Axosomatic spiking may be due to a) increased synaptic excitability caused by increased amounts of acetylcholine, b) increased sodium influx (abnormal permeability, c) depletion of intracellular potassium. Intense and prolonged axosomatic spiking may lead to spread (involvement of distant normal neurons) and a generalized seizure may develop.

of ionic premeability and b) decreased threshold of the resting potential (J. W. Woodbury, 1969).

The resting membrane potential of the neuron is maintained by energy derived from high-energy phosphate bonds provided by a) the cytochrome system, b) Krebs cycle and, to a lesser degree, c) glycolysis. Hypoxia gives rise to membrane instability which may lead to seizure activity (anoxic convulsions). A hypoxic factor has been presumed in Pentylenetrazol (Metrazol®) convulsions; this drug leads to acute astrocytic swelling which impairs capillary cerebral blood flow (DeRobertis et al., 1969).

Chemical changes occurring during epileptic seizures are closely related to the neurocellular energy metabolism and to ictal alterations of cerebral blood flow. Major convulsions are associated with a steep rise of cerebral blood flow, oxygen consumption, carbon dioxide production and glucose consumption; according to Plum et al. (1968), these values increase between 50 to 500 percent. The cortical oxygen and carbon dioxide tension increases if there is sufficient ventilation (Aizawa et al., 1965); the cerebral glucose concentration decreases while there is an enormous increase of the lactate concentration (King et al., 1967).

The old concept of a cerebral vasoconstriction during a grand mal seizure (Foerster, 1926; Spielmeyer, 1927) has been refuted by Penfield's (1932) demonstration of increasing cerebral blood flow in the ictal and post-ictal phase.

With regard to the *chemical changes related to the termination of seizures*, the role of gradually increasing neuronal hypoxia has been emphasized (Meyer and Portnoy, 1959). According to this view, the brain would simply run out of fuel during a convulsion. This concept, however, hardly explains the rather abrupt termination of a grand mal seizure and the extremely brisk transition from pronounced electrical activity to sudden flatness, which is noted synchronously in cortical as well as in deep structures. Efron (1961) has postulated an active type of inhibition in the termination of seizures and the development of a post-ictal paralysis. Such an active inhibition may be of chemical as well as of electrical nature (Levy and O'Leary, 1965). The nature of the former remains obscure since, according to Tower (1965),

TABLE I

SOME BIOCHEMICAL CAUSES AND MECHANISMS OF EPILEPTIC SEIZURES
(after Tower, 1960)

	Causes and mechanisms	*Therapy*
A) *Acetylcholine metabolism*	Cholinesterase-inhibitous (Nerve gases, Insecticides, organic phosphates)	Anticholinergics (Atropine etc.) Pyridoxine 2-aldoxime methiodide (PAM)
B) *Electrolyte metabolism*	1) Energy-rich-phosphate depletion (Anoxia, dinitrophenol, cyanide, hypoglycemia) 2) Hyperventilation, CO_2-withdrawal 3) Adrenalectomy	Adenosinetriphosphate Acetazolamide Deoxycorticosterone, Aldosterone
C) *Amino acid metabolism*	1) Pyridoxine deficiency (dietary, "dependency") 2) Pyridoxine deficiency (chemical: hydrazides, antimetabolites) 3) Ammonia 4) Methionine sulfoximine	Pyridoxine Pyridoxine Gamma-amino-butyric acid (Arginine) Methionine
D) *Oxidative metabolism*	1) Anoxia 2) Heavy metals (lead, etc.) 3) Cyanide 4) Fluoroacetate Fluorocitrate 5) Hypoglycemia (Insulin, 2-deoxyglucose)	(Oxygen) BAL, Versene Sodium nitrite Sodium thiosulfate Monoacetin (Glucose)

no transmitter substance with unequivocal inhibitory function has been demonstrated (although the inhibitory function of GABA has been frequently discussed).

A *variety of biochemical disturbances* leading to seizures are shown in Table I. The large bulk of neurobiochemical data concerning basic epileptic mechanisms might be compared with a mosaic, the "gestalt" of which is still poorly delineated. Abundant details of knowledge are still fragmentary and there is presently no universal neurobiochemical concept of epilepsy. Most of the discussed neurobiochemical epileptogenic mechanisms pertain to acute convulsions rather than to chronically recurrent epileptic seizures which stand in the foreground of clinical epileptology.

3) *Electrophysiology*

a) The variety of cerebral electrophysiological phenomena. A short glimpse at the extremely condensed presentation of neurobiochemical changes in epileptic activity shows clearly how the chemical and electrical elements are intimately interwoven. The electrical manifestation is easily documented by a tracing which is often the most impressive datum to the beholder but its secondary and epi-phenomenal character is undubitable. It is the biochemist alone who is capable of searching for the primordial disturbances leading to the discovery of nosological entities.

Table II presents a brief view of the better known electrophysiological phenomena. This shows clearly that the electroencephalogram (EEG) is but one of several different types of neuronal electrical discharges.

b) The EEG or macroelectroencephalogram. The EEG represents the *"noise" of the brain* in which the minute "clicks" of individual responses to single stimuli merge into the rhythmical oscillations generated by huge cellular contingents. This noise, in general, reveals more about the physiological or abnormal condition of the brain than the evaluation of the response to individual signals may yield. Thus, the EEG permits indirect inferences on the level of awareness in a given person and, moreover, on the presence of certain focal or diffuse lesions. In this context, the occurrence of *sudden discharges* (*"spikes" or "sharp waves"*) is most informative concerning the presence of an epileptic disorder and its presumable cerebral localization. Table III lists the most common epileptic discharges in the EEG; the great diagnostic value lies in the fact that these discharges occur in the interictal interval, either spontaneously or facilitated by certain activating procedures (hyperventilation, intermittent photic stimulation, certain neuropharmacological activations).

The sudden and abrupt rise of voltage in conjunction with a spike discharge has been thought to express the *hypersynchrony* of firing epileptic neurons. It would be erroneous, however, to conceive epileptic activity simply as "paroxysmal hypersynchrony." Desynchronization or flattening of the macro-EEG-activity has

TABLE II

ELECTROPHYSIOLOGICAL PHENOMENA
MICRO-ELECTROPHYSIOLOGY

1) *Axo-somatic spike-potential*
(The "spike" of the micro-electrophysiologist)
An all-or-none-response of the membrane, 0.5-1.5 msec, 70-85 millivolts, caused by a rapid succession of depolarization-repolarization of the membrane with concomitant chemical changes.

2) *Slow membrane potential variations*
Graded potentials, recorded from the neuronal membrane, 10-20 msec and longer, 5-20 millivolts.
a) *Depolarization wave*
Gradual decrease of the membrane potential, usually facilitating or triggering axosomatic spikes (may accompany seizure discharges in the macro-EEG).
b) *Hyperpolarization wave*
Gradual augmentation of the membrane potential, almost always inhibiting axo-somatic spikes.
c) *Excitatory post-synaptic potential (EPSP)*
A depolarization wave triggered synaptically from a different neuron.
d) *Inhibitory post-synaptic potential (IPSP)*
A hyperpolarization wave triggered synaptically from a different neuron.

3) *Apico-dendritic potential*
Slow graded responses, about 100-500 msec and about 0.5-3 millivolt, recorded from cortical surface.
Presumed to play an eminent role as source of the macro-EEG

MACRO-ELECTROPHYSIOLOGY

1) *Electroencephalogram (Macro-EEG)*
The continuous "noise" of the brain, derived from various cellular sources but chiefly from apical dendrites, recorded from the scalp, cortex (electrocorticogram) or deep structures (depth-EEG). Average amplitudes, 10-100 microvolt on the scalp, 100-1000 microvolt over the cortex, higher in seizure discharges.
a) *EEG in the usual (clinical) frequency range (0.5/sec to about 60/sec)*
Comprises the basic (alpha) rhythm and a wide range of physiological and abnormal patterns including epileptic discharges (the "spike" of the electroencephalographer).
b) *"DC phenomena": ultra-slow frequency range*
Recorded from scalp, cortex depth, requires DC amplifiers.
Contingent negative variation (CNV), recorded from vertex, associated with readiness to perform motor acts. Amplitude around 10 micro V.
Negative DC phenomena with seizure bursts
Positive and negative phenomena during cerebral anoxia
c) *Ultra-fast frequency phenomena*
Physiological activity of cerebellar cortex (around 200-300/sec.)
Frequencies of 500 to 1000/sec during initiation of clinical seizure activity.
d) *Spreading depression*
A poorly understood slow (0.5 mm/sec) spread of depressed cortical electrical activity following strong electrical stimulation of the cortex and biochemical changes.

2) *Evoked responses*
Electrical response to visual, auditory or somesthetic stimuli, recorded from the scalp over the corresponding cortical projection area (or, especially in auditory stimulation, from the vertex as an area of secondary convergence of afferent stimuli).
Consisting of 5 chief components (P1, N1, P2, N2, P3) in a latency range from 20-250 msec (more delayed over the vertex), reaching about 5-15 microvolt.
Averaging techniques usually required in order to extract "signal" from "noise."

TABLE III

EPILEPTIC DISCHARGES IN THE EEG

Spike
(random single spike)

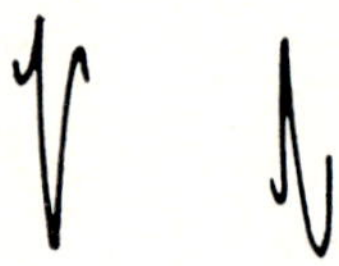

Short duration (10–70msec), mostly focal, often in bilateral synchrony, seldom in generalized synchrony.

Classical interval seizure discharge. Epileptogenicity limited in children (only 40–80% having clinical seizures).

Sharp wave
(random sharp wave)

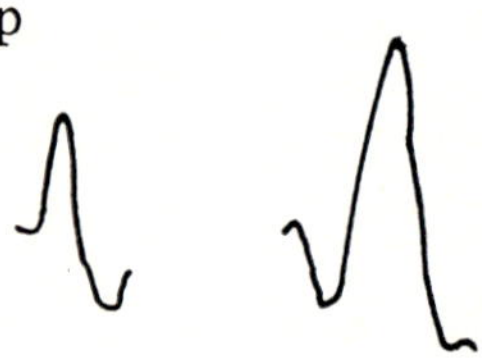

Longer duration (80–150msec and longer), focal, sometimes in bilateral-temporal synchrony, very seldom generalized.

Typical interval seizure discharge in temporal lobe epilepsy (anterior temporal region). Epileptogenicity limited in children.

Small sharp spike.

A low voltage spike, very inconspicuous and easily missed in the EEG reading.

An interval finding, almost exclusively seen in adults, mostly in drowsiness and sleep. Fairly widespread, bilaterally shifting, chiefly in temporal leads, sometimes heralding a temporal lobe focus. Epileptogenicity limited (50% or even less).

(TABLE III, *Continued*)

Multiple spikes

a.) 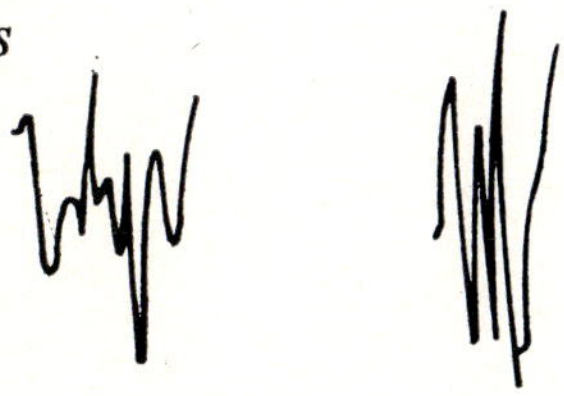

b.) 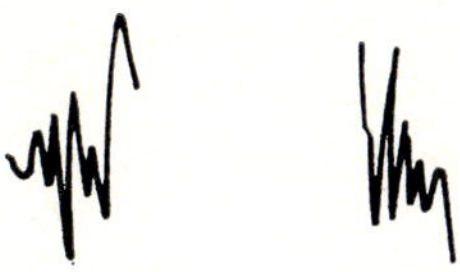

Burst of fast spikes, (frequency from 20–60/sec) often of moderate voltage (b.) Mostly a bilateral or generalized–synchronous discharge. Very common in Common generalized epilepsy (sleep), hypsarrhythmia and Lennox-Gastaut syndrome.

Runs of rapid spikes

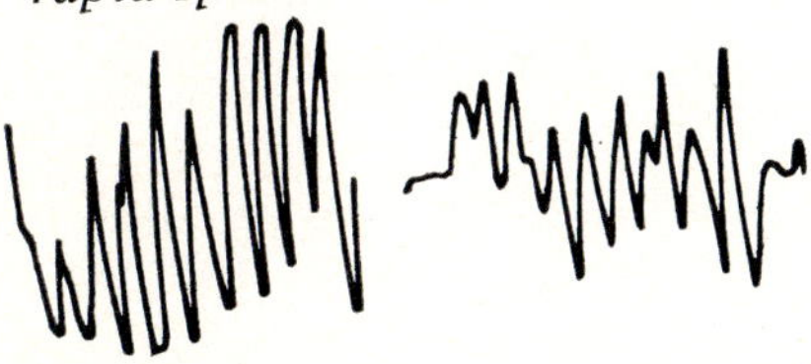

More sustained and slower than multiple spikes, mostly 10–20/sec, most often bilateral-frontal.
Typical in Lennox-Gastaut syndrome.

Spike-wave complex, classical (3/sec)

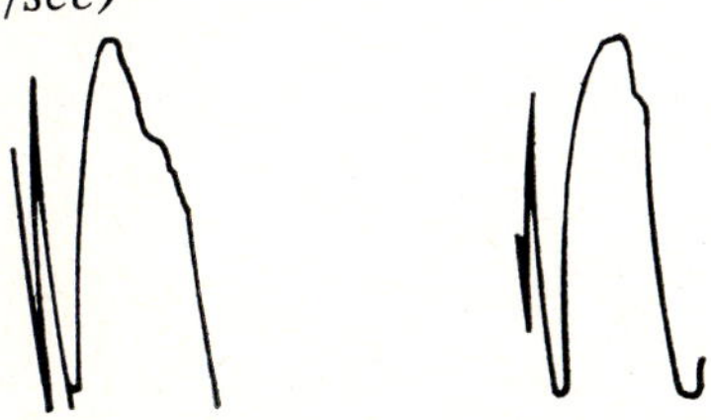

In generalized-synchrony or bilateral-anterior bursts. When sustained for more than 5 seconds, association with clinical petit mal very likely.

Typical finding in Common generalized epilepsy (Petit mal or petit mal and grand mal), easily activated with hyperventilation. Seldom in Lennox-Gastaut syndrome. Discharge seen mainly from age 4–20 years.

(TABLE III, *Continued*)

Slow spike-wave complex (1–2.5/sec)

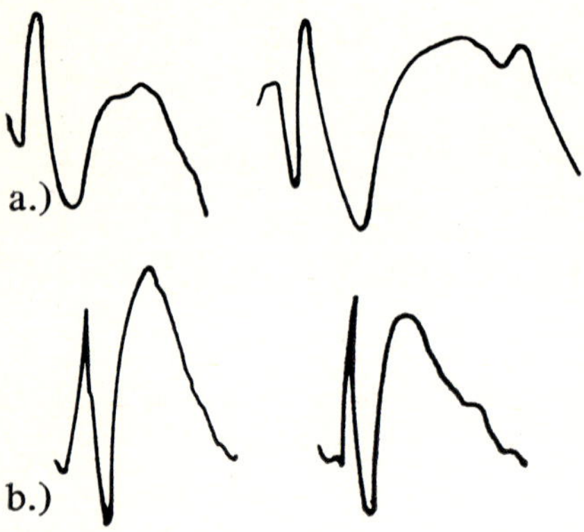

Most commonly in bilateral or generalized synchrony, seldom focal. Often in very prolonged bursts. Spike-component may be slow (a.) or fast (b.).

Typical interval finding in Lennox-Gastaut syndrome. The discharge tends to disappear in adulthood.

Fast spike-wave complex (4–5/sec)

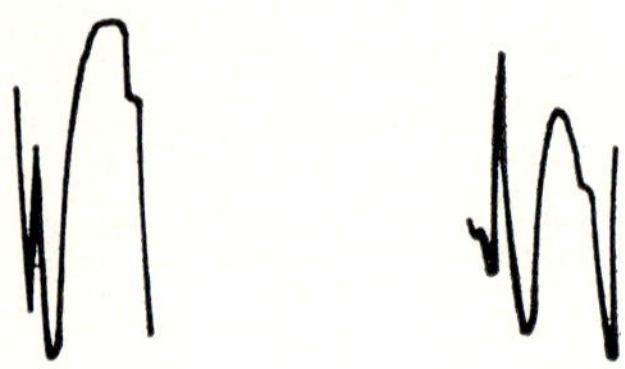

In bilateral-anterior or generalized-synchronous brief bursts.

Typical interval finding in a subgroup of Common generalized epilepsy (grand mal only, often with flicker-sensitivity in the EEG). Seen throughout adolescence and adulthood.

(Small) fast spike-wave complex (6/sec)

In bilateral-posterior brief bursts seldom generalized, often very small and inconspicuous.

Mainly in adults, most common in light and moderate drowsiness. Epileptogenicity limited (around 50% may have sporadic grand mal).

also been observed in certain forms of temporal lobe automatisms and might be related to certain electrophysiological properties of the amygdaloid nucleus (Feindel and Gloor, 1954; Jasper, 1964). Such *"electro-decremental seizures"* with sudden generalized ictal flattening of a thus far spike dominated EEG tracing of high voltage are also common in infantile spasms with hypsarrhythmia.

The pragmatic value of the EEG is great despite the fact that the basis of this electrophysiological phenomenon is still poorly understood. When we look upon the variety of micro-electrophysiological events (Table II), there is general consensus that the all-or-nothing axo-somatic spike of the single nerve cell contributes very little to the macro-EEG whereas slower potential variations are apparently of much greater significance. The role of the apico-dendritic graded potentials in the genesis of the has been stressed by Clare and Bishop (1955), Tasaki et al. (1954), and Purpura and Grundfest (1956). The graded postsynaptic responses to presynaptic stimulation may also contribute to the macro-EEG; these phenomena were reported in the spinal cord by Brock, Coombs and Eccles (1952) and, in the brain, by Phillips (1956). Very little is known about the possible role of glial potentials (Schadé, 1964; Orkand, 1969; Trachtenberg and Pollen, 1970; Prince, 1971).

From the historical viewpoint, the advent of clinical electroencephalography (Berger, 1929) and the demonstration of epileptic discharges by means of this technique (by Fischer, 1933, in the experimental animal; by F. A. Gibbs, H. Davis and W. G. Lennox, 1935, in human epileptics) have initiated a new era of epileptology. A large bulk of work stemming from the pre-EEG era has been subsequently reduced to merely historical value. Imaginatively used with refined techniques, electroencephalography will give further and deeper insights into epileptic conditions. Unfortunately, the greatest threat to its prestige has arisen from the large host of inadequately trained electroencephalographers.

4) The epileptogenic focus

It is a logical thought that epileptic activity with its electrical and clinical concomitants must originate from a primordial focal disturbance with or without local morphological changes.

The epileptogenic focus has been the topic of a large number of studies. Neurons located within a focus behave differently from healthy nerve cells and show the following characteristics (Schmidt and Wilder, 1968): 1) Autonomous and sustained paroxysmal discharge which can be influenced from outside by synaptic activity, 2) Increased electrical excitability, 3) Sustained cortical surface electrical negativity (in comparison to surrounding normal cortex), 4) Initiation of volleys of very-high frequency-impulses (700-1000/sec) by a sudden depolarization of the resting membrane potential, and 5) The ability to induce secondary epileptogenic foci in synaptically related areas. One could add to these characteristics 6) The abnormally synchronized type of neuronal discharge (Creutzfeldt, 1969).

In other words, the neurons located within an epileptogenic focus are hypersensitive. Such excessive sensitivity has been ascribed to a reduced number of dendritic synapses leading to partial de-afferentation (Ward, Jr., 1961; Westrum et al., 1964) after a relationship between denervation, supersensitivity and epilepsy had been recognized by Cannon (1939). Matsumoto and Ajmone Marson (1964) have emphasized the instability of the epileptogenic neurons. Other authors, especially Prince (1966), have stressed the afferent influences on the epileptic neuron; accordingly, depolarization shifts of the epileptic neuron would be synaptically driven.

The topical application of convulsive drugs (strychnine, penicillin, ouabain), in cortical or subcortical regions of the acute experimental animal has been the basis for the genesis of epileptic activity and its spread. In the chronic experiment, alumina cream has been most commonly used in order to imitate the pathological process of scar formation with gradual development of an epileptogenic focus (Fig. 2). Cats and monkeys have been most often used for this type of experimental work but there is no doubt that every species is potentially utilizable since even in lower animals, epileptic activity has been demonstrable (Servit, 1959, 1970).

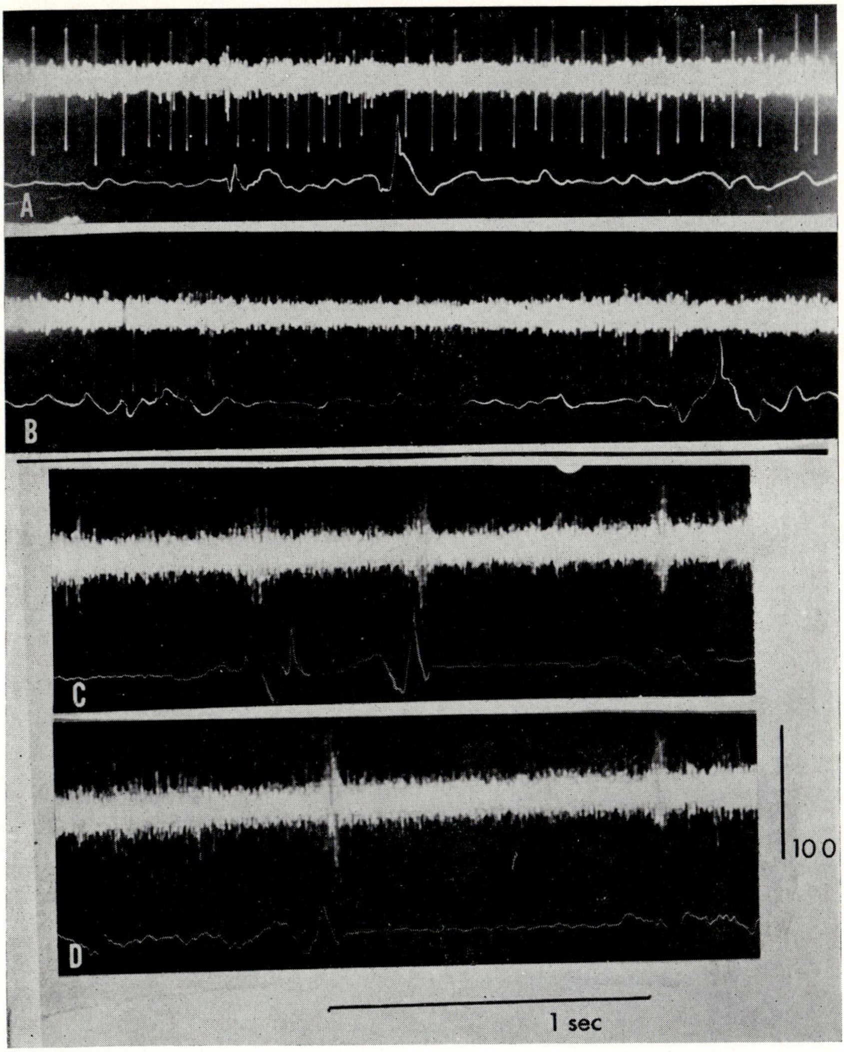

FIGURE 2. Single unit (extracellular), multi-unit and cortical macro-EEG recording in Macaca mulatta, obtained from the vicinity of a deep experimental scar focus (alumina cream) in the temporal lobe. a) (top) upper tracing: Single unit activity. Lower tracing: cortical EEG near the site of electrode penetration. In b) depression of single unit activity is noted during the occurrence of macro-EEG spiking. c, d) Upper tracing: Multi-unit burst activity. Lower tracing: depth EEG near the focus; a few mm from the site of the micro-recording (Courtesy of Dr. G. Gücer and Dr. A. Earl Walker, Baltimore).

In clinical epileptology, the role of the epileptogenic focus, its relationship to cerebral topography and clinical seizure manifestations, its re-activation by cortical stimulation, its neuropathological substratum and its surgical removal has been the main subject of the work of Penfield and Jasper (1954).

5) Propagation of epileptic activity

There is good reason to presume that an epileptogenic focus transmits abnormal impulses into adjacent or more distant areas. The hyperexcitability of the primary focus may be partially counter-balanced by inhibitory action within the focus (Goldensohn and Purpura, 1963; "surround inhibition" of Prince and Wilder, 1967) and temporarily depressed by long duration cyclical changes in excitability (Prince, 1971).

Projection and propagation of seizure discharges may principally employ the following different mechanisms: a) by intracortical diffusion, b) by volume conduction of potential fields ("ephaptic" conduction) or c) along conducting pathways ("synaptic" conduction). The synaptic mechanism has proved to be by far more important than the ephaptic one. According to Jasper (1969), potential fields might have only a facilitating action . . . "though this may be of great importance for cells in the subliminal fringe."

The general rules according to which epileptic spread develops from various epileptogenic structures have been studied for many years by A. Earl Walker and his associates (Faeth et al., 1956; Poblete et al., 1959; Lichtenstein et al., 1959; Walker and Udvarhelyi, 1965; Udvarhelyi and Walker, 1965; Walker, 1970). This work has placed the emphasis on the existence of "low and high threshold areas" with greater or lesser susceptibility to the bombardment with epileptic activity. Older work by Dusser de Barenne and McCulloch (1939) on the propagation of strychnine spikes led to the concept of "strychnine neuronography" but has left only temporary imprints on the research work dealing with epileptic spread.

Spread of epileptic discharges may eventually lead to *secondary epileptogenic foci* (Morrell, 1960, 1969). This development may give rise to a "*mirror focus*" contralaterally on the homologous site via commissural pathways. This mechanism is better understood in the experimental animal than in man.

6) Generalization of epileptic activity

Generalization of epileptic activity frequently denotes the final stage following an avalanche of progressive propagation. In clinical terms, this development is typefied by a focal seizure followed by gradual transition into a full-blown grand mal attack.

In contrast to this crescendo-type of development stands the generalized seizure activity of sudden bilateral onset. This type of abruptly commencing seizure is clinically seen in the classical petit mal absence and also in grand mal seizures with no initiating focal onset and subsequent buildup.

Such generalized-synchronous seizure discharges epitomized by the classical 3/sec spike-wave pattern of the petit mal absence have been thought to originate in a "common central (midline subcortical) pacemaker" (Jasper and Kershman, 1941). Widespread neocortical responses to rhythmical slow electrical stimulation of the intralaminar portion of the thalamus ("recruiting response") were demonstrated in the cat by Morison and Dempsey (1942) and, in 1947, Jasper and Droogleever-Fortuyn elicited 3/sec spike-wave-like activity in the cat by 3/sec electrical stimuli applied to the intralaminar thalamus.

This work (confirmed in later studies by Ingvar, 1955, and Pollen et al., 1963) represents the experimental basis for a primary generalized type of epilepsy termed "*centrencephalic*" (Penfield, 1952; Penfield and Jasper, 1954).

Centrencephalic seizures such as petit mal and grand mal (with no focal onset) were presumed to involve the "*centrencephalic system*" consisting of thalamocortical circuits integrating both hemispheres; this hypothetical system was felt to be intimately related to the function of consciousness. Although conceived as a subcortico-cortical interrelating mechanism (Penfield, 1957), the role of the thalamus was overemphasized and, in epileptology, the thalamus was widely assumed to be the focal origin of generalized-synchronous seizure discharges.

Further experimental work (Jung, 1949; Starzl et al., 1953; Sager et al., 1959; Okuma et al., 1961; Pradhan and Ajmone

Marsan, 1963; Walker and Udvarhelyi, 1965; Marcus and Watson, 1966, 1968; Marcus, 1972) have cast much doubt on the primary role of the thalamic level as the origin of generalized seizure activity. Gloor (1968, 1969) has provided further evidence against the leading role of the thalamus in his studies of the effect of intracarotid pentylenetetrazol (Metrazol®) in the human. Jasper himself (1969) admitted the lack of anatomical identification of a centrencephalic system.

7) Precipitating mechanisms of epileptic discharges and seizures

At the cellular level with the continuous dynamic fluctuations of excitatory and inhibitory presynaptic action upon epileptic neurons, the existence of precipitating and inhibitory mechanisms is readily understood.

Various chemical and neural mechanisms of precipitating and inhibitory nature have been identified and the character of convulsive and anticonvulsive drugs is strongly related to their excitatory and inhibitory properties. These properties may be sometimes confusing as it is the case with strychnine; its blocking action on inhibitory mechanisms ("inhibition of the inhibition") was theorized by Sherrington and experimentally demonstrated by Bradley, Easton and Eccles (1953). In clinical electroencephalography, alkalosis induced by hyperventilation (for clinical purposes introduced by Foerster, 1924) plays an eminent part as a precipitating mechanism.

Among neural mechanisms, the circadian waking-sleeping cycle has been proposed as a prominent factor in the determination of clinical seizures (Janz, 1953, 1962, 1969). The role of arousal ("dyshormia") has been stressed by Niedermeyer (1966, 1970, 1972) with regard to generalized-synchronous seizure discharges.

Afferent-sensory mechanisms as triggering factors of electrical seizure discharges and clinical seizures are not too uncommon in human epilepsy and a whole chapter will deal with these mechanisms. All of these various precipitating factors have been reviewed by Gastaut and Tassinari (1966) and will be discussed in Chapter 6.

Some of these seizure-triggering afferent mechanisms have

been regarded as evidence of *"reflex epilepsy."* Most of the early experimental work was based on the enhanced regional sensitivity to somato-sensory stimuli, following the application of strychnine on the post-central sensory cortex (Baglioni, 1909; Amantea and Martino, 1927; Clementi, 1929). The validity of this concept will be discussed in Chapter 6.

8) Inhibitory mechanisms of epileptic discharges and termination of seizures

Inhibitory pathways have been demonstrated in every level of the CHS; this bulk of work has been recently reviewed and summarized by Eccles (1969). It is reasonable to assume that well functioning inhibitory systems are essential in the prevention as well as in the termination of epileptic seizures.

Negative feedback circuits act upon the motor neurons of the spinal cord (Renshaw, 1941) and on the Purkinje cells of the cerebellum via the inhibitory action of basket cells (Eccles et al., 1966), outer stellate cells and Golgi cells (Hamori and Szentagothai, 1966); even the Purkinje cells themselves have been shown to give rise to inhibitory action (Ito and Yoshida, 1966). The wealth of cerebellar inhibitory mechanisms might have some significance in the termination of seizures as it will be discussed later.

Other important negative feedback mechanisms have been demonstrated in the hippocampic basket cells acting upon the adjacent pyramidal cells (Kandel, Spencer and Brinley, 1961), in the ventrobasal thalamus (Andersen, Eccles and Sears, 1964) and in the neocortical level (Stefanis and Jasper, 1964).

These inhibitory systems are based upon two different mechanisms; a) post-synaptic inhibition, acting via hyperpolarization of the post-synaptic membrane, occurring rather selectively in higher CNS levels, and b) pre-synaptic inhibition (Frank and Fuortes, 1957) which acts on excitatory fibers and exerts an indirect inhibitory effect on the neuron. This mechanism is rather ubiquitous in peripheral and lower CNS levels.

Thus, the brake pedal is applied on excessive excitatory action in multifold ways. Linked with these neural pathways are neural transmitter substances with inhibitory action; their complex action in various CNS levels has been discussed by Eccles (1969).

The occurrence of single spikes in the EEG may be followed by a slow wave and a *rhythmical spike-wave pattern* may develop as it is seen in the petit mal seizure. While the spike corresponds to a depolarization shift in the single neuron which fires in a rapid series of axo-somatic spikes, the following slow wave is accompanied by a hyperpolarization shift increasing the membrane potential and inhibiting further axo-soma-spikes (Pollen, 1964; Weir and Sie, 1966). Hence the slow wave apparently prevents a single spike discharge (in the macro-EEG) from turning into a train of repetitive spikes which could readily generate local or widespread motor activity or even a grand mal. The *inhibitory nature of the slow wave* had been stressed in earlier studies by Jung and Toennies (1950) ("Bremswelle").

The termination or arrest of seizure activity might depend on a variety of mechanisms. Inhibitory influences are likely to emanate from the cerebellum (Dow, 1965). The electrical stimulation of this structure never gives rise to seizures and, according to Jung (1949), the cerebellum does not participate in the epileptic activity induced by electroshock in the cat. Ablation of the cerebellum is followed by intensified and prolonged induced seizures in various animals (Dow, 1965). Therefore, the role of the cerebellum and its functional breakdown ought to be considered in the genesis of grand mal status epilepticus (Niedermeyer, 1959, 1960; see also Chapter 7).

9) Neuropathological aspects

The primary neurobiochemical disturbance within an epileptogenic focus is frequently associated with morphological changes which are due to specific and often progressive brain diseases or residual brain damage with scar formation. The description of expanding and atrophic epileptogenic lesions by Penfield and Jasper (1954) has set new standards in this domain which are still valid. This is particularly true for the *residual lesions of birth and infancy* which have been subdivided as follows: a) abnormal head growth in infancy (often with occlusion of large arteries), b) meningocerebral cicatrix formation at birth, b) local microgyria, d) incisural sclerosis impinging on the temporal lobe (which will be discussed in the chapter on temporal lobe epilepsy), e) brain cysts and vascular occlusions and f) cerebral atrophy secondary to meningo-encephalitis.

A different neuropathological approach dealt with *secondary cerebral pathology due to grand mal seizures and associated cerebral ischemia.* The sclerosis of field h_1 (Sommer's sector) of the hippocampus had been well known in the 19th century (Bouchet and Cazauvielh, 1825; Sommer, 1880; Pfleger, 1882; Osler, 1888) and it was felt that this lesion might constitute the cause of otherwise unexplained epilepsies (Sommer, 1880). The secondary nature of this disturbance was emphasized by Pfleger (1882), Alzheimer (1907), Spielmeyer (1933) and especially by Scholz (1951) who studied the changes caused by electro-convulsions in the cat. It was shown that, in addition to the hippocampic sclerosis, other typical anoxic changes were demonstrable in the brain involving mainly the cerebellum (Purkinje cells) and, less commonly, neocortical regions, where microgyria ("ulegyria") and lobar sclerosis may develop. Areas of relatively poor blood supply appeared to be preferentially affected.

More recently, Peiffer (1963) and, in this country, Malamud (1966), have re-emphasized the role of secondary lesions (caused by Grand mal-induced cerebral hypoxia) and their significance in the pathogenesis of temporal lobe epilepsy.

In most recent years, however, this type of approach is vanishing and modern neuropathology has concentrated on the *electron-microscopic studies of structures poisoned by convulsants* and the concomitant changes seen in the epileptic neuron. This work is joining forces with neurobiochemists and electrophysiologists. The recent reviews of Pope (1969) and Peiffer (1970) give testimony of these changes in the neuropathological orientation.

The selective vulnerability of structures like the field h_1 of the hippocampus or Purkinje cells could be due to biochemical rather than to vascular properties; these ideas might resurrect the concept of *pathoclisis* of C. and O. Vogt (1937) according to which certain cerebral areas show a selective and presumably biochemical affinity to certain disease processes.

CHAPTER 2

TYPES OF EPILEPTIC SEIZURES

1) Introductory remarks

THE VARIETY OF epileptic seizures is determined by the following principal factors:

a) Localization of the involved cerebral area
b) Age of the patient
c) Basic epileptic condition (often age determined).

On the other hand, the etiology of the seizure disorder (tumor, trauma or infantile residual lesion) has little or no influence on the type of seizures.

The relationship between cerebral localization and the corresponding focal character of the seizures has been the topic of earlier masterful descriptions, especially in the work of Penfield and Jasper (1954). It is only natural that a neurosurgeon and a neurophysiologist (both of them neuroscientists of highest rank) would choose the approach of cerebral-clinical correlations in the light of the functional anatomy of the brain. From the viewpoint of the practicing neurologist, pediatrican, or general practitioner, however, the factors of age and the hitherto underrated factor of the basic epileptic condition are of utmost importance with regard to prognosis and therapy.

For this reason, the description of the variety of seizures will be rather short and cursory while most of the emphasis will be placed upon the age-determined types of seizure disorders and the basic epileptic conditions.

The recognition of the type of seizure may, of course, lead to the detection of the primarily affected cerebral region and this may be a significant diagnostic step in the localization of a circumscript lesion. In other cases, the correct analysis of the type of seizure will be helpful in the determination of the basic epileptic condition. The EEG demonstration of inter-ictal seizure discharges (or ictal episodes) is usually instrumental from the diagnostic viewpoint.

All of the listed types of focal seizures may be nothing but the prelude of an ensuing full-blown grand-mal-convulsion. The focal seizure may then become the warning of an imminent major seizure and, in the case of an initiating strange perceptive experience, the term *aura* has been widely used. It is important to recall that an aura as such is nothing but a certain type of a focal seizure.

A satisfactory *classification of epileptic seizures* is extremely difficult. A strict neurophysiological basis for such a classification (Ajmone Marsan, 1961) may prove to be impractical in clinical work. Gastaut et al. (1964) and, more recently, Gastaut (1970) and Merlis (1970) have proposed an "International Classification of Epileptic Seizures," somewhat complex and cumbersome in its original form but perfectly acceptable (in a condensed abstract shown in Table IV). Stress must be laid on the fact that there are *unclassifiable seizures* of a nebulous and protean semeiology which even the experienced observer cannot place into a defined category.

2) *Grand mal*

The *tonic-clonic sequence* of generalized convulsive activity in a grand mal seizure represents a maximal epileptic response of the brain. Grand mal seizures are not precisely uniform since certain variations in the strength of the attack are likely to exist. (Rodin et al., 1966; Petsche, 1968 and Rodin, 1970). The major convulsion may be generalized from the start or the final stage of a primary focal attack. Subtle focal signs at the beginning of the convulsion (for instance a slight adversive movement of the head or a conjugated eye movement to one side), however, are often irrelevant.

TABLE IV

INTERNATIONAL CLASSIFICATION OF EPILEPTIC SEIZURES

Part One: Classification after Gastaut, 1970

I. PARTIAL SEIZURES (seizures beginning locally)
- A. Partial seizures with elementary symptomatology (generally without impairment of consciousness)
  1. With motor symptoms (includes Jacksonian seizures)
  2. With special sensory or somatosensory symptoms
  3. With autonomic symptoms
  4. Compound forms
- B. Partial seizures with complex symptomatology (generally with impairment of consciousness) (temporal lobe or psychomotor seizures)
  1. With impairment of consciousness only
  2. With cognitive symptomatology
  3. With affective symptomatology
  4. With "psychosensory" symptomatology
  5. With "psychomotor" symptomatology (automatisms)
  6. Compound forms
- C. Partial seizures secondarily generalized

II. GENERALIZED SEIZURES (bilaterally symmetrical and without local onset)
  1. Absences (petit mal)
  2. Bilateral massive epileptic myoclonus
  3. Infantile spasms
  4. Clonic seizures
  5. Tonic seizures
  6. Tonic-clonic seizures (grand mal)
  7. Atonic seizures
  8. Akinetic seizures

III. UNILATERAL SEIZURES (or predominantly)

IV. UNCLASSIFIED EPILEPTIC SEIZURES (due to incomplete data)

INTERNATIONAL CLASSIFICATION OF THE EPILEPSIES

Part Two: Classification after Merlis, 1970

I. GENERALIZED EPILEPSIES
  1. Primary generalized epilepsies (includes petit mal and grand mal seizures)
  2. Secondary generalized epilepsies
  3. Undetermined generalized epilepsies

II. PARTIAL (FOCAL, LOCAL) EPILEPSIES (includes Jacksonian, temporal lobe, and psychomotor seizures)

III. UNCLASSIFIABLE EPILEPSIES

Grand mal is the *most common of all seizure manifestations and may occur in all epileptic conditions* except for the first six months of life when insufficient cerebral myelination prevents the brain from a synchronous all-out display of epileptic activity. Febrile convulsions occurring after at least 6 months denote the first grand mal manifestations in life but these convulsions appear to be somewhat mitigated and irregular in the tonic-clonic sequence. It will be shown that the limitation to grand mal seizures and absence of partial types of attacks is common in benign types of seizure disorders.

Grand mal is associated with *deep coma* which gradually resolves after the attack. Seizure-induced falls from heights (scaffolds, into moving machinery) and loss of control of motor vehicles are well known hazards; *true emergency situations very seldom develop* from a single grand mal since the ictally suppressed respiratory function quickly returns after the seizure which usually lasts 50 to 90 seconds. Asphyxia from obstructed airways (food, dentures) rarely materalizes; prolonged postictal apnea is rather unique; the case of Nelson and Ray (1968) had a history of electric trauma and presumably an oblongata-type of respiratory disturbance.

Acute skeletal complications such as fractures of vertebrae and luxation of the mandible have often been reported in electrically induced grand mal convulsions (psychiatric electroshock treatment) and exceptionally occur in spontaneous grand mal seizures.

Tongue biting and subsequent wounds or scars along the lateral margin of the tongue provide almost convincing evidence of the grand mal character of an attack; the attempt of prevention (placing a padded object between the rows of teeth) at the onset of the seizure is of controversial value. This symptom is often absent, especially in grand mal of focal onset (Janz, 1969). *Urinary incontinence* depends on the degree of filling of the bladder; fecal incontinence is uncommon. The initiating epileptic cry (a contraction of the diaphragm) is usually muffled while foaming from the mouth is the result of hypersalivation.

A detailed description of the tonic-clonic motor characteristics (as presented by Ruttner, 1944) would exceed the frame of this book. Most recently, Gastaut and Broughton (1972) have beautifully documented the clinical-ictal semeiology and the concomitant electrophysiological events of the typical grand mal seizure (see Fig. 3).

The *focal initiation of a grand mal attack* can be derived from the type of preceding motor, sensory, autonomic, emotional or

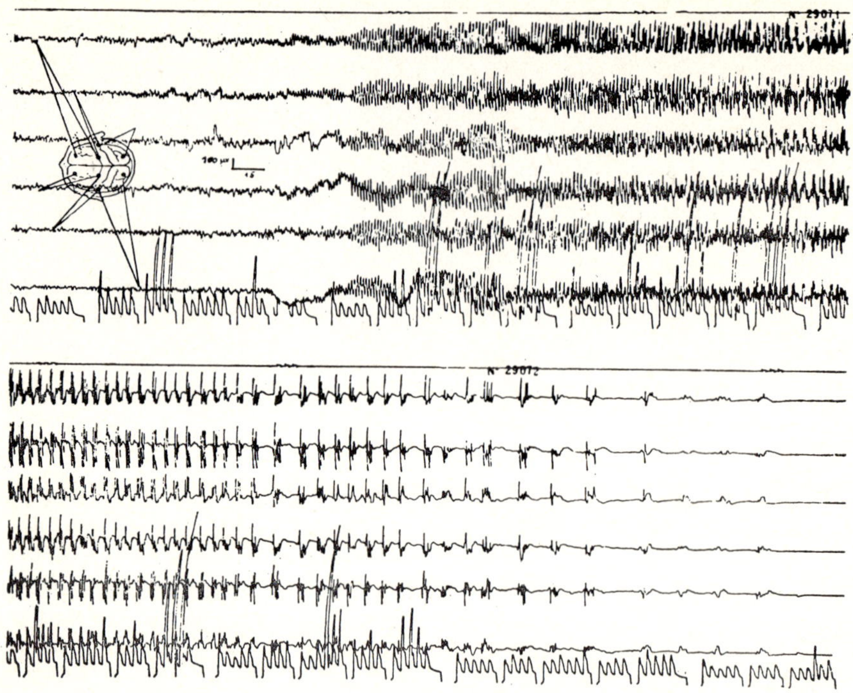

FIGURE 3. The EEG correlates of a generalized tonic-clonic convulsion (grand mal), obtained in a curarized patient and hence almost free of superimposed muscle activity. The bottom channel of this continuous recording shows the deflections of a frequency analyser (after W. Grew Walter). The seizure activity is characterized by fast spiking of increasing amplitude during the tonic phase; note transition into repetitive bursts of spikes (mixed with weak persistent muscle potentials) during the clonic phase (lower portion of the recording). Prior to the seizure, unremarkable EEG activity is noted (upper part); the termination of the convulsion is characterized by general voltage depression. (Taken from H. Gastaut and R. Broughton: EPILEPTIC SEIZURES, Thomas, Springfield, 1972, with kind permission of the authors.)

mental phenomena. In such cases, the grand mal simply indicates the full generalization of an originally focal epileptic event. The initiating "*aura*" must be understood in terms of a brief focal seizure; such short-lasting sensations must be carefully separated from *warnings* or *premonitions* of an imminent grand mal. Warnings may consist of a special type of headache or emotional tension and may last for hours.

3) *Petit mal*

Petit mal is a well delineated type of seizure with classical EEG characteristics; Its clinical signs, however, are often subtle and inconspicuous. A *brief absence* with mild impairment of consciousness usually lasts 5 to 30 seconds and is associated with slight myoclonic activity (mostly limited to eye lid flutter) as well as postural (retroflexion of head) and autonomic changes (pallor, change of respiratory and pulse rate etc.). No falls and no other dramatic manifestations occur.

Petit mal seizures never start prior to the age of 3 years and are *most common in the age range from 4 to 16 years.* Thereafter, a sharp decline occurs. Persistence of the attacks into the third decade is uncommon, further persistence into adult life very rare.

Petit mal is *readily diagnosed and documented by the EEG;* hyperventilation may precipitate an absence in less than 30 seconds and the generalized-synchronous 3/sec spike-wave pattern is extremely impressive (Fig. 4a) although it could be confused with somewhat similar ictal EEG changes in other epileptic conditions and especially in the Lennox-Gastaut syndrome (Niedermeyer, 1972). The generalized character of the EEG abnormalities and the lack of inter-ictal or preceding focal discharges indicate the role of primary generalization but, in a minority of the cases, primary cortical or deep midline foci may be present and the generalization of secondary character ("seconday bilateral synchrony") (Fig. 4b).

The incidence of petit mal epilepsy is lower than it is generally presumed; Gibbs and Gibbs (1952) arrived at a figure of around 10 percent in their huge sample of 11,000 epileptics but this figure might be much lower in the material of most seizure clinics; even in a purely pediatric population of epileptics, the figure of 10 percent may not be reached.

The concept of a petit mal triad (Lennox, 1945) has been generally abandoned since one element, the akinetic petit mal falls in a different clinical category (Lennox-Gastaut Syndrome), where also the cases of petit mal variant belong. More will be said concerning the differential diagnosis of petit mal in the discussion of Common generalized epilepsy and the Lennox-Gastaut syndrome.

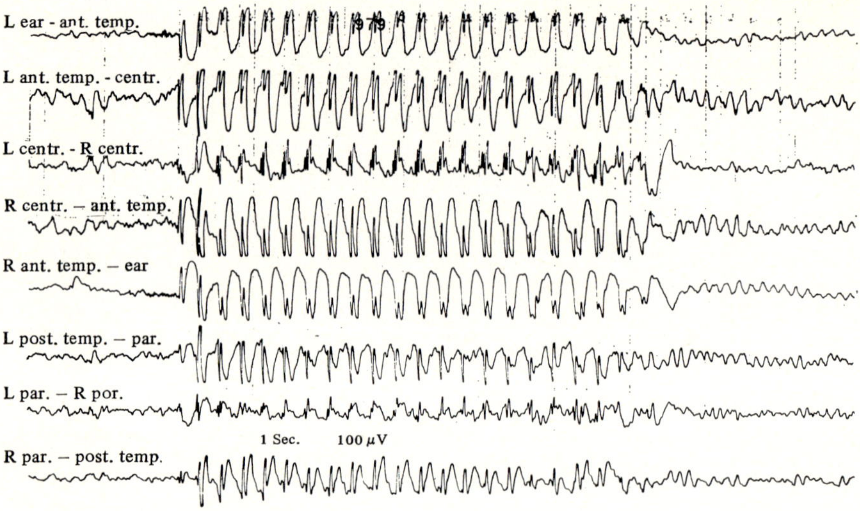

FIGURE 4. a) The EEG of a clinical petit mal absence, recorded in a five-year-old girl. Generalization of the spike-wave activity appears to be primary and immediate (although an EEG tracing can never rule out with absolute certainty the possibility of a hidden focal onset). The record is unremarkable prior to the onset of the seizure and almost immediately returns to normalcy with the termination of the spike-wave activity.

4) *Psychomotor seizures*

The wide variety of ictal signs and symptoms of psychomotor seizures will be *discussed under the heading of temporal lobe epilepsy*. These automatism like or subjectively consciously experienced types of seizures (with a vast range of weird appearing hallucinatory perceptions) stem from temporal lobe foci. Hence we are dealing with a partial type of epileptic manifestation.

5) *Myoclonic seizures*

These very brief but frequently repetitive seizures consist of rapid, usually bilateral-synchronous movements of the extremities (with flexor predominance), face and, more seldom, of the trunk musculature. Their semeiology and electrophysiological concomitants have been studied in great detail by Halliday (1967) and by Gastaut and Broughton (1972).

These seizures may be *due to a wide variety of etiologies*

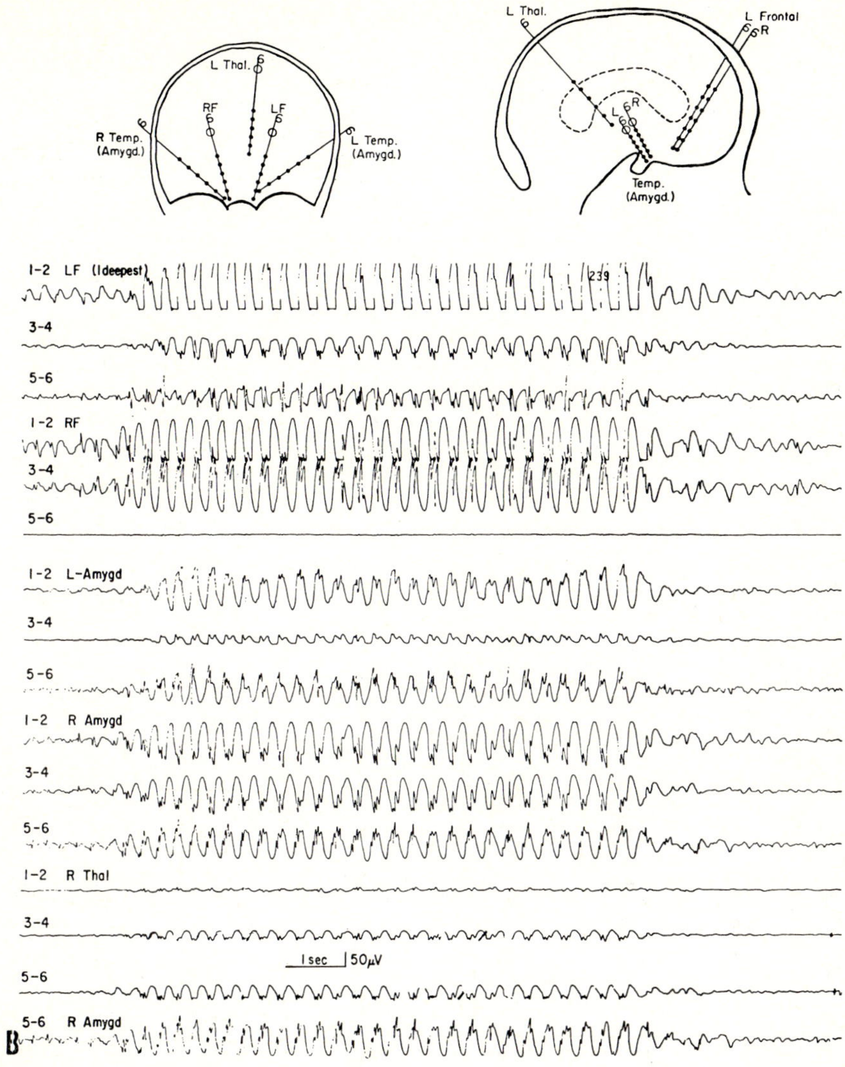

FIGURE 4. b) Depth EEG recording obtained from a 15-year-old boy with petit mal, ill-defined automatisms and, earlier in life, grand mal (#930545). A subclinical burst of 3-4/sec spike-wave complexes is initiated by local spike-waves in the depth of the right frontal lobe. This right frontal onset proved to be a consistent finding. The thalamic and limbic regions participate in the spike-wave activity but nothing suggests a thalamic or limbic origin of the discharge. The patient was markedly improved after a partial right frontal lobectomy. This is a good example of *secondary bilateral synchrony.*

(Essential hereditary myoclonus epilepsy, lipidosis of the CNS, acute encephalitis, subacute sclerosing panencephalitis, acute cerebral anoxia, Creutzfeldt-Jakob's encephalopathy, spongiform encephalopathy, renal insufficiency with uremia) and occur in various epileptic conditions (common generalized epilepsy, Lennox-Gastaut syndrome, hypsarrhythmia).

In Tay-Sachs' disease and in acute cerebral anoxia, the myoclonus may be startle-induced or stimulus sensitive in general.

According to Rodin et al. (1971), Metrazol induced myoclonus is associated with extremely high EEG frequencies (around 1000/sec) which are most prominent in the brain stem reticular formation. A continuous (rather than burst like) high frequency discharge in the reticular formation was noticed when a grand mal attack developed.

Occasional myoclonus in the morning hours may herald an imminent grand mal in patients with common generalized epilepsy; some children with petit mal have an unusually strong accompaniment of myoclonic phenomena.

Myoclonic seizure are based on bilateral or generalized-synchronous seizure discharges and no cortical or deep focus is demonstrable. Certain types of myoclonic conditions are not associated with EEG abnormalities: Hartung's form of benign essential hereditary myoclonus and the physiological violent muscle jerks which occur in the state of falling asleep after strenuous muscular activity.

6) Focal motor and other focal seizures

These seizures will be discussed in Chapter 5 under the heading of "Epilepsy due to hemispheric lesions other than temporal."

7) Hemiconvulsions

Hemiconvulsions must be separated from focal motor seizures. This type of seizure is common and almost completely limited to infancy and early childhood (Gastaut et al., 1962). Tonic or clonic elements may prevail and some of these attacks could be termed "*hemiclonic seizures.*"

Some children with hemiconvulsions fall into the category of the Lennox-Gastaut syndrome.

8) Atonic-akinetic seizures

These seizures are characterized by a *sudden vehement fall* which is often traumatizing (see Fig. 16, 17). The fall may occur in any direction; naturally, a fall in forward direction is likely to lead to facial and cranial trauma. Protective headgear is therefore a necessary preventive measure. The attacks are frequent and may occur several times in one day.

These seizures are most common in children from age 2 to 10 years; in some cases, the attacks persist through adolescence and early adulthood. Almost all of the sufferers from atonic-akinetic seizures fall into the category of the Lennox-Gastaut syndrome in which institutionalization of the progressively mentally defective patient may become a necessity.

Synonymous terms are static seizures (Hunt, 1922), akinetic petit mal (Lennox, 1945; Doose, 1964), "akinetic seizures" (Bridge, 1949), "myokinetic seizures" (Sorel, 1964), "atonic seizures" (Gastaut et al., 1966) and "myoclonic-astatic petit mal" (Kruse, 1968).

9) Tonic seizures

Epileptic seizures with tonic movements must be separated from the tonic type of posturing seen in decerebrate and decorticate patients or so-called mesencephalic and cerebellar fits in which the tonic movements represent a release phenomenon.

The truly epileptic type of tonic seizures may be divided into the axial type (head, neck) and the rhizomelic type involving the limbs (Chatrian, 1971).

Tonic seizures with brief extension of the limbs are very common in children and adolescents with Lennox-Gastaut syndrome. These attacks may become very frequent during sleep but the clinical ictal manifestations may be so subtle that the seizures are often overlooked or ignored. Sleep EEG recordings are particularly helpful in the detection of this type of seizure which is associated with a run of rapid spikes bilaterally and mainly over frontal areas. More minute details of these attacks have been described by Gastaut et al. (1963), Chatrian (1971) and Gastaut and Broughton (1972).

Another type of tonic seizures may occur in childhood and adulthood; these seizures are often asymmetrical and consist of extension of one or both arms, extension in one and flexion in the other arm, clawing of one or both hands and similar variations. This type of epilepsy is *focal and involves chiefly the supplementary motor region* in the interhemispheric fissure; it will be discussed under the heading of epilepsy due to hemispheric lesions (Mesio-frontal epilepsy, Chapter 5). Some of these cases are characterized by *sensitivity to startle.*

The *tonic brain stem attacks* of Mumenthaler and Altermatt (1967) are *unilateral and painful* with unimpaired consciousness. Vascular and neoplastic brain stem lesions but also multiple sclerosis may be the cause; there are no ictal EEG changes (Matthews, 1958; Ambrozy, 1964). These attacks may or may not be of epileptic nature.

10) Clonic seizures

In addition to massive myoclonic jerking, attacks of rapidly repetitive clonic muscular activity in all extremities and facial muscles may occur in the Lennox-Gastaut syndrome (Gastaut et al., 1966, Niedermeyer, 1972).

The rapid clonic activity is less vehement than in myoclonus and the locomotor effect is smaller. The frequency of the clonus does not slow down in the final stage of the seizure as is the case in the clonic phase of a grand mal.

11) Head nodding attacks

This seizure type is almost limited to *infantile spasms* (*hypsarrhythmia*) of infancy in which condition it occurs very often. These attacks are a special form of myoclonus and are usually seen in a series of repetitive head nodding motions.

12) Jackknifing and salaam attacks

These seizures are confined to *infantile spasms* (hypsarrhythmia) and will be discussed in Chapter 4.

CHAPTER 3

THE ETIOLOGIES OF EPILEPTIC CONDITIONS

1) Introductory remarks

EVERY HUMAN BEING and every animal is a potential epileptic. Epileptogenic stimuli have to be sufficiently strong in order to precipitate seizures even in individuals with no spontaneous seizures. For many years, induced seizures have represented an armamentarium in the therapy of schizophrenic and manic-depressive psychoses after the introduction of Metrazol®—convulsions (Meduna, 1933) and electroconvulsions (Cerletti and Bini, 1938).

Every type of cerebral pathology or insult to the brain could give rise to epileptic seizures, either acutely or after some delay due to the epileptogenic effect of secondary scar formation. In the following, the more commonly encountered causes of epilepsy will be discussed. This formulation indicates that a list of etiologies will always be incomplete because of the abundance of causes and the changing aspects of pathology and medicine. New diseases and syndromes are being discovered; certain conditions have moved into the foreground while others are more seldom seen than in the past. Even the advent of new drugs and toxic substances has to be taken into account. Moreover, the acute epileptic condition with myoclonic jerking in a comatose state after partial resuscitation from respiratory or cardiac arrest is the result of improved techniques of resuscitation, since these patients used to die acutely.

Irrespective of all etiologies, epileptic manifestations are not limited to chronically recurrent seizure events due to a residual epileptogenic scar or a slowly progressive lesion; seizures may occur acutely as the accompaniment of an acute cerebral disease. This notion of *acute epilepsy* has been scarcely discussed in the past and deserves greater clinical attention. In the case of acute seizures in an infectious disease with encephalitis, in a severe stroke or in the acute stage of a craniocerebral trauma, the treatment of the basic disease must remain in the foreground. Such epileptic seizures are simply a concomitant neurological sign which requires anticonvulsive therapy only if the seizure activity remains severe, unabated and threatening to develop into a status epilepticus.

Some epileptic etiologies and conditions are acute epilepsies by their very nature: neonatal seizures fall into this category and all of the predominantly myoclonic seizure manifestations which occur in acute cerebral anoxia (usually following cardiorespiratory arrest and incomplete resuscitation). The most common etiologies of epileptic seizures and their relationship to the age of onset are shown in Table V.

2) The etiological role of genetic factors

In bygone days many physicians were inclined to regard all epilepsy as inherited. This view is, of course, a gross distortion of the reality but the fact remains that even in well documented acquired epileptogenic lesions, the presence of a genetic component as a contributory factor cannot be ignored. This additional genetic element in acquired epilepsies has been conceived as "*threshold genes*" in the work of Metrakos and Metrakos (1960, 1961, 1970); the idea of a combined action of hereditary and acquisitional factors dates back to Stauder (1935).

More obvious and undisputed is the genetic factor in seizure disorders caused by a well defined genetic disease ("disease genes" after Metrakos and Metrakos, 1961). This is exemplified by a number of cerebral diseases due to inborn errors of metabolism on a genetic basis and will be discussed somewhat later in this chapter (Fig. 5).

There still remains the crucial question concerning *epilepsy*

TABLE V

THE MOST COMMON CAUSES OF EPILEPTIC SEIZURES ACCORDING TO AGE OF ONSET OF SEIZURES (listed in order of importance)

First week

1) Perinatal trauma
2) Perinatal anoxia
3) Cerebral malformations (atrophy, porencephaly etc.)
4) Hypocalcemia
5) Hypoglycemia

Second week

1) Hypocalcemia
2) Cerebral malformations
3) Early CNS infection (E. Coli, Staph., Herpes simplex virus)
4) Extracranial infection (pneumonia, gastro-enteritis)
5) Perinatal trauma
6) Perinatal anoxia
7) Kernicterus

3rd week to 3 months

1) CNS infection (H. influenzae, and others)
2) Cerebral malformations
3) Subdural collection following CNS infection
4) Inborn errors of metabolism (Tay-Sachs and others)

4 months to 2 years

1) FEBRILE CONVULSIONS (triggered by upper respiratory disease; predominantly genetic)
2) CNS infection
3) Cerebrovascular disorder (arterial occlusion, venous thrombosis)
4) Residual scars of earliest CNS insults (mostly with cerebral palsy)
5) Inborn errors of metabolism (phenylketonuria, Tay-Sachs and others)

NOTE: Minor seizures at this age tend to occur as Infantile Spasms (Hypsarrhythmia)

3 - 10 years

1) Residual scars of early CNS insults (in severe cases: Lennox-Gastaut syndrome)
2) Genetic: Common generalized epilepsy (presenting as petit mal)
3) CNS infection
4) Trauma
5) Lead poisoning (residual, ingestion around age 2)
6) Inborn errors of metabolism

(Brain tumor uncommon)

11 - 20 years

1) Genetic: Common generalized epilepsy (petit mal plus grand mal)
2) Trauma
3) Residual scars of early CNS insults (in severe cases: Lennox-Gastaut syndrome)
4) A-V malformation
5) Brain tumor (in general, onset of seizures not very common in this decade)

21 - 40 years

1) Trauma
2) Brain Tumor
3) Chronic alcoholism
4) A-V malformation
5) Residual scars of early CNS insults
6) Vasculitis (systemic lupus erythematosus)

41 - 60 years

1) Brain tumor
2) Chronic alcoholism
3) Trauma
4) Cerebral arteriosclerosis
5) Neurosyphilis

above age 60

1) Cerebral arteriosclerosis
2) Brain tumor (primary or metastatic)

At all ages: CAUSE FREQUENTLY REMAINS UNKNOWN

In subtropical and tropical countries: always consider intracranial parasites. Even malaria may be followed by epileptic seizures.

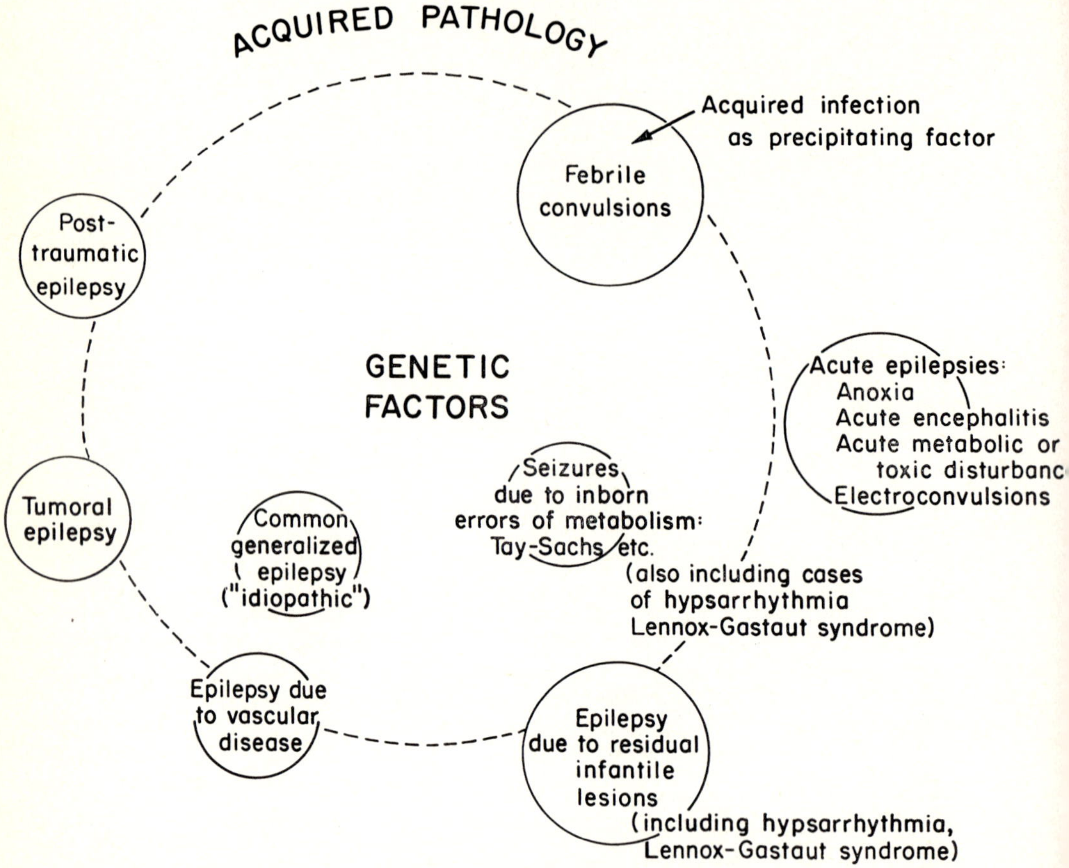

FIGURE 5. Schematic presentation of genetic factors and acquired pathology and their contributory role in various types of seizure disorders. Common generalized epilepsy (a cerebral disturbance with no evidence of pathology) and inherited brain diseases with seizures (such as Tay-Sachs disease and other inborn errors of metabolism) are shown as disorders based on genetic defects. Febrile convulsions appear to be predominantly determined by genetic factors. Note the small contributory role of genetic factors and obviously acquired brain diseases. "Threshold genes" (according to J and K. Metrakos) partly determine the occurrence of epileptic seizures in acquired cerebral pathology.

as a disease entity in the absence of any other plausible epileptogenic etiology such as brain damage, toxic or metabolic alterations. This poses the question as to whether certain genes may bring forth an epileptic condition totally detached from any demonstrable cerebral pathology. A "disease *per se*" would mean —in Greek—"idiopathic" and there have been indeed endless attempts to provide evidence for (or to disprove) the existence of an idiopathic type of epilepsy. The intricacies of this problem will be discussed later under the heading of "common generalized epilepsy."

3) *Inborn errors of metabolism*

The demonstration of a primary genetic biochemical defect in several diseases of the CNS denotes a remarkable change of pathological concepts. In recent years, a growing list of such diseases have been identified. Most of these disorders manifest themselves in infancy or childhood. The CNS is quite often involved and, in some of these diseases, the CNS affection stands in the foreground. It is obvious that epileptic manifestations may arise in these disorders.

A discussion of the biochemical basis of these disorders would not only exceed the scope of this book but, in some instances, would become outdated in a short period of time. For this reason, only the better known conditions with a high incidence of epileptic seizures will be mentioned in the following.

a) VARIOUS FORMS OF LIPIDOSIS. The most representative disorder in this group is *Tay-Sachs' disease,* in previous years termed *amaurotic idiocy* but, more recently recognized as nosological entity on its biochemical basis. An accumulation of a particular ganglioside (GM_2) has been demonstrated (Svennerholm, 1964), presumably due to the absence of a lipid hexosaminase. An autosomal-recessive gene causes the disease; Jewish individuals are almost exclusively affected. Loss of vision, progressive mental defects, general spasticity and rigidity develop rapidly after about the third month of life; the cherry red macular changes are usually seen in the second half of the first year. At this time, *tonic convulsions and spasms develop, usually induced by startling auditory stimuli* (loud noise). The infants die around the age of 2 years.

Other forms of cerebral lipidosis begin somewhat later in life (between the age of 1 to 10 years). The *late infantile form* (Bielschowsky, 1913) has been distinguished from *juvenile* (Batten, 1903, 1914; Vogt, 1905; Spielmeyer, 1906) and *later forms* (Kuf's type); convulsive manifestations include myoclonus, often prolonged, and tonic spasms with severe cyanosis (Pampiglione and Lehovsky, 1968). A marked driven spike response in the occipital leads with rhythmical low-frequency photic stimulation is helpful in the EEG diagnosis of the late infantile form (Pampiglione and Lehovsky, 1968). The pace of the downhill course is somewhat slower; spasticity, tremor, speech disturbance and loss of vision with optic atrophy are some of the clinical characteristics. More recently, all of these forms have been lumped together under the heading of juvenile cerebroretinal degeneration (Freeman and McKhann, 1969).

Convulsions may also occur in the acute infantile form of Gaucher's disease which is thought to be a cerebroside lipidosis with cerebral involvement. Head retraction, bulbar paralysis and a decerebrate state characterize this disease which is more common in Jews than in other races.

b) Amino-acidurias. The best known example of a deranged amino acid metabolic defect is phenylketonuria. More than one fourth of the affected children develop epileptic seizures such as major convulsions and myoclonus. Less common are seizures in the more rapidly advancing *maple syrup urine disease*. Seizures may occur in the advanced stage of ocular cerebral renal dystrophy (Lowe et al., 1952) with a disturbance of the renal production of ammonia. The complex biochemical-nutritional *therapy* of these disorders cannot be presented in this context.

The reader would gain very little from a long list of all known inborn errors of metabolism with cerebral implications; it is self-evident that many or most of these diseases could give rise to convulsive disorder.

c) Principles of Classification. A valuable principle of subdivision for biochemical degenerative CNS afflictions lies in the separation of *gray matter vs. white matter disease* as proposed by Freeman and McKhann (1969). Predominant *gray matter disease is more likely to lead to dementia and epilepsy* whereas predominent white matter disease gives rise to long tract signs. Tay-Sachs' disease and the subsequently discussed essential hereditary myoclonus epilepsy are representative examples of gray matter disease which are very eloquent in the EEG and produce severe paroxysmal EEG abnormalities. On the other hand, typical white matter diseases such as the leucodystrophies (metachromatic, sudanophilic type, globoid type also called Krabbe's disease, Alexanders disease, Pelizaeus-Merzbacher's disease) are of only mildly epileptogenic character and their effect on the EEG is much less significant.

Appendix

PYRIDOXIN-DEFICIENCY. In the absence of apparent brain damage, the nutritional deficiency of Vitamins B_6 (pyridoxin) results in severe and even fatal convulsions in neonates and infants (Reilly et al., 1953; Coursin, 1964). Pyridoxin dependency may develop in fetal life and occur on a *genetic basis* (Hunt, Jr., 1954; Waldinger and Berg, 1963). Large doses of Vitamin B_6 (exceeding the usual therapeutic range) constitute the only effective treatment in these rare cases. Pyridoxin is also helpful to prevent toxic convulsive responses in long-term *isoniazid treatment* of tuberculosis (Reilly et al., 1953); 50 mg/day is the ordinary dosage in the adult.

4) Essential hereditary myoclonus epilepsy (Lafora-Unverricht-Lundborg)

This progressive encephalopathy is due to an autosomal recessive gene and occurs as a variety of sub-entities according to the severity of the clinical picture. Therefore, essential hereditary myoclonus epilepsy can be subdivided as follows:

a) The type described by Lafora and Glueck (1911) with the most rapid progression
b) Unverricht's form with a slightly more protracted and milder course (Unverricht, 1891)

c) Lundborg's form with considerably less severe cerebral defects (Lundborg, 1913).

The disease usually begins between age 6 and 16 years. *Subtle or more conspicuous myoclonic twitching and jerking* is noticed in the facial musculature, trunk and limbs; grand mal seizures occur in varying intervals. *A cerebellar syndrome with intentional tremor and dysmetria* develops with comparatively slight involvement of the postural equilibrium (minor vermis component). Dysarthric changes are due to mild myoclonic interference with the speech musculature. Pyramidal tract involvement may be present and a mixture of spasticity and rigidity (basal ganglia component) may ensue. Gradually progressive *dementia* may be associated with some degree of juvenile behavior disorder.

In the further course, cerebellar intentional tremor and myoclonic jerking may become inseparably intermingled and this combination could be classified as *intentional myoclonus* (Lance and Adams, 1963; described in cases of post anoxic myoclonus). Violent jerks may throw the patient to the floor. Death occurs between age 15 and 30 years (or later in Lundborg's form).

Neuropathological changes are widespread but the cerebellum-brain stem region (Guillain-Mollaret's triangle, consisting of the cerebellar dentate nucleus, the inferior olive and the red nucleus) is predominantly involved. The affected regions are the seat of Lafora bodies which, according to Harriman and Millar (1955), have the properties of an acid polymucosaccharide. For this reason, essential myoclonus epilepsy might represent a *mucopolysaccharidosis of the brain.* Consanguinity may be instrumental in the materialization of the genetic defect. From the biochemical viewpoint, this disease should be separated from the various types of mucopolysaccharidosis with secondary or induced brain involvement (Hurler's, Hunter's, Sanfilippo's, Morquio's and other syndromes, associated with gargoylism and other severe body defects).

The EEG is of considerable diagnostic value in myoclonus epilepsy. Figure 6 shows a mixture of cerebral and myogenic spikes which is almost diagnostic. In most cases, there is also a very marked enhancement of seizure discharges and myoclonic activity with intermittent photic stimulation whereas sleep attenuates the abnormalities.

Normal EEG findings are obtained in the autosomal-dominant form of *Hartung's type of hereditary myoclonus epilepsy.* This benign disorder does not lead to dementia. Frequent myoclonic jerking occurs; these discharges evidently feed into the anterior horn cells and the lower motor neuron while the lack of upward discharges to the cortex accounts for the normalcy of the EEG.

Similar to the Lafora-Unverricht-type is the *Dyssynergia cerebellaris myoclonica* (*Hunt*) with more prominent cerebellar symptomatology in addition to myoclonus.

In all of these forms of essential hereditary myoclonus epilepsy, there is *no effective treatment* and the prognosis depends mercilessly on the pace of progression of the biochemically induced brain lesions.

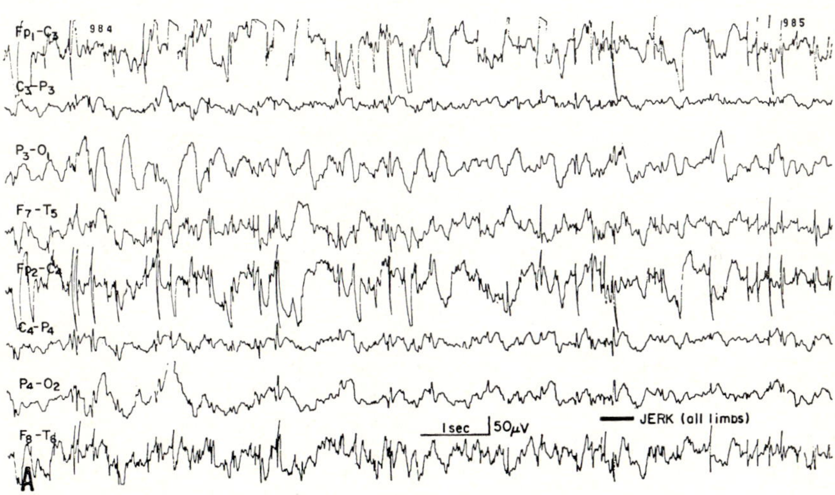

FIGURE 6. a) EEG of a 17-year-old male patient diagnosed as Lafora-Unverricht-Lundborg's essential hereditary myoclonus epilepsy (#1346267). The patient is awake and resting. Note the abundant bilateral-frontal or generalized spike activity. The fastest single spikes over anterior regions are most likely to be myogenic but authentic cerebral spikes are also seen. There is a rather unimpressive EEG concomitant of a brief myoclonic body jerk.

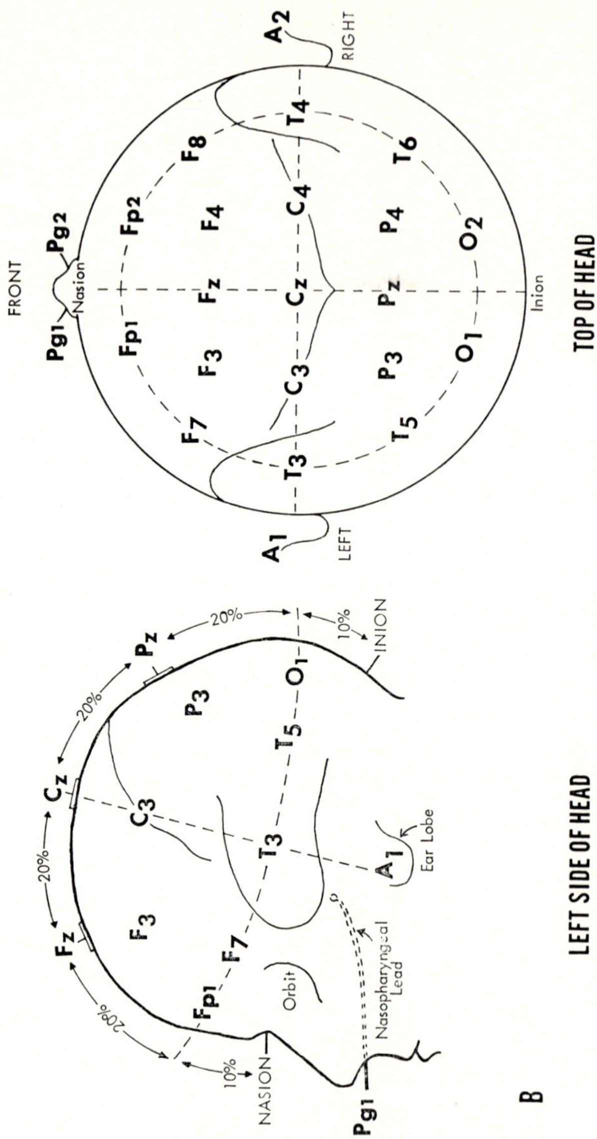

FIGURE 6. b) Demonstration of the electrode placement according to the International Electrode System (used in most of the scalp recordings shown in this book).

5) Prenatal, perinatal and post-natal infantile brain damage

Acquired brain damage during fetal life and early infancy is one of the most common causes of epilepsy, which often manifests itself for the first time with considerable delay, not infrequently even in adulthood. The pathology of the residual cerebral impairment is manifold and can be divided into various types of insult.

a) Prenatal brain damage. Developmental disturbances of the CNS during fetal life may lead to a gamut of cerebral malformation ranging from encephalomalacic porencephalies to gross monstrosities like schizencephalies and anencephaly or hydranencephaly. From the epileptological viewpoint, *microgyria* is the most important type of regional cortical damage which is very frequently associated with the formation of an epileptogenic focus. *Prenatal infection* should also be taken into account; rubella is seldom followed by seizures whereas intrauterine infection with syphilis and toxoplasmosis are more likely causes of epilepsy.

Chromosomal aberrations such as Down's syndrome (mongolism) are associated with epilepsy only in conjunction with additional cerebral pathology.

Tuberous sclerosis is a genetically transmitted neuroectodermal disorder giving rise to hamartoma-like growths which, in homozygous gene carriers, severely affect the CNS. Neoplastic glial masses commonly give rise to grand mal convulsions in such cases. Facial adenoma sebaceum is the most significant sign among the multiple cutaneo-visceral lesions. *Sturge-Weber's* syndrome with extensive facial nevus and intracranial calcifications is usually associated with focal or major convulsions.

b) Perinatal brain damage. Cerebral birth trauma may be divided into *birth anoxia* and *mechanical trauma with bleeding.* A strong contributory factor to perinatal pathology is *prematurity.*

All of these cerebral insults may lead to convulsive disorders which may be present early in the neonatal period or may be delayed into childhood or even adulthood. Neonatal convulsions may be the expression of the acute cerebral injury while delayed recrudescence, recurrence or onset of seizures, is likely to be the result of cicatrix formation. Many of these cases are associated with forms of *cerebral palsy* such as the hemiplegic, diplegic, quadriplegic, dyskinetic (basal ganglia-type) and atonic variety. Pathology may reach from local damage to mesial portions of the temporal lobe ("incisural herniation" of Earle et al., 1952; frequently believed to be one of the most important causative mechanisms of temporal lobe epilepsy) to multicystic encephalomalacia. The incidence of epilepsy in various forms of cerebral palsy and the role of the EEG in the prognostication has been the subject of intensive studies by Perlstein and Gibbs (1949; see also Gibbs and Gibbs, 1964).

c) Postnatal brain damage. Epileptic seizures of the neonatal period are not necessarily the result of morphological damage to the brain. Frequent and mild causes are *transient electrolyte disturbances* (often the result of early extracerebral infection such as otitis, pneumonia or gastroenteritis) with hyponatremia and hypocalcemia in the first place, or the etiologically poorly understood states or neonatal hypoglycemia. Meningoencephalitic infections will be dealt with in the following section.

Kernicterus is caused by hyperbilirubinemia which injures the basal ganglia and other cerebral structures. Fetal erythroblastosis secondary to Rh-incompatibility and related conditions are the most common causes. This condition is a frequent cause of the dykinetic or choreo-athetoid form of cerebral palsy and concomitant epileptic seizures are not uncommon.

6) Infectious diseases (encephalitis)

Infectious processes of the CNS may develop as early as intrauterine life (toxoplasmosis, syphilis) or, as it has been recognized more recently, during the passage through the birth canal in the case of the herpes genitalis virus (a variety of herpes simplex) which leads to a severe destructive neonatal encephalitis; convulsions may be associated with these diseases. More common, however, are meningeal infections of bacterial etiology in the neonatal period and infancy. *Neonatal convulsions* and especially those occurring between the age of 2 weeks to 3 months (Massa and Niedermeyer, 1968) are frequently caused by *meningitis.* Escherichia coli and, somewhat later, Hemophilus influenzae are the most common causative agents. The seizures provide evidence for a concomitant encephalitic affection. After initial improvement due to appropriate antibiotic treatment, a return of temperature elevation, irritability and convulsions may signal a *postmeningitic subdural collection* of fluids which requires tapping through the fontanelle or surgical evacuation with removal of the membrane. The prognosis is guarded or dubious as far as recurrent post-meningo-encephalitic seizures are concerned.

Tuberculous meningitis contracted in infancy or early childhood may result in a severe consecutive convulsive disorder, especially when tuberculostatic treatment was started with excessive delay. *Measles* is often accompanied by a parainfectious encephalitis frequently associated with acute epileptic manifestations and followed by postinfectious epilepsy in conjunction with neurological and mental deficits; massive preventive immunization will reduce considerably this cause of epilepsy. Parainfectious encephalitis with convulsions may also occur in *mumps, German measles* (very seldom), *chickenpox* and as a complication of *smallpox vaccination.* These convulsions accompany the acute cerebral disease but are unlikely to persist in a residual postencephalitic state. Convulsions in the first stage of *exanthema subitum* (*roseola infantum*) are very common in the absence of further substantial encephalitic involvement. The strong linkage of acute convulsions with this benign disease suggests that the mechanism is *different from simple febrile convulsions* which will be discussed later. Postinfectious epilepsy does not develop after roseola.

Nonspecific infections and particularly acute upper respiratory ailments may lead to severe cerebral complications associated with coma, hemiplegia and hemiconvulsions in the affected extremities. Hyperthermia is common in this condition which is rare and confined to the age range from 6 months to 2 years. *Thrombosis of the superior sagittal* (*longitudinal*) *sinus* is most frequently encountered as the substrate of this condition which has been termed *H.H.E.-syndrome* (Gastaut et al., 1957). This abbreviation stands for hemiconvulsion hemiplegia as the acute manifestations, and epilepsy as the usual sequel of the severe cerebral lesions. The prolonged character or the rapid succession of the hemiconvulsions in the acute state often necessitate a status epilepticus type of treatment.

In *subacute sclerosing panencephalitis* (*SSPE*), major convulsions are a rare event but *repetitive myoclonic jerking* is one of the most characteristic clinical manifestations. The etiology of this disease has been clarified by the demonstration of the measles virus in obviously prolonged and slow action. Almost rhythmically recurrent irregular slow and sharp bursts in all leads are the main characteristic of the EEG which, in this disease, is of almost specific diagnostic value (except for the initial and the terminal stage). Many of these periodical bursts are accompanied by widespread and sometimes asymmetrical brief jerks of the extremities; the myoclonus, however, may be overshadowed by a periodically recurrent brief loss of muscular tone with slight buckling of the knees and dropping of the head when the patient is standing. Childhood and early adolescence delineate the usual age range of this disease which is mostly fatal; some cases may be arrested (attempts with antiviral agents have not been crowned with success thus far) or come to a spontaneous standstill with severe residual cerebral deficits. Anticonvulsant medication is of no use in this condition.

Primarily neurotropic viruses may give rise to acute or post-encephalitic convulsions and may occur at any age. In this country, St. Louis encephalitis and the various types of equine encephalitis (Eastern, Western and Venezuela type) are predominantly mild and of little epileptological interest. The Far East of Asia is plagued by the extremely severe Japanese encephalitis (B encephalitis) and the Siberian *spring-summer encephalitis* which is the main and principal cause of *Epilepsia partialis continua* (*Koshevnikov's syndrome*). In the post-encephalitic stage, the involvement of either the motor cortex or deeper structures (basal ganglia, thalamus) leads to continuous repetitive clonic movement limited to a particular muscular segment. This type of constant focal seizure activity tends to defy anticonvulsive therapy. Causes of epilepsia partialis continua reported outside Russia are, in most instances, not as clearly defined and less protracted than the Siberian post-enphalitic cases with year-long and almost indefinite continuation of the segmental clonus. *Von Economo's* encephalitis (lethargic or epidemic encephalitis) has virtually disappeared for the last 40 years; post encephalitic cases are characterized by Parkinsonism. I had the rare opportunity to see a patient in whom temporal lobe epilepsy developed simultaneously with the postencephalitic Parkinson syndrome. The presumed viral etiology of this enigmatic disease (which is believed to still exist in a district of Mongolia) has never been proven.

Herpes simplex encephalitis is a focal type of encephalitis which involves predominantly the limbic portions of the temporal lobe before the viral infection becomes more diffuse. Epileptic seizures may occur in this condition which is more common in adults (in 64% of the cases according to Haymaker et al., 1958). The neonatal type of infection has been mentioned farther above. Fatal outcome is very frequent but not necessarily the rule. Another limbic type of viral encephalitis is *rabies* which, however, is not associated with seizures.

In *neurosyphillis,* grand mal and focal seizures are often seen and may occur in both *general paresis* and the *meningo-vascular forms* of syphillis.

A special paragraph will be devoted to Creutzfeldt-Jakob's encephalopathy which was generally considered a rapidly progressive degenerative brain disease until a viral etiology was demonstrated by Gibbs, Jr., and Gajdusek, 1969. The pathogenesis of *multiple sclerosis* is still obscure; inflammatory changes have been suggestive of an infectious agent. Epileptic seizures are a rare symptom of this disease. (Bronisch and Rauch, 1947; Drake and Macrae, 1961; Hopf et al., 1970; Trouillas and Courjon, 1972). A special variety of tonic seizures may occur in the absence of concomitant ictal EEG changes (Matthews, 1958; Matthews, 1962; Joynt and Green, 1962).

Acute allergic phenomena may be associated with grand mal convulsions in very rare cases when acute edematous changes affect the brain (F. Kennedy, 1962, 1938; H. Stevens, 1965).

Non-purulent cerebral parasitic agents may be an important cause of seizures (the purulent brain infections caused by parasites will be briefly discussed in connection with brain abscess). *Cerebral cysticercosis* is most notorious as an epileptogenic disorder, especially in Latin American and South Eastern European countries as well as on the Iberian peninsula (Moniz et al., 1932; Asenjo, 1961). According to Arseni and Cristescu (1972), seizures occurred in 60 percent of their patients and focal seizures were more common than grand mal.

7) Craniocerebral trauma

The concluding remarks on the foregoing discussion of infectious diseases and epilepsy apply also to a certain degree to traumatic causes of seizures. There is indeed a valid distinction between convulsions occurring in the acute traumatic stage and posttraumatic epilepsy.

Major convulsions occurring in the acute stage of the craniocerebral trauma denote that the head injury caused some neuronal irritation. This type of parenchymatous impairment would be hardly attributable to an uncomplicated cerebral concussion.

Trauma induced epileptic manifestations may be divided as follows:

a) Immediate seizures. Grand mal attacks may occur during the first 2 or 3 seconds following an acute head injury. A. E. Walker (1949) has ascribed this causation of seizures to a direct mechanical stimulation of cerebral structures with low epileptogenic threshold. Rowbotham (1964) found evidence of such early seizures in approximately 1 percent of the victims of acute head injuries.

b) Early epileptic responses to acute traumatic cerebral pathology. These attacks develop during the first 24 to 48 hours in severely traumatized patients with cerebral contusion, intracerebral hematoma or brain laceration. A more diffuse concomitant cerebral edema may give rise to grand mal seizures whereas focal seizures prevail in local edematous responses to the cerebral lesion (Jennett, 1962).

c) Early posttraumatic epilepsy. These seizures develop after the acute traumatic phase, i.e. between one week and 3 months following the trauma. Early posttraumatic tissue changes are evidently the cause of these attacks.

d) Late posttraumatic epilepsy. This type of epilepsy is

due to the development of scarring processes in the brain with an onset of seizures later than 3 months and generally not later than 2 years after the injury. Cerebral laceration is the most frequently encountered original traumatic condition and a brain dura cicatrix causes particularly strong epileptogenic neuronal irritation. This is *the most common type of trauma induced epilepsy* and its prevalence increases considerably in wartime. According to A. E. Walker (1949), parietal wounds are "more prone to have a complicating epilepsy than frontal, temporal and occipital injuries."

e) FRONTAL (FRONTOTEMPORAL) POSTTRAUMATIC EPILEPSY WITH SLOW SPIKE-WAVE COMPLEXES IN THE EEG. This rare complication of severe closed crainiocerebral trauma acquired either in childhood, adolescence or adulthood is characterized by a particularly recalcitrant seizure disorder which may necessitate surgical treatment (Niedermeyer; A. E. Walker, and Burton, 1970). Slow spike wave complexes and runs of rapid spikes in the EEG suggest a close relationship to the Lennox-Gastaut syndrome which will be the topic of more detailed discussions; the type of seizures (usually grand mal and psychomotor automatisms) do not show the variety seen in the Lennox-Gastaut syndrome and mental deficits are milder or absent in the posttraumatic form which has a markedly delayed onset of seizures, usually several years after the injury.

f) EPILEPTIC SEIZURES ASSOCIATED WITH CHRONIC SUBDURAL HEMATOMA. In this type of epilepsy, the trauma is merely an indirect cause of the seizures. Grand mal and/or focal seizures are no rare events and caused by the irritative effects of the hematoma.

The *course of posttraumatic epilepsy* in general is thought to be favorable in 75 percent of the cases; the attacks become less and less frequent and eventually disappear after several years under adequate anticonvulsive medication (Courjon, 1969). Patients with seizures in the acute traumatic stage are usually better off and the vast majority of these patients do not develop late cicatricial epilepsy. According to A. E. Walker and Jablon (1961), among patients with open head wounds and eventual development of posttraumatic epilepsy, in 8.3 percent the first seizure occurred during the first week after the trauma. The evaluation of the prognosis is often hampered by the fact that a patient may have financial gain from the persistence of the seizures; for this reason, information obtained from the patient may be misleading (A. E. Walker and Erculei, 1970).

The long interval between trauma and the onset of late posttraumatic seizures makes one wonder if the *EEG* could be used *as prognostic guideline* concerning future development of posttraumatic epilepsy. Unfortunately, the EEG has not fulfilled early hopes in this regard and the occurrence of focal or widespread spikes in the first weeks and months after the injury could be more confusing rather than prognostically contributory. Such spikes may or may not herald the development of posttraumatic epilepsy; in children and adolescents, such spikes seen in the first weeks after the injury are mostly innocuous. On the other hand, the first late posttraumatic attack may appear without preceding warnings in serial EEGs. The reason for this discrepancy is poorly understood, especially when one recalls the excellent prognostic value of the EEG after acute encephalitis.

The anticonvulsive treatment of posttraumatic epilepsy follows the general principles (to be discussed in a separate chapter); the surgical removal of brain dura scars and other forms of traumatic pathology will prove to be worthwhile in some cases. Of considerable practical interest is the question of *preventive anticonvulsive therapy* following severe head injuries and especially after cerebral lacerations. There is no clear cut answer to this question. While Rowbotham (1964) recommends the prophylactic use of phenobarbital or Dilantin® in such cases, Kristiansen et al. (1969) feel that this type of preventive treatment is worthless.

8) Intracranial tumors

Approximately ⅓ of the cases of intracranial tumors are associated with epileptic seizures; this figure rises to around 50 percent when tumors of the cerebral hemispheres are considered separately (Hess, 1970).

From the epileptological viewpoint, intracranial neoplasms

are a common cause of seizures when the onset of the attacks falls into the age range from 25 to 60 years. In peace time when the incidence of posttraumatic epilepsy is greatly reduced, brain tumors may advance to the first place among the causes of seizures when the onset falls in the above mentioned period of life. This, however, also depends on regional factors as it will be pointed out in the following discussion of alcoholism which, in certain areas, becomes the leading cause of seizures in middle adulthood. While the role of brain tumors in the causation of seizures in adult life can hardly be exaggerated, such worries about a neoplastic etiology should be soothed by the physician in the case of seizure in infancy and childhood. At this life period when proneness to epilepsy reaches a peak, brain tumors represent one of the least frequent causes. It is part of the physician's competence and art (one should not be ashamed to use this word), to assess cases of childhood epilepsy as to whether the diagnostic pursuit of the possible tumoral etiology is worthwhile at all. *A dull and lengthy diagnostic routine scheme for the exclusion of a brain tumor in every child with seizures would be ill advised.*

The histopathology of the tumor is a strong determining factor concerning the occurrence or absence of seizures. The greatest epileptogenicity is seen in oligodendrogliomas which are associated with seizures in 90 percent of the cases (Hess, 1970). Other tumors with high epileptogenicity are astrocytoma (69%), glioblastoma (34%), meningeoma (37%) and metastatic neoplasms (41%).

Another determining factor in tumor epilepsy is the seat of the neoplasm. Frontal tumors are most likely to lead to major convulsions (30-40%) but this figure is not strikingly different from other hemispheric regions (15-35%). Major motor status epilepticus is more likely to occur in frontal rather than in other hemispheric tumors (Janz, 1962). Focal motor seizures are very common in tumors of the central region but this type of focal seizure is also surprisingly often noted in frontal tumors (Hoefer et al., 1946; Hess, 1970). Epileptic manifestations of temporal lobe tumors will be discussed in a separate chapter on temporal lobe epilepsy; may it suffice to point out that olfactory and gustatory hallucinations as a part of temporal lobe attacks are more common in tumoral etiologies rather than in residual and other causes of temporal lobe epilepsy (Bingley, 1958; Hess, 1970). There are, however, no types of seizure which could be regarded as characteristic for a brain tumor.

Deep seated tumors involving lateral ventricles, basal ganglia and thalamus *are less epileptogenic* than hemispheric neoplasms. *Tumors located between third* ventricle and posterior fossa are *epileptogenic only under exceptional circumstances* although Millichap et al. (1962), reported the occasional occurrence of major convulsions in posterior fossa tumors in children. *Diencephalic epilepsy* (Penfield, 1929) in hypothalamic tumors with paroxysmal alterations of the autonomic nervous system is an unproven entity; such attacks may occur in temporal lobe epilepsy but also in non-epileptic conditions.

It is obvious that the *treatment* of tumor-induced epilepsy is surgical, but anticonvulsive medication proves to be helpful following surgery. The medication will be gradually tapered off in the course of one to several years according to the severity of the presurgical epileptic condition and the patient's general postsurgical condition.

9) Brain abscess

Brain abscesses develop following acute purulent encephalitis which leads to confluence of pus and formation of a capsule. The abscess will subsequently cause perifocal edema and, for this reason, both the infectious-inflammatory nature and the space occupying character of the brain abscess have to be taken into consideration.

Brain abscesses are caused by a) penetrating craniocerebral wounds with laceration and infection of brain tissue, b) infections in the neighborhood (middle ear and inner ear, nose and paranasal sinuses, teeth), c) distant infections with metastatic brain involvement, usually located within the chest (pleural empyema, lung abscess, bronchiectasy, acute or subacute endocarditis) and d) congenital heart disease with inadequate tissue oxygenation and subsequent infection. Some brain abscesses are never etiologically clarified and termed "cryptogenic."

Epileptic manifestations are very frequently observed in brain abscesses and may be first clinical sign of cerebral involvement. Grand mal and focal motor seizures are most often observed; this is partially determined by the localization of the process. It is possible that the use of penicillin has increased the incidence of seizures in cases of brain abscess since the convulsive action of penicillin could become manifest by passing through the blood-brain barrier which is perhaps more permeable under the unusual condition of a purulent cerebral infection.

The symptomatology and differential diagnosis of brain abscesses cannot be discussed in this condensed subchapter. Subdural empyema and intracranial venous thrombosis or thrombophlebitis have to be considered in evidently infectious conditions; the brain abscess is less likely than other purulent intracranial affections to give rise to stormy hyperthermias. A delta focus in the EEG is helpful in the diagnosis but angiography is superior and the brain scan almost invariably yields a positive uptake in the area of the abscess.

The emergence of *seizures in a child or infant with congenital heart disease* (and especially with a cyanotic type of cardiac disease) is often *the first manifestation of a brain abscess* although other types of cerebral complications of congenital heart disease may also give rise to epileptic attacks (Tyler and Clark, 1957, 1958; Kalyanaraman et al., 1968).

In addition to purulent bacteria, intracranial *fungus infection* may also lead to abscess formation (actinomyces, nocardia asteroides); brain abscesses in tropical countries may be due to schistosoma affection or similar parasites; convulsions are frequently associated with the cerebral disease.

The combination of antibiotic and surgical *therapy* has been the subject of numerous studies. Postsurgically, recurrent epileptic seizures are not uncommon and the epileptogenic focus may differ from the site of the abscess; we observed temporal lobe epilepsy following the removal of an ipsilateral parietal abscess.

Status epilepticus may be the medically embarrassing cause of death of an undiagnosed case of brain abscess.

10) Cerebrovascular disorders

a) Cerebral arteriosclerosis and similar diseases. The acute or gradually progressive development of ischemic zones in the brain due to *cerebrovascular disorders* is the *most common cause of epilepsy with onset in late adulthood.* Arteriosclerosis (atherosclerosis) is most frequently the pathological substrate of the vascular disease.

This type of convulsive disorder may be divided into *seizures in patients with major cerebrovascular accidents* (CVAs, strokes) and those with no evidence of such events. As to the stroke patients, the seizure may a) occur acutely during the stroke, b) develop as a consequence of the destructive vascular lesion due to subsequent scar formation (Barolin and Scherzer, 1963) or c) precede or usher in the vascular catastrophe ("vascular precursive epilepsy"; Barolin et al., 1971).

Another type of vascular epilepsy *manifests* itself *independently from any major stroke like event.* There is reason to believe that *the hippocampus might be instrumental in this type of seizure disorder.* This limbic region depends chiefly on the vertebrobasilar supply route via the posterior cerebral artery and partly on the internal carotid system via the anterior chorioidal artery; this creates a very vulnerable watershed area (Schröder, 1962). A second and probably less important watershed area lies in the hippocampus between the posterior blood supply and the internal carotid-middle cerebral artery system. Moreover, the rake-like distribution of the small arterial vessels supplying the hippocampus (Lindenberg, 1957) contributes to the local proneness to vascular lesions. The very frequent EEG finding of minor slow and somewhat sharp activity in the anterior temporal mid temporal leads in almost symptom-free mild arteriosclerotics might be attributable to presumed minor vascular lesions of the hippocampus. In possibly predisposed individuals, these small disturbances may assume epileptic properties and give rise to overt seizures. The majority of these patients have a mild or moderately severe type of seizure disorder. Grand mal attacks and psychomotor automatisms are the most common seizure manifestations.

The acute hemiplegic *stroke* may be accompanied by an almost *status like succession of focal motor seizures* in the affected half of the body and even frank status epilepticus may occur. A special type of rather mild but constantly repetitive focal motor clonic twitching may linger on for many hours; this seizure activity is usually accompanied by a unilateral or focal rhythmically repetitive larke spike discharge in the EEG ("pseudoperiodic lateralized epileptiform discharge": Chatrian et al., 1964; Markand and Daly, 1971). This discharge is often seen in a rather surprisingly posterior localization; Naquet and his co-workers (1966, 1969) have related this electrical-clinical syndrome to a *watershed-type* of CVA in the bordering zone between the territories of the middle cerebral and the posterior cerebral arteries. Such watershed type strokes are due to a critical decline of the systemic blood pressure or deteriorating cardiac output.

Arteriosclerosis is not the sole type of pathology in cerebrovascular epilepsy but it is certainly the most frequently encountered one (it must be admitted, of course, that convincing proof of this type of underlying vascular disease can be but seldom provided and that the diagnosis remains somewhat hypothetical in most cases). According to Fischer (1959), *about 4 percent of patients with presumed cerebral arteriosclerosis* requiring a clinical neurological workup *suffer from epilepsy of late onset.* The EEG is most frequently characterized by anterior temporal spikes or sharp waves (Niedermeyer, 1961; Takahashi, et al., 1962; Gibbs and Gibbs, 1964).

In middle adulthood, major convulsions may occasionally be due to a severe or malignant type of arterial hypertension; cases with primary kidney disease will be discussed separately. Another cause of vascular disorder is the group of collagen diseases. The associated arteriitis (vasculitis) may lead to major convulsions in some cases of lupus erythematosus and, very seldom in other collagen diseases. *In systemic lupus erythematosus, grand mal seizures may be the initial manifestation of the disease* (Randow et al., 1965).

In children, adolescents and young adults, acute or chronically recurrent epileptic seizures (grand mal or focal) may be due to vascular lesions caused by *Sickle cell anemia* (SS hemoglobinopathy) (Baird et al., 1964). In most of these cases, convulsions occur in conjunction with other neurological complications (Portnoy and Herion, 1972).

b) Intracranial aneurysms and arteriovenous malformations. In acute subarachnoid hemorrhages from ruptured intracranial aneurysms (Bifurcation, Forbus-type or fusiform type), epileptic seizures may be observed in a minority of the cases (10-20%); such an occurrence usually plays no major role in the general management of the patient. Consecutive seizures are almost unheard of.

Arteriovenous malformations of the cerebral hemispheres are *very often associated with grand mal or focal seizures.* The onset falls most commonly into the age from 10 to 35 years; mild subarachnoid hemorrhages may also occasionally occur. This cause of seizures is not rare and should be considered in the diagnostic workup, especially in the above mentioned age range (Fig. 7).

11) Creutzfeldt-Jakob's encephalopathy

Creutzfeldt (1920) and Jakob (1921) reported cases of a progressive CNS disease with characteristic neuropathological changes in cortex, brain stem and spinal cord level. One of the most consistent clinical signs proved to be *myoclonic* jerking. Kirschbaum, a contributor of some of the earliest case reports (1924), has recently reviewed the nosological outlines of this disease (1968). There is reason to presume that a similar syndrome known as *spongiform encephalopathy* (Jones and Nevin, 1954) may in fact represent the same disease. The myoclonic activity is usually associated with a very typical EEG pattern of almost rhythmically repetitive spikes or sharp waves (Abbott, 1959; Fig. 8a).

In recent years, this disease has attracted much attention following the transmission from man to the chimpanzee (Gibbs, Jr., and Gajdusek, 1969). The myoclonic activity in the affected

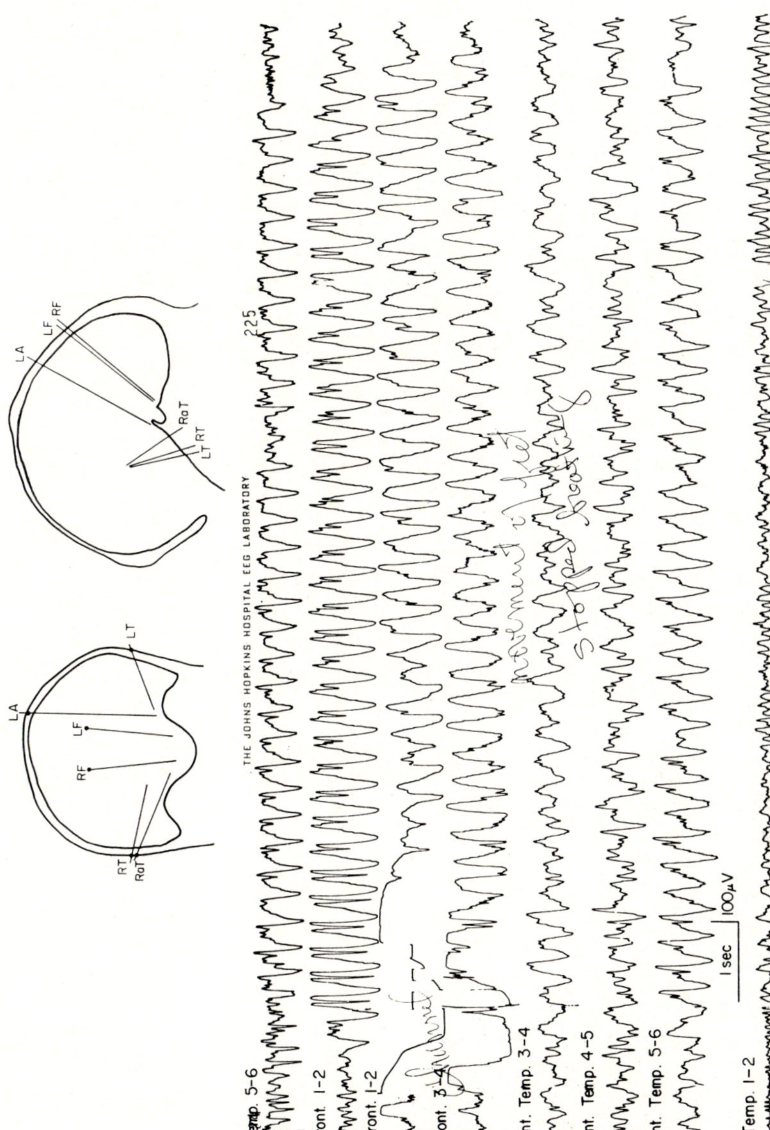

FIGURE 7. Depth EEG recording of a 33-year-old female patient with a history of grand mal, petit mal absences and atonic-akinetic falling spells (onset of seizures at age 13). Note deep left frontal predominance of 3/sec spike wave discharges.

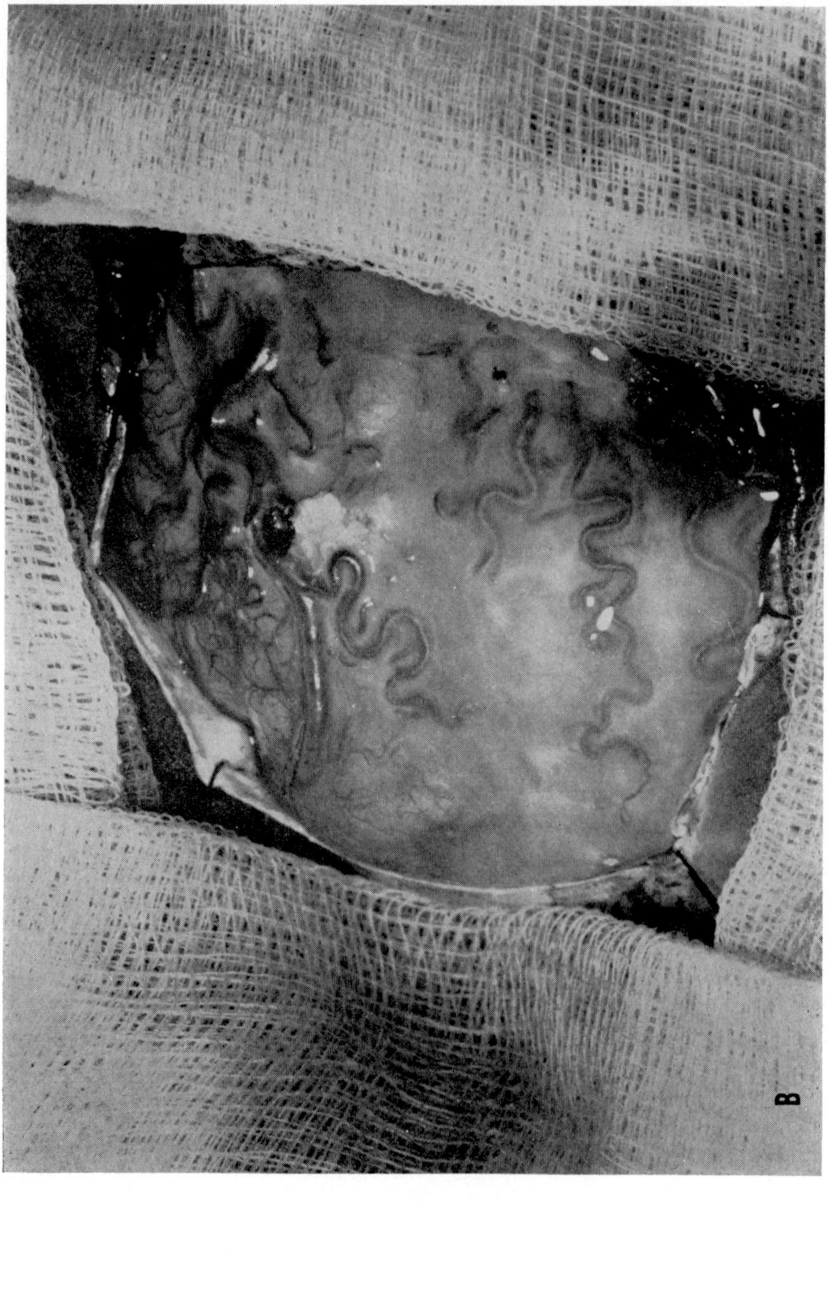

FIGURE 7. b) Same patient. On the basis of angiographic evidence, a left frontal craniotomy is carried out (Dr. A. Earl Walker) and reveals a cortical arterio-venous malformation. Left frontal lobectomy has failed to reduce the frequency of the major and minor seizures.

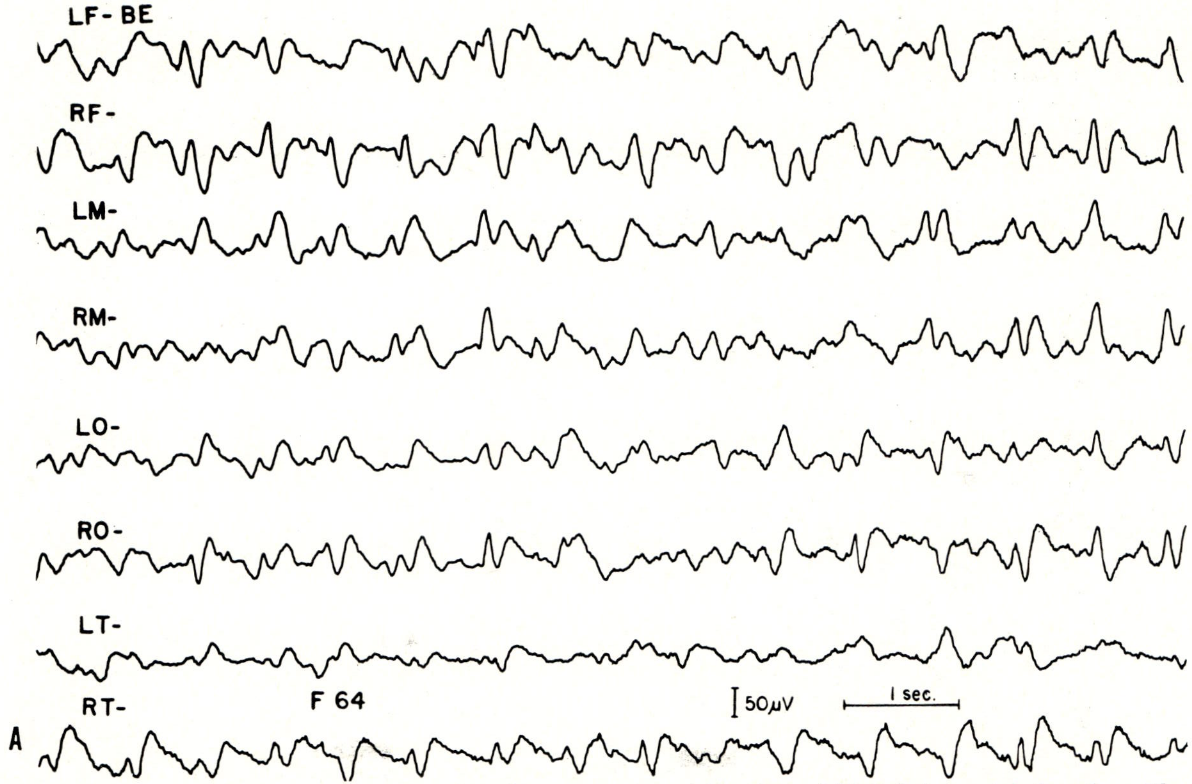

FIGURE 8. a) Electroencephalogram taken from a patient with Creutzfeldt-Jakob encephalopathy. The record is slow, disorganized and shows fairly rhythmical sharp activity of bilateral-anterior predominance (resembling "triphasic waves"). (Reprinted from K. A. Kooi: FUNDAMENTALS OF ELECTROENCEPHALOGRAPHY, New York, Harper and Row, 1971, with the author's and publisher's kind permission.)

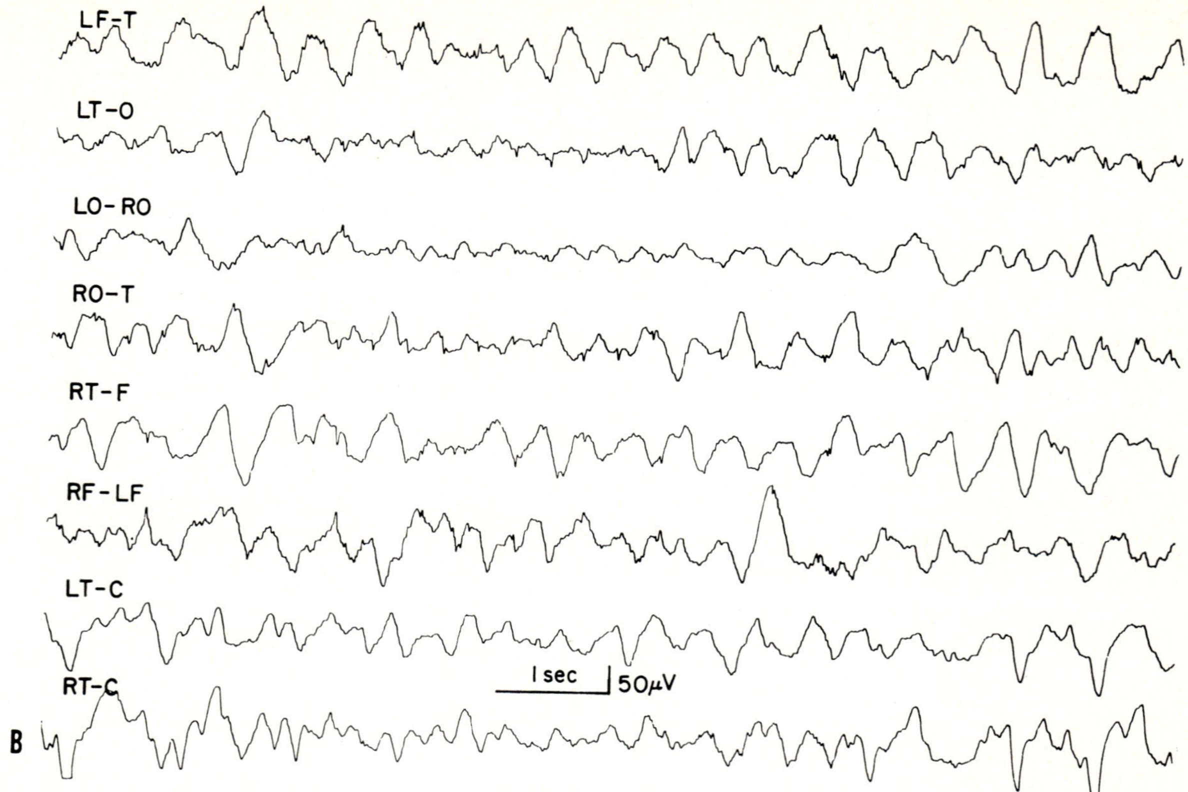

FIGURE 8. b) EEG of a 3½ year old female chimpanzee, recorded 13 months after experimental intracerebral inoculation with brain material from a patient with clinical-pathological evidence of Creutzfeldt-Jakob encephalopathy. At the time of the recording, the animal was in a stuporous state with constant tremor, ataxia and frequent myoclonis jerking of all limbs and head. The EEG was characterized by diffuse 2-4/sec activity of medium to high voltage. Frequent myoclonic jerking never altered the tracing and there was no evidence of any spike or sharp wave activity. These data were obtained in collaboration with Dr. C. J. Gibbs, Jr.; Dr. R. Marsh, and Dr. D. C. Gajdusek, U.S. Department for the Study of Slow and Latent Virus Infections, Patuxent, Maryland; Laboratory for slow and latent virus infections, National Institute for Neurological Diseases and Stroke, National Institutes of Health, Bethesda, Maryland.

chimpanzee is unaccompanied by spike discharges (Niedermeyer et al., 1972; Fig. 8b). In addition to the demonstrated viral etiology, additional predisposing genetic factors may exist in man.

Progressive mental decline associated with recurrent myoclonus in a middle aged or aged individual is the diagnostic hallmark of Creutzfeldt-Jakob's encephalopathy; long tract signs, ataxia and repetitive bilateral-synchronous seizure discharges provide further evidence for this diagnosis. Neurosyphilis may imitate this picture (even the EEG characteristics as I found recently); the good response to penicillin stands in stark contrast to the steady progression and lack of therapeutic response in Creutzfeldt-Jakob's disease.

12) Renal insufficiency and other metabolic or toxic encephalopathies

Acute and especially *chronic kidney disease* may give rise to epilepsy; grand mal attacks are the most common epileptic manifestation. The etiology varies; chronic glomerulonephritis, nephrosis, polycystic kidney disease and obstructive nephropathy could be the primary cause of the secondary cerebral involvement. Arterial hypertension may or may not be present. This type of renal epilepsy is more common in children, adolescents and young adults. Renal failure giving rise to uremia in older patients is often associated with frequent myoclonic jerking (Fig. 23).

In renal insufficiency, the EEG becomes frequently abnormal and characterized by excessive slowing; these EEG *abnormalities are often enhanced during and after hemodialysis* (Kennedy et al., 1963). In some of the patients (perhaps those with individual predisposition), seizures may develop in the wake of hemodialysis. Prill et al. (1969), observed seizures in ⅓ of their patients with renal insufficiency. According to these authors, ". . . acute changes in circulatory regulation, water and electrolyte balance always preceded the cerebral seizures." Even status epilepticus may occur (Prill et al., 1969).

Eclampsia gravidarum (or *intra partum*) constitutes a still poorly understood syndrome with combined renal, cerebral and hepatic involvement; arterial hypertension is a common feature.

The observed seizures are true grand mal convulsions and may occur in rapid succession. Coma may ensue and may lead to a potentially dangerous emergency situation. Recovery in the postpartum phase is the rule; residual brain damage may become epileptogenic but consecutive "*posteclamptic epilepsy*" (Ledermair and Niedermeyer, 1954) with grand mal as well as focal seizures is a rare event.

Hepatic encephalopathy is associated with a severe progressive brain syndrome and striking EEG changes (slowing with triphasic wave formation). Although the sharp component of these triphasic waves reveal a paroxysmal element, overt *seizures are much less common in hepatic insufficiency than in renal failure.*

Severe and extensive burns are sometimes followed by a cerebral syndrome (*burns encephalopathy*). This complication develops about 3 to 10 days following the burns and the EEG may become abnormal (Petersen et al., 1964). Acute convulsions as well as consecutive epilepsy may materialize (Hughes et al., 1972).

Toxicity and acute poisoning must be regarded as a cause of acute convulsions in various types of drug overdoses or ingestions of poisons; this will be discussed under the heading of the diagnosis of acute convulsions. *Barbiturate withdrawal* and especially the abrupt discontinuation of the intake of short-acting and ultrashort acting barbiturates *in hitherto seizure free addicts* leads to convulsions in more than 50 percent of these individuals (Kalinowsky, 1942), usually after 48 hours from the onset of abrupt withdrawal; generalized bursts with spikes in the EEG are the rule in this stage (Isbell, 1950; Wulff, 1959; Wikler and Essig, 1970). An acute schizophrenia-like psychosis frequently follows after a few days. Nonbarbituric sedatives and hypnotics can give rise to a similar syndrome after sudden withdrawal.

Long term psychiatric treatment with phenothiazines (especially chlorpromazine, Thorazine®) leads to generalized paroxysmal burst activity in the EEG (Bente and Itil, 1954) and, in some patients, grand mal attacks develop (Schlichther et al., 1956; Itil, 1970). As to chronic psychiatric patients, spontaneous major convulsions may also develop *after prolonged use of electroconvulsive treatment* (electroshock) and *after prefrontal lobotomy.*

Chronic lead poisoning (*lead encephalopathy*) is frequently associated with major convulsions. This condition is practically confined to early childhood and to areas with substandard housing. Flakes of lead paint are ingested by toddlers under such circumstances. Mental deterioration, moderate to severe EEG abnormalities, ataxia, papilledema, convulsions and lethargy may be seen when the serum lead level reaches dangerous values exceeding 0.1 mg per 100 ml. In children, the encephalopathy becomes manifest before other signs of lead toxicity develop (peripheral neuropathy with prominent wrist drop, anemia with stippling of erythrocytes, hypertension and colicky abdominal pain).

Legislative measures have greatly reduced the incidence of lead poisoning by making illegal the use of lead-containing paints.

As far as intrinsic intoxications are concerned, the central form of *intermittent porphyria* could be a cause of sporadically recurrent major convulsions in association with other signs of acute cerebral impairment.

Endocrine disturbances as the cause of epileptic seizures are rare unless states of hypoglycemia are listed in this group. *Hypoglycemia-induced convulsions* sometimes occur in spontaneous states of lowered blood sugar (hyperinsulinism, islet cell tumors, ketotic hypoglycemia) or in states of hypoglycemic coma due to excessive dosages of, or "overshooting" responses to, the therapeutic administration of insulin or other hypoglycemia-inducing agents. In studies based on therapeutic insulin coma (Sakel cure) in schizophrenics, grand mal seizures were noted in 3 percent of the induced comatose states whereas massive myoclonus occurred in 90 percent of the comas (Poiré, 1969). In spontaneous hypoglycemic states, transient cerebral impairment, fainting and coma must be distinguished from epileptic manifestations which, of course, may also develop in these conditions.

Hypoparathyroidism with states of severe *hypocalcemia* is a rare cause of major convulsions which then occur in addition to the usual tetanic carpopedal spasms. These latter were sometimes believed to be cerebral or epileptic phenomena but the primary role of the peripheral nerve under the influence of hypocalcemia and blood alkalosis has been well established (Alajouanine, Contamin and Cathala, 1958). Mixed tetanic and epileptic types of attacks provided the basis for spasmophilia of infants; this condition was much discussed in earlier years and often confused with other types of infantile epilepsies. True spasmophilias have disappeared from the scenery just as much as their once ubiquitous basic condition, namely *ricketts* or *states of vitamin D deficiency.*

Clinically more important are *convulsions due to neonatal hypocalcemia.* Their occurrence between the fourth and fourteenth day post partum has been related to alimentary causes (artifical milk).

Hyperparathyroidism caused by malignant bone disease and other etiologies can give rise to neurological complications. We recently observed the occurrence of seizures in association with visual field cuts and abundant interictal spiking over the occipital regions.

Extremely severe states of *adrenocortical insufficiency* are associated with cerebral impairment and epileptic seizures which are obviously caused by the electrolyte imbalance. Accordingly, *hyponatremic states* are occasionally associated with acute convulsions and play a rather important role as a cause of seizures in neonates.

13) Chronic alcoholism (Alcohol epilepsy)

Alcohol epilepsy is caused by a *transient metabolic disturbance in chronic alcoholics;* this disturbance is almost completely limited to the *acute state of alcohol withdrawal.* Grand mal seizures are probably the only seizure manifestations of alcohol epilepsy. The attacks usually occur between 6 and 30 hours after the last drink (Victor and Brausch, 1967), for instance in the wake of a prolonged bout of drinking. Monday is a day of predilection for such events. The occurrence of truly metabolic alcohol seizures at the height of a drinking spree is a matter of controversy. Chronic epileptics may find consolation in alcoholic beverages; this linkage of a preexisting convulsive disorder and subsequent alcoholism must be separated from metabolic alcohol epilepsy.

According to Victor and Brausch (1967) and Victor (1970), the proneness to epileptic seizures constitutes the first phase of a biphasic process of withdrawal. According to these authors, flicker sensitivity with photomyoclonic responses is coupled with the transient proclivity to major convulsions. In this stage, the magnesium blood level is lowered while the arterial pH shifts to alkaline values in the range of 7.45 to 7.55. The second stage may or may not materialize; this stage consists of the well known symptomatology of the delirium tremens with a peak onset of 72 to 96 hours after cessation of drinking.

At the time when the patient is referred to electroencephalography, a low voltage fast but essentially normal tracing is usually obtained; this type of record is most common in chronic alcoholics. The state of increased sensitivity to flickering light is evidently very short-lived. Abnormal EEG findings with focal or generalized spikes suggest that one is dealing with an epileptic who has happened to become an alcoholic. This represents a fundamental difference from transient metabolic character of true alcohol epilepsy.

Epileptic seizures due to alcoholism are usually seen in patients of low socioeconomic status; malnutrition may be a contributory factor. According to my personal impression, an additional element of arterial hypertension is very common; blood pressure values are usually very labile in this stage. Almost all of the cases fall into the age range from 25 to 60 years. In the slum areas of North American cities, alcohol epilepsy is likely to constitute the most common etiology of seizures starting during adulthood in male individuals.

The *treatment of alcohol epilepsy* is nothing but the treatment of chronic alcoholism. The use of anticonvulsive medication has been rightly discouraged since chronic alcoholics fail to take the tablets with the required regularity. During sprees of heavy drinking, the patients will completely forget the intake of their medication and an additive element of phenobarbital withdrawal may make things worse. Some of these patients might sell phenobarbital on the market for illicit drugs.

The physician must be aware of other complications of alcoholism. The *delirium tremens* frequently follows in the wake of alcohol withdrawal seizures; liver disease is a faithful companion of this condition and *hepatic encephalopathy* may suddenly develop. This development is usually reflected by dramatic changes in the EEG characterized by marking slowing and triphasic waves. The above mentioned *hypertensive component* requires appropriate treatment. The development of headaches and progressive lethargy deserves particular attention; a *chronic subdural hematoma* is often caused by most trivial head injuries in chronic alcoholics. The occurrence of focal seizures or hemiparesis are very suggestive in this direction. Ataxia, cranial nerve deficits and loss of recent memory are likely to herald *Wernicke's encephalopathy* caused by vitamin B_1 deficit.

14) Anoxic convulsions

Convulsions caused by cerebral anoxia have been well documented by experimental studies (Noell and Kornmüller, 1944; Ward, Jr., 1947; Gellhorn and Heymans, 1948; Noell, 1948; Ajmone Marsan and Fuortes, 1949; Gänshirt and Zylka, 1952). These seizures are characterized by tonic extension of the extremities and opisthotonic posturing. This type of tonic seizure has been thought to be a release phenomenon of the brain stem in a decerebrate state (Sherrington, 1898). In the human, an initially flat EEG in association with tonic posturing was demonstrated by Niedermeyer (1956) in cerebral anoxia caused by suicidal hanging. Gastaut, Naquet and Fischer-Williams (1958) have emphasized the distinction between tonic anoxic attacks with flat or featureless EEG tracings and authentic epileptic phenomena with typical spiking in various cerebral levels.

In recent years, *acute anoxic convulsions with predominant myoclonic manifestations* have become a more common sight in intensive care units. These patients usually have a *history of respiratory or cardio-respiratory* (more seldom cardiac) *arrest* due to various causes such as general anesthesia, other types of toxicity, broncho pulmonary disease, myocardial infarction etc. While immediate death can be avoided by improved techniques of resuscitation, many of these patients remain comatose and eventually succumb to a cerebral type of death caused by irreversible anoxic brain damage associated with cessation of the

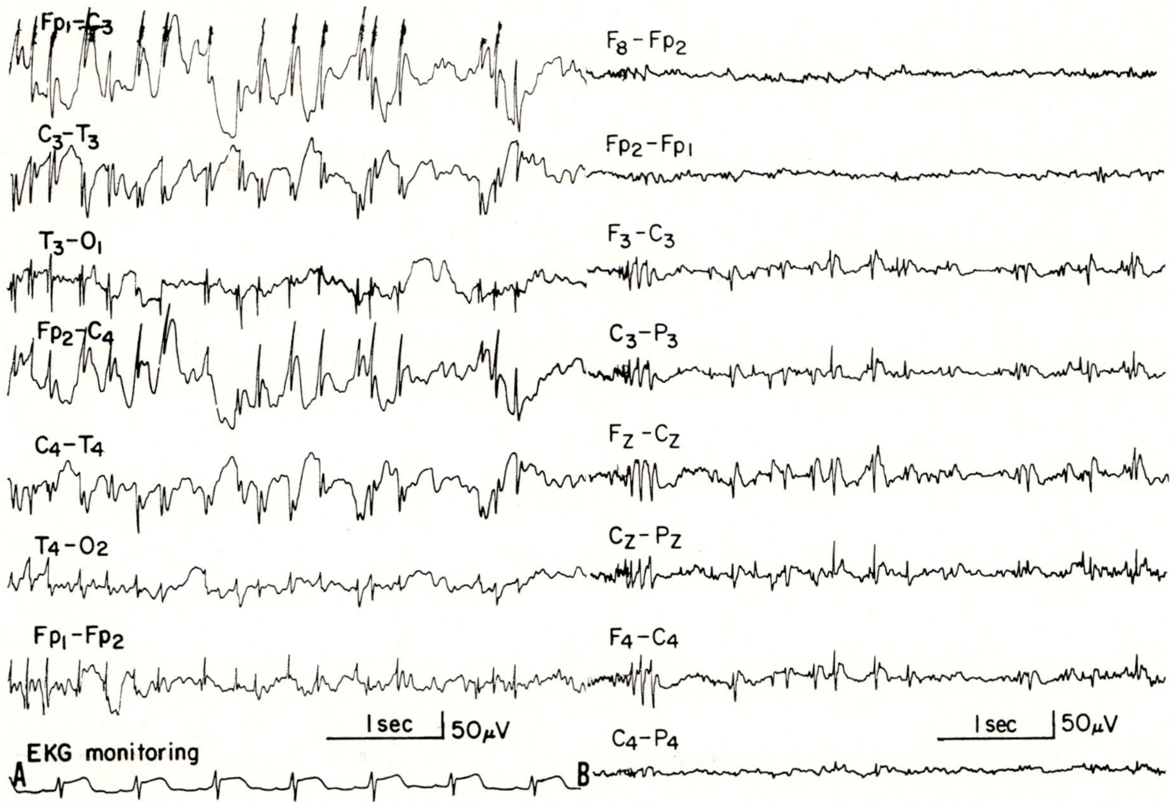

FIGURE 9. a) (left) Comatose patient, 22 years old. History of acute cerebral anoxia. Almost continuously repetive generalized-synchronous spikes, often accompanied by symmetrical generalized myoclonus. b) The same patient, two months later, awake, with severe intentional myoclonus. Note maximum of spikes over the vertex with spread into frontal and central areas. The patient has remained disabled through the following two years because of the intractable intention-myoclonus.

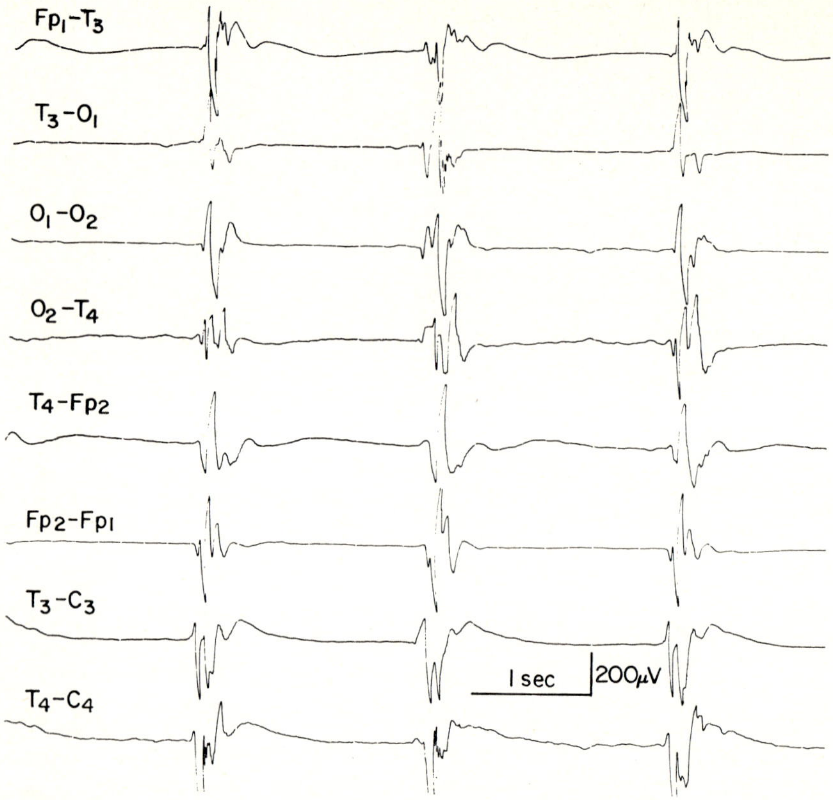

FIGURE 10. Comatose 57-year-old patient with constantly repetitive myoclonus after a severe anoxic episode. Note the alternating polyphasic spikes, generalized-synchronous against a flat background, occasionally associated with generalized myoclonus.

cerebral bioelectrical activity. Some of these patients exhibit abundant myoclonic jerking of the limbs, facial and trunkal muscles; these jerks may or may not be stimulus sensitive. In this stage, the EEG shows repetitive generalized spike activity (Madison and Niedermeyer, 1970, Fig. 9, 10). The prognosis is extremely grave for adults and somewhat less gloomy for children. If recovery from the comatose state occurs, massive myoclonus may persist, usually in conjunction with intentional movements ("intention myoclonus"; Lance and Adams, 1963). This type of myoclonus is usually refractory to therapeutic attempts which should include stereotaxic coagulation within the cerebello-thalamic-cortical system.

CHAPTER 4

AGE-DETERMINED EPILEPTIC CONDITIONS: CLINICAL PICTURE AND COURSE

1) Introduction

TYPE OF SEIZURE, focal origin of the cerebral discharge and etiology of the underlying cerebral disturbance are important determinants of a seizure disorder but, in many cases, these three factors alone will not provide the physician with sufficient comprehension of the disorder's special character. The age of the patient has great influence on the course of the epilepsy; this is particularly true for the first two decades of life and especially for infancy and early childhood. In other words, the factor of age determines certain epileptological entities, or epileptic conditions which may appear monolithic in spite of a wide variety of etiologies and probably also despite inconsistencies in the topography of cerebral involvement.

The common denominators of such an age-determined epileptic condition are a) certain types of seizures, b) certain characteristics of the course of prognosis, and c) certain EEG patterns. Later in life, the primarily involved area may become the predominant factor which gives a specific flavor to the type of epilepsy; this creates the hallmarks of temporal lobe or frontal lobe epilepsy (Chapter 5).

The physician's therapeutic approach to the seizure disorder will be shallow and often futile when he ignores the special character of such epileptic conditions.

There is, in general, a factor of enhanced seizure susceptibility in infancy and childhood. The well known fact that epileptic phenomena are more common in children than in adults has been linked with the process of cerebral maturation. On the basis of experimental work in kittens, Purpura (1964) has stressed the hyperexcitability of the immature hippocampus, but his observations ". . . by no means exhaust the possible mechanisms underlying the development of seizures in immature animals." We are still far away from a satisfactory understanding of the heightened proclivity to seizures in the early periods of life.

2) *Neonatal convulsions*

Seizure disorders occurring during the first three months of life show many similarities as far as the type of seizure and the EEG changes are concerned. The introductory de-emphasis of the etiology, however, is somewhat out of place in this type of epilepsy since etiological considerations are of considerable diagnostic, therapeutic and prognostic value. Hence, neonatal convulsions are likely to show wide varieties in their course when compared with the subsequently discussed conditions (hypsarrhythmia, febrile convulsions, Lennox-Gastaut syndrome, etc.).

The *type of seizure* are rather poorly defined in the neonatal period. The seizures consist of mixed tonic and clonic elements whereas the classic sequence of a tonic and a clonic stage fails to materialize. Tremulous and jerky movements shift from one side to the other or from one limb to the next (Bridge, 1949; Ribstein and Walter, 1958; Ford, 1960; Vizioli, 1962; Craig, 1963; Massa and Niedermeyer, 1968); Bamberger and Matthes (1959), however, separate generalized and grand mal like neonatal seizures from focal attacks. *The convulsive state is not always readily distinguished from normal neonatal motor actiivty.* This has been pointed out by highly experienced observers such as Dreyfus-Brisac and Monod (1964); in some of their cases, the EEG alone could determine the ictal states because of the subtle character of the behavioral changes. This is particularly true for prematurely born neonates (Bridges, 1949; Dreyfus-Brisac and Monod, 1964) who are interestingly less prone to neonatal seizures than full-term babies. In addition to the tonic and clonic manifestations, the occurrence of sudden eye opening, paroxysmal blinking, abnormal cry and sudden chewing motions can also be helpful in the clinical recognition of neonatal seizures (Minkowski and Sainte Ann-Dargassies, 1956). Kellaway (1971) divides neonatal and infantile seizures into a) tonic, b) clonic, c) atonic, d) autonomic, and e) automatism like seizures.

The *length of the seizures* compensates for the mild and inconspicuous character of the clinical ictal manifestations. Thus, neonatal convulsions often assume status like character without presenting with the clinical severity of status epilepticus of mature age.

The electroencephalogram often shows ictal changes; because of the long duration of the convulsive episodes, the electroencephalographer has a good chance to see the tracing during the ictal state. Rhythmical discharges with a well developed or hidden spike component are very typical in this condition; the frequency often varies. According to Kellaway (1971), the onset of a neonatal seizure is always focal in the EEG (Fig. 11); onset of the discharge in the temporal lobe is most common, followed by an occipital onset. Widespread and multifocal spiking may be seen in neonates with frequent brief tonic and clonic seizures (Fig. 12). Interictal EEG abnormalities are usually diffuse and often completely absent.

From the *etiological viewpoint, perinatal brain damage* and *birth anoxia* are the most important causes of convulsions occurring in the earliest segment of the newborn period, i.e. the first week of life (Massa and Niedermeyer, 1968). During the ensuing weeks, *infection* represents the most frequent cause. Among intracranial infections, E. coli and staphylocci give rise to purulent meningitis in a slightly earlier stage than the more commonly involved *Hemophilus influenzae*. After good initial response to antibiotic therapy, the baby may become listless again with return (or first occurrence) of convulsions; this development is suggestive of a *post-meningitic subdural collection* requiring diagnostic subdural taps and frequently neurosurgical evacuation with stripping of the membrane. *Viral infections* also must be taken into account, especially the highly destructive Herpes simplex encephalitis due to infections with herpes genitalis from the passage through the birth canal. *Extracranial infections* may

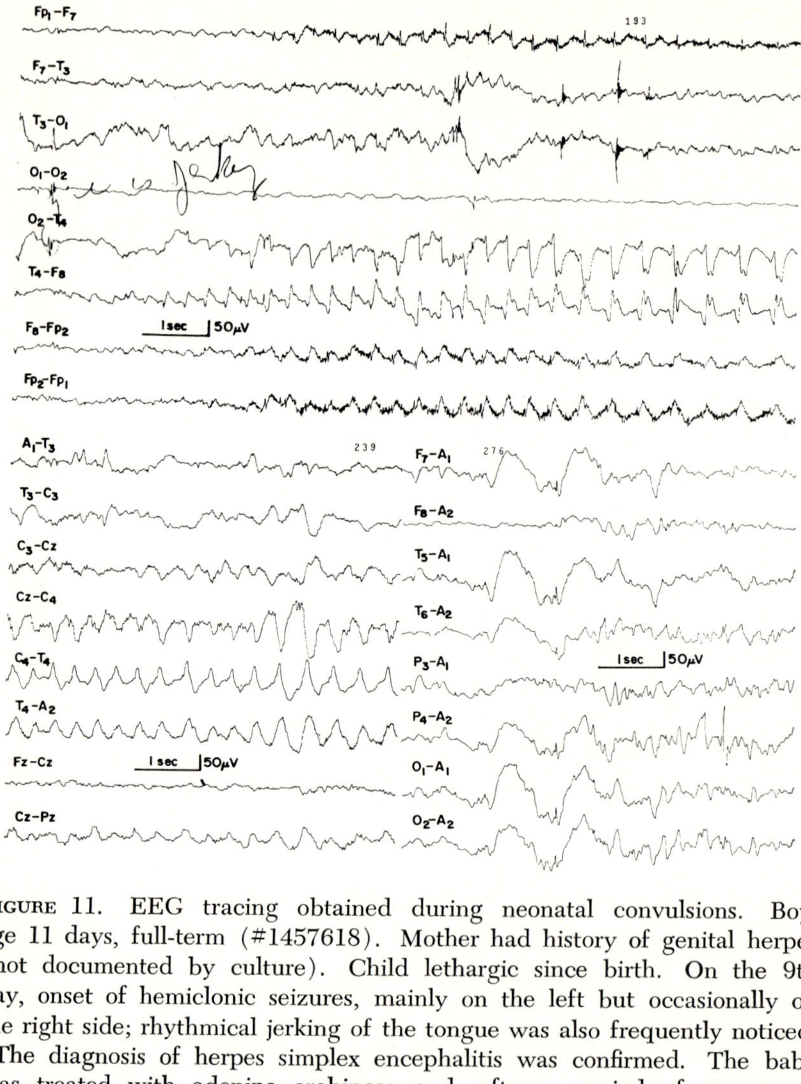

FIGURE 11. EEG tracing obtained during neonatal convulsions. Boy, age 11 days, full-term (#1457618). Mother had history of genital herpes (not documented by culture). Child lethargic since birth. On the 9th day, onset of hemiclonic seizures, mainly on the left but occasionally on the right side; rhythmical jerking of the tongue was also frequently noticed. (The diagnosis of herpes simplex encephalitis was confirmed. The baby was treated with adenine arabinose and, after a period of coma and convulsions, recovered from the acute disease with severe mental deficits.) a) (upper tracing) Onset of a left sided clonic hemiconvulsion; with jerking of tongue note rhythmical spiking starting over right temporal area. b) (lower tracing, left) Record taken during a left sided hemiconvulsion; note right central maximum of rhythmical slow activity with a sharp component. c) (lower tracing right) Widespread single spikes in the inter-ictal interval.

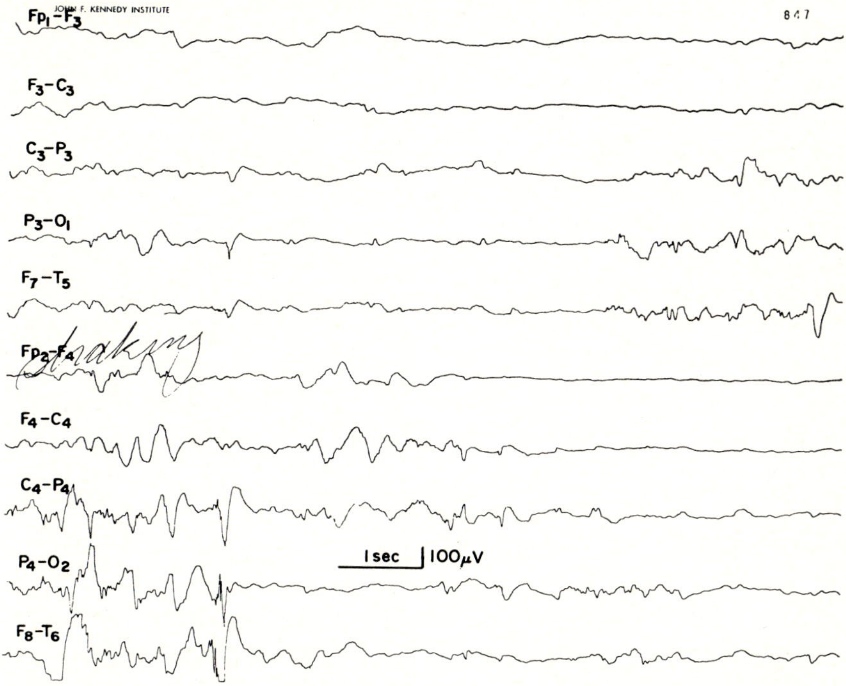

FIGURE 12. Electroencephalogram of a 10-weeks-old girl (#1484654) with almost constantly repetitive brief convulsions since birth (with irregularly mixed tonic and clonic elements). Note stretches of markedly depressed voltage between irregular bursts of slow activiy mixed with spikes.

also give rise to seizures, especially gastroenteritis with dehydration, pneumonia, bronchiolitis and otitis media; in these cases, there is an intervening metabolic element which chiefly accounts for the convulsions.

Metabolic disturbances are further causes of neonatal seizures; hypocalcemia, hyponatremia, hypernatremia, hypoglycemia and hypomagnesemia require the appropriate therapy (Freeman, 1970); a rare cause is pyridoxine dependency and a therapeutic trial is worthwhile.

Various types of *noninfectious morphological brain damage* encompass conditions such as the above mentioned cerebral anoxia at birth and perinatal brain injury; other conditions are cerebral malformations, Sturge-Weber syndrome, kernicterus, arterial or venous occlusions, cerebral atrophies, etc. *In a large number of cases of neonatal seizures, the etiology remains obscure* in spite of a thorough diagnostic workup.

THERAPY. It has to be kept in mind that neonatal convulsions represent the acute type of epilepsy caused by a florid or active (rather than residual) cerebral or metabolic disturbance. It is needless to say that the properly diagnosed disorder requires primordial therapeutic attention. Adequate antibiotic therapy of a bacterial meningitis, evacuation of a subdural collection and correction of disturbances in the glucose or electrolyte level are of utmost importance. Sustained clinical seizure activity is preferably treated with phenobarbital, i.m. or orally administered at a dosage of 5 to 10 mg/kg per day; intravenous administration requires slow and cautious injection (over several minutes) in order to avoid respiratory depression. Because of this complication, the use of intravenous diazepam (Valium®) is not as safe as it is in the treatment of status like seizure episodes or frank status epilepticus in children or adults. According to Freeman (1970), paraldehyde i.v. is safe and effective but could produce pneumonitis in a newborn because of its pulmonary excretion.

PROGNOSIS. Initial mortality may reach 25 to 42 percent (Burke, 1954; Craig, 1960; Prichard, 1964) or may be as low as 2.5 percent (Massa and Niedermeyer, 1968). These differences might be due to the type of material. Normal EEG findings in the interictal period suggest a good prognosis according to Rose and Lombroso (1970) who feel that such infants have an 86 percent chance of normality; flat records are presumed to be incompatible with normal development. Metabolic disturbances and extracranial infections are most likely to be followed by normal development and absence of further seizures, whereas neuropsychiatric sequelae and recurrence of seizures are most common in infants with morphological brain damage (Massa and Niedermeyer, 1968). This indicates that the prognosis of neonatal seizures is, in general, rather guarded and depends strongly on the type of underlying brain disease.

3) *Infantile spasms* (*Hypsarrhythmia*)

Infantile spasms constitute the epitome of an age-determined epileptic condition occurring between the age of 4 months to approximately 24 months. In recent years, the electroencephalographic term "hypsarrhythmia" (Greek: *"hypselos"* means *"high,"* indicating the high voltage of the EEG in addition to the lack of rhythmicity) has been used more frequently. The term "West's syndrome" is also in use since West described the symptomatology in his own child in a letter to the editor of "Lancet" (1841) and consulted one of England's leading authorities, Charles Clarke, who had already seen a number of such cases.

Infantile spasms have unmistakable ictal-clinical and electroencephalographic characteristics while there is a multitude of possible etologies. The most common type of seizure is the *salaam spasm* which consists of an anteroflexion of the upper part of the body. The movement is of tonic rather than clonic character and its execution may be moderately slow or moderately rapid; it resembles an oriental salutation. This impression is derived from watching the infant being held in somebody's arms or in a sitting position. The frequently used term "jackknifing seizure" is also correct and conveys the observer's impression from watching the baby in a supine position (Fig. 13, 14). These brief attacks usually repeat themselves several times in short salvos.

In similar manner, repetitive *massive myoclonic jerking* may be observed, especially involving the head (*head nodding attacks*). These seizure manifestations have prompted terms like "spasmus nutans" (Newnham, 1849), "Blitz- Nick- und Salaam-Krämpfe" (Zellweger, 1948) or "Propulsive Petit Mal" (Janz and Matthes, 1955). In very rare instances, the seizure manifestations are lateralized or confined to one half of the body.

The *electroencephalogram* shows a mixture of irregular high voltage slow activity, faster frequencies and copious intermixed single and multiple spikes or sharp waves; the seizure discharges may be generalized and fairly synchronous or widely scattered with a maximum over posterior regions. This impressive blend of irregular high voltage activity and widespread seizure dis-

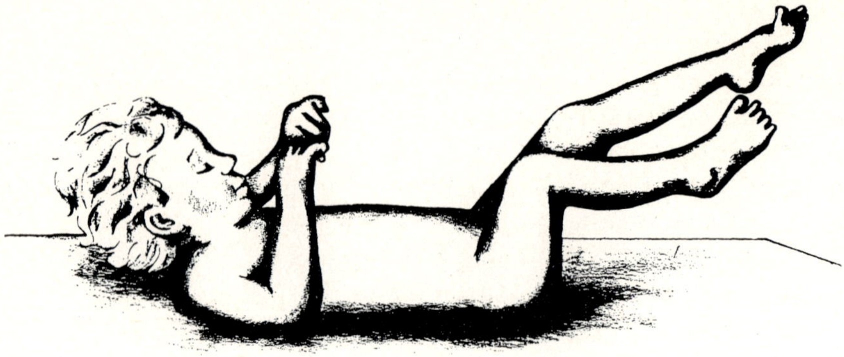

FIGURE 13. Infant with hypsarrhythmia. Jackknifing seizure occurring while in supine position.

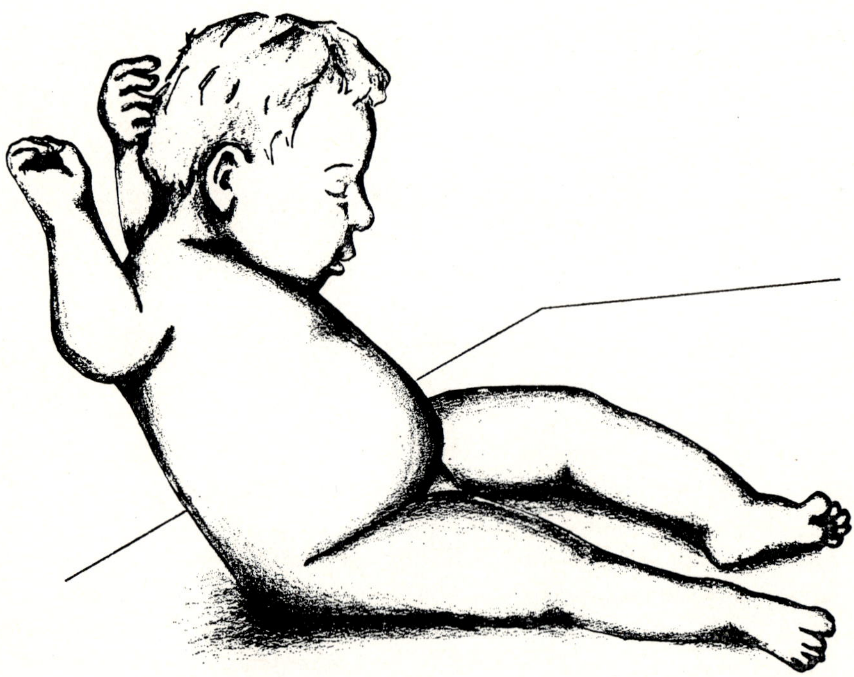

FIGURE 14. Infant with hypsarrhythmia. Jackknifing seizure occurring while sitting, associated with "salaam"-like flexion of the trunk.

charges has prompted the term *"hypsarrhythmia"* which is now frequently used for the designation of the clinical condition. The hypsarrhythmic characteristics of the EEG become more evident in the sleep tracing when bursts of generalized spikes are followed by brief stretches of depressed voltage in all leads (Fig. 15). Clinical seizures may also be associated with general depression of electrical activity. At other occasions, clinical seizures are seen in conjunction with massive seizure patterns or with no appreciable change of the tracing.

The clinical and electrical signs of infantile spasms do not materialize prior to the age of four months. With the emergence of the spasms, *the mental development of the infant ceases to progress* and a delay of the developmental milestones is noticed. Within one year, the infant may be profoundly mentally retarded. The patients may be divided into a) babies with normal development up to the age of 4 to 6 months when the first attacks occur, and b) babies with evidence of brain damage at birth, neonatal seizures and initial delay of the mental development. In the latter case, the infantile spasms are engrafted on a pre-existing cerebral impairment. In primary infantile spasms, the often unusually pretty face of the baby and a limitation of facial expressivity were stressed by some observers (Zellweger, 1948; Bamberger and Matthes, 1959).

The *diagnosis of infantile spasms is very easy for the experienced physician* who is aware of the uniqueness of the seizure manifestations and the EEG characteristics. Some parents tend to interpret the jackknife attacks as the expression of painful abdominal colic or as a startle response to unexpected stimuli. *Every delay in the correct diagnosis may be of dire therapeutic consequences.*

The diagnosis of infantile spasms is not an etiological diagnosis. It was said before that this is a polyetiological condition and, in a large number of infants (or even in the majority of the cases), the cause will remain undetermined. In general, the search for the primary cause may be somewhat academic since the treatment is essentially directed to the infantile spasms as such. If the diagnostic search reveals an inborn error of

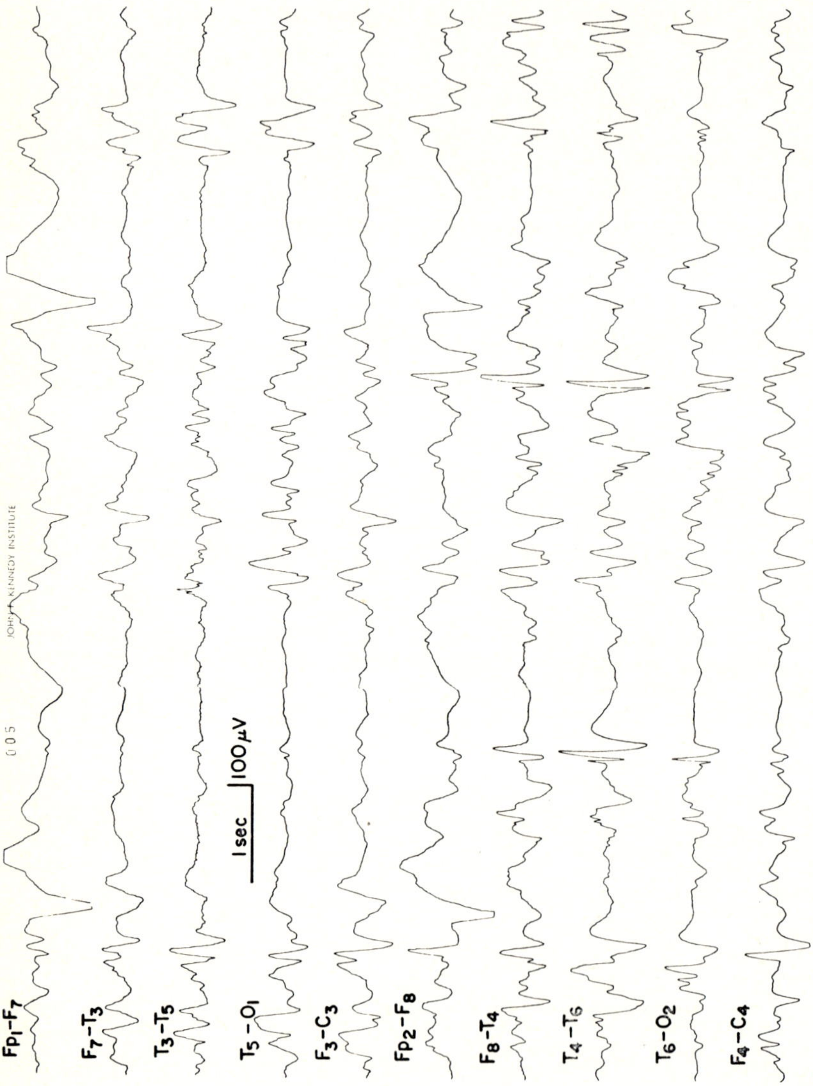

FIGURE 15. Girl, age 2 years, 10 months; history cf infantile spasms since first year of life; presently decerebrate. The EEG shows the picture of hypsarrhythmia with moderately well synchronized bursts of very high voltage, intermixed spikes and brief stretches of voltage depression. This patient died one month later. Autopsy revealed diffuse cortical atrophy in both cerebral hemispheres and hypoplasia of the cerebellar vermis.

metabolism such as phenylketonuria, the delay of a truly etiological therapy will become tragically manifest. If an intracranial neoplasm is found, chances are that this tumor is just a manifestation of tuberous sclerosis which usually gives rise to typical cutaneous changes.

THERAPY. Therapeutic efforts with the usual anticonvulsants fail completely; for this reason, infantile spasms were thought to be the worst form of seizure disorder in childhood. The introduction of *ACTH* (Sorel and Dusaucy-Bauloye (1958), represents one of the great therapeutic achievements in epileptology; the effect of this pituitary hormone may also be obtained by *corticosteroids*. The neural mechanisms of this hormone and its anticonvulsive action in infantile spasms are unknown. In other types of epilepsy, its effect is dubious. One could argue that infantile spasms are not ordinary epileptic manifestations and perhaps are extremely enhanced and internally triggered startle mechanisms brought forth by the impairment of inhibitory cerebral structures. The tendency of ictal flattening in the EEG also underscores the unique position of infantile spasms in epileptology. There is, however, no reason to place this condition outside the field of epilepsy; many babies with hypsarrhythmia had unequivocal epileptic neonatal manifestations first, and later (following the period of infantile spasms) develop other forms of indubitable epilepsy.

The original treatment of Sorel and Dusaucy-Bauloye (1958) consists of 5 to 10 units of ACTH daily in 2 week courses with one-week-intervals; this dosage was later increased from 40 to 80 units/day (ACTH gel i.m.) in a 6 weeks course, followed-up by long-term treatment with steroids, for instance prednisolone (40-50 mg/day). This treatment is gradually tapered off over several months.

Nitrazepam (Mogadon®) has been introduced more recently on the basis of the work of Liske and Forster (1963), Markham (1964), Gibbs and Anderson (1965), Gastaut et al. (1966) and Weinmann (1966). It cannot be used in the United States because of strict F.D.A. regulations. According to Doose (1970), the optimal dosage lies between 0.5 to 1.0 mg/kg/day. Drowsiness is the most common side effect.

The effectiveness of ACTH steroids and nitrazepam lies in the range of 50 to 70 percent; in Doose's opinion, the nitrazepam treatment is not inferior to the hormonal therapy. In almost 50 percent of the cases, full suppression of the attacks occurs and the EEG normalizes. *Diazepam* (Valium®) is chemically closely related to nitrazepam (as a benzodiazepine) and can be used in this country, but its effectiveness is inferior in the treatment of infantile spasms. Its combination with ACTH is advisable, whereas the use of barbituates and hydantoines (in combination with the specific therapies) does not yield any better results. Another type of treatment consists of *ketogenic diet* recommended by Livingston (1954) for poorly controllable forms of epilepsy in infancy and childhood.

The treatment with ACTH, steroids or benzodiazepines must be started without any delay as soon as the diagnosis of infantile spasms has been made.

Prognosis. The prognosis depends on two main factors: a) a pre-existent neonatal or infantile convulsive disorder with concomitant cerebral impairment is associated with poorer results of the treatment than a primary type of infantile spasms with a period of normal development during the first months of life, and b) every delay of the start of the appropriate treatment makes the outcome more dubious.

In the unfavorable cases, the seizure disorder and the EEG changes will exacerbate after some initial response to treatment. After the age of 2 years, the ictal and electrical character of infantile spasms disappears and, in the poorly responsive cases, other types of seizures and other types of electrical seizure discharges enter the scenery. The generalized hypsarrhythmic pattern may turn into focal or multifocal spiking but, in most of these cases, the slow spike-wave complex starts to predominate. This indicates a transition into the Lennox-Gastaut syndrome which will be discussed later.

Even in very favorable responses with steady improvement of the intellectual abilities, the possibility of recurring seizure disorder later in childhood or adolescence must always be taken into account. One has to keep in mind that the earliest reports of the modern type of treatment are not older than 15 years and the follow-up periods are still fairly short. Whatever type of epilepsy may recur in later years, it is unlikely to interfere with the mental development as badly as in infantile spasms and the Lennox-Gastaut syndrome.

4) Febrile convulsions

Convulsions triggered exclusively by fever usually occur in the age from 6 months to 3 years; they very seldom present earlier but are not so rare between 3 to 5 years of age. The onset falls into the range from 6 to 24 months. Febrile convulsions are the most common and also the most benign type of all epileptic conditions. The true incidence is difficult to estimate but is thought to exceed 5 percent of the total population (compared with an overall incidence of 0.5% "hard core" epilepsies).

The convulsions themselves are of unequivocal epileptic nature and usually exhibit the tonic-clonic sequence of grand mal seizure, although in a clearly attenuated manner. The attacks may last from the usual duration of a grand mal (1 to 1½ minutes) to 10 or 20 minutes; longer lasting seizures are unlikely to be simple febrile convulsions. The academic clinician almost never observes these attacks, and he needs the assistance of the general practitioner or pediatrician for an adequate discussion of the ictal features. The seizures occur at the very beginning of the temperature rise, often before the parents are aware that the child has contracted a febrile illness.

Trivial upper respiratory tract infections are the usual cause of febrile convulsions. Infantile seizures associated with fever could be due to genuine cerebral involvement with edema, meningo-encephalitis or venous thrombosis; *these seizures caused by febrile brain disease must be strictly separated from simple febrile convulsions.* Even a mild and short-lasting infection such as *exanthem subitum* (roseola) is very often associated with convulsions but this is probably attributable to a rudimentary encephalitic component. The same is true for convulsive reactions after smallpox vaccination and immunization for pertussis. Table VI demonstrates the main differences between febrile convulsions and seizures due to febrile brain disease.

TABLE VI

DIFFERENCES BETWEEN FEBRILE CONVULSIONS AND SEIZURES DUE TO FEBRILE BRAIN DISEASE

	Febrile convulsions	*Seizures in febrile brain disease*
Typical age range	6 months to 3 years (seldom 5 years)	Mainly 0 to 3 years
Genetic predisposition to seizures	May be strong	Mostly minor or insignificant
Type of seizure	Tonic-clonic (modified or attenuated grand mal)	Tonic-clonic (grand mal-like) or hemiconvulsions
Duration of seizure	Mostly 1-3 minutes, seldom prolonged	Often prolonged, 10 minutes to hours, status-like or in rapid succession
Clinical setting in which seizures occur	At the onset of a febrile disease, mostly upper respiratory illness, often coinciding with the first sharp rise of temperature	In a variety of CNS infections (encephalitis, meningo-encephalitis), intracranial venous thrombosis, cerebro-vascular accidents of infancy. Also in exanthema subitum and after vaccination (smallpox) but usually less severe.
Type of underlying cerebral pathology	None	Various types of inflammatory and vascular changes, in milder cases limited to edema
Post-ictal neurological deficit (Todd's paralysis)	Very uncommon	Common and often mixed with pathology-determined neurological defect
EEG	Rapidly normalizes after convulsion, normal interval tracings in 80-90%	Abnormal throughout febrile episode, abnormal in interval (except for mild encephalitis)
Anticonvulsive medication	Not necessary (neither for acute convulsions nor for prevention of further seizures)	Acutely needed (preferably diazepam, phenobarbital), long-term-treatment required afterwards (except for mild encephalitis)
Prognosis	Excellent in the vast majority (especially those with normal interval EEG's)	Guarded. Neurological defects and further seizures common

There is some evidence of *genetic predisposition* to febrile convulsions (Schmidt, 1958; Metrakos and Metrakos, 1961; Schuman and Miller, 1966) which may be indeed the mildest type of genetically determined epilepsy; this view, however, is not generally accepted. Other authors have laid more emphasis on acquired cerebral disturbances. The seizure-precipitating action of hyperthermia is virtually limited to infancy and early childhood; *brisk changes of the water and electrolyte balance* (Millichap et al., 1960) may play a very important part. Physicians witnessing febrile convulsions are sometimes impressed by the manner in which the seizure develops out of a chill with violent shivering and one wonders if the physiological mechanism of shivering may "get out of control" by excessive neuronal spread. Strong vagotonic mechanisms have been proposed by Gastaut and Gastaut (1957) on the basis of marked oculo-cardiac reflex excitability.

The *electroencephalogram* secured in the inter-ictal interval is usually normal (80-95% of the cases) and the presence of seizure discharges is suggestive of a more complex seizure disorder which, later in life, will change to afebrile convulsions due to residual brain disease. This underscores the prognostic significance of the EEG.

In a large number of cases, only one or two febrile convulsions ever occur; a history of more than 4 attacks and with extension beyond the age of 4 years raises the suspicion of future afebrile convulsions. These considerations are very important with regard to therapeutic measures.

THERAPY. The therapy of febrile convulsions is at least as controversial as the physiopathogenesis. The question is simply ". . . to treat or not to treat"; in other words, the use of anticonvulsants vs. a *laissez-faire* philosophy. The answer should be partly determined by the attitude of the parents who may have a very strong desire for the installation of therapy or a strong aversion. The physician must therefore take his time to discuss the question unhurriedly.

There is no cogent reason for insisting on anticonvulsive therapy since a total of perhaps 2 to 4 febrile convulsive episodes may be expected in the course of the self-limited disorder. There is also no convincing evidence of a brain damaging effect of a single febrile convulsion (see further discussion on the concept of "secondary temporalization"). Some pediatricians start medication only after the second febrile convulsion hoping that the first one will remain a single event. The occurrence of febrile convulsions in several members of a family and especially the fact that some of them developed afebrile convulsions later in childhood or adolescence would speak in favor of active therapy. *Phenobarbital is the treatment of choice*; at this early age, general irritability is not a common side effect as it is later in childhood; a total of 16-32 mg/day for an infant of 6 to 12 months will be sufficient and gradual slight increases will be made over the following years. The treatment may be tapered off at the age of 4-6 years provided that the EEG has remained normal and that there is no incidence of a febrile seizures in other family members. Much higher dosages (60-100 mg/day, 3-4 mg/kg/day) have been advocated by Faerø et al. (1972) who attempt to build up a constant serum concentration level of more than 1.6 mg/100 ml.

The benign character of febrile convulsions ought to be pointed out to the parents after the first episode but one has to agree with Livingston (1963) that no full guarantee can be given to the parents concerning eventual complete seizure freedom. This clearly shows that a physician's humane qualities are tested in this condition in which there is no simple "yes or no" answer to the question of therapy.

The prognosis is excellent in about 80 to 95 percent of the patients; these are the cases of true simple febrile convulsions with seizure freedom achieved before school age, whereas the remaining 5 to 15 percent may be considered retrospectively as epilepsies initially camouflaged as febrile convulsion.

5) The Lennox-Gastaut syndrome

Like infantile spasms, the Lennox-Gastaut syndrome is characterized by typical seizure manifestations and fairly specific EEG abnormalities, for which a large number of etiological brain disorders may account. Perhaps 1/5 of the patients have infantile spasms with hypsarrhythmia as infants and then develop the signs of the Lennox-Gastaut syndrome. The age range for the onset of this epileptic condition usually lies between 1 and 10 years; onset in the second decade of life is much less common. The characteristics of the syndrome gradually change to other types of epilepsy during or after the third decade of life.

In contrast with infantile spasms, the Lennox-Gastaut syndrome has been recognized as a clinical epileptological entity in more recent time. The ictal seizure manifestations are obviously too diversified (as will be pointed out later) to impress the clinician directly as an entity; the observation of typical EEG changes in these cases was necessary in order to establish the common characteristics of this syndrome. Gibbs et al. (1939) noticed the severity and poor prognosis of the seizure disorder in patients with slow spike wave complexes (called "*petit mal* variant" by these authors) in comparison with the classical 3/sec spike-wave complexes in patients with typical petit mal and a more benign type of epilepsy. Lennox (1945, 1960) gave a detailed account of the clinical and ictal symptomatology of these patients; Gastaut and his co-workers (1966) contributed most valuable further information for which reason the term "Lennox-Gastaut syndrome" has been suggested (Niedermeyer, 1968, 1969). It is also known as "Epilepsie myokinétique grave" (Sorel, 1964) and as "Lennox syndrome"; more about the terminological aspects may be found in a "revisitation" of the syndrome by Gibbs (1971) and Gastaut (1971).

Almost all types of seizures may occur in the Lennox-Gastaut syndrome but some of them are diagnostically very suggestive or nearly specific. Most important in this regard are the *atonic-akinetic seizures* or *drop spells* (Fig. 16, 17). These attacks are of very short duration and lead to a vehement and frequently traumatizing fall. These and the following types of seizure are more explicitly presented in Chapter 2. Very typical are brief *tonic seizures* with extension of all limbs, limited to sleep and easily overlooked because of their unimpressive manifestations; sleep EEG tracings will often lead to their detection. *Massive myoclonus* and very rapid *clonic attacks* are common. In addition, there are types of seizure which may also occur in other forms of epilepsy. *Grand mal* attacks occur, at least once in the majority of the patients; the major convulsions may take place at the onset of the seizure disorder without ever recurring again. *Petit mal absences* and *certain variants of petit mal* (Gastaut et al., 1966) may occur; *psychomotor automatisms* are rather predominant in

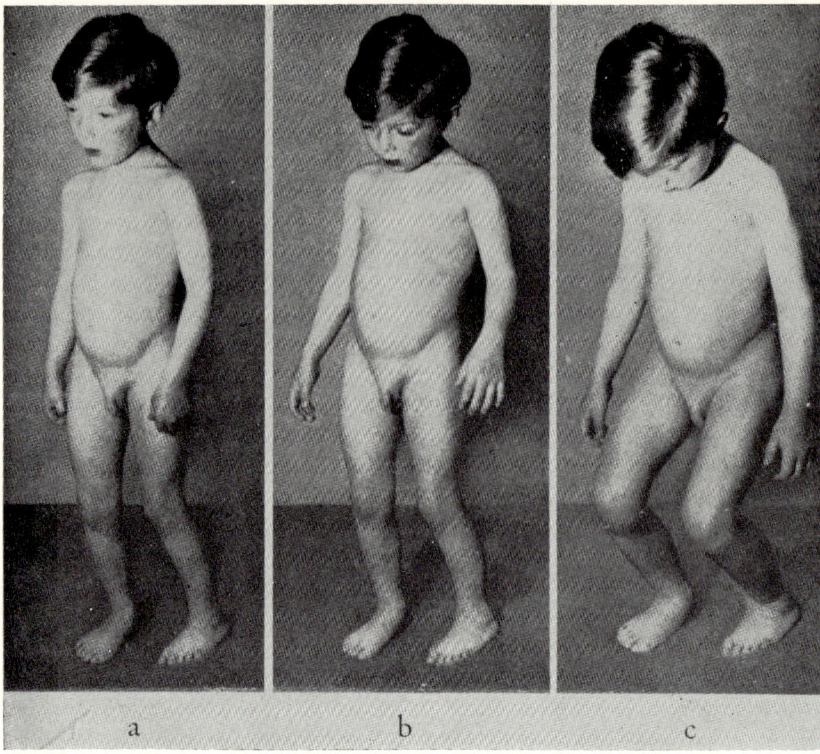

FIGURE 16. Cinematographic demonstration of the onset of an atonic-akinetic seizure in a 5-year-old boy. Note buckling of knees. In this instance, the attack was aborted and no fall materialized. (Reprinted with friendly permission from Prof. Dr. Doose: *Arch. Psychiat. Nervenkr.*, *205*:632, 1964.)

some patients; *focal-motor, hemiconvulsive and adversive* attacks are not seldom seen whereas *petit mal status* (*ictal stupor*) is one of the least common manifestations.

In the diagnostic workup, the *electroencephalogram* is very important. Above all, the slow spike-wave complex, frequent fast multiple spike discharges and "runs of rapid spikes" are instrumental findings in the EEG evaluation (Fig. 18-20). Further details have been presented by Niedermeyer (1969, 1972). In the vast majority, the EEG abnormalities are fully or predominantly generalized. A more extensive workup is not merely of

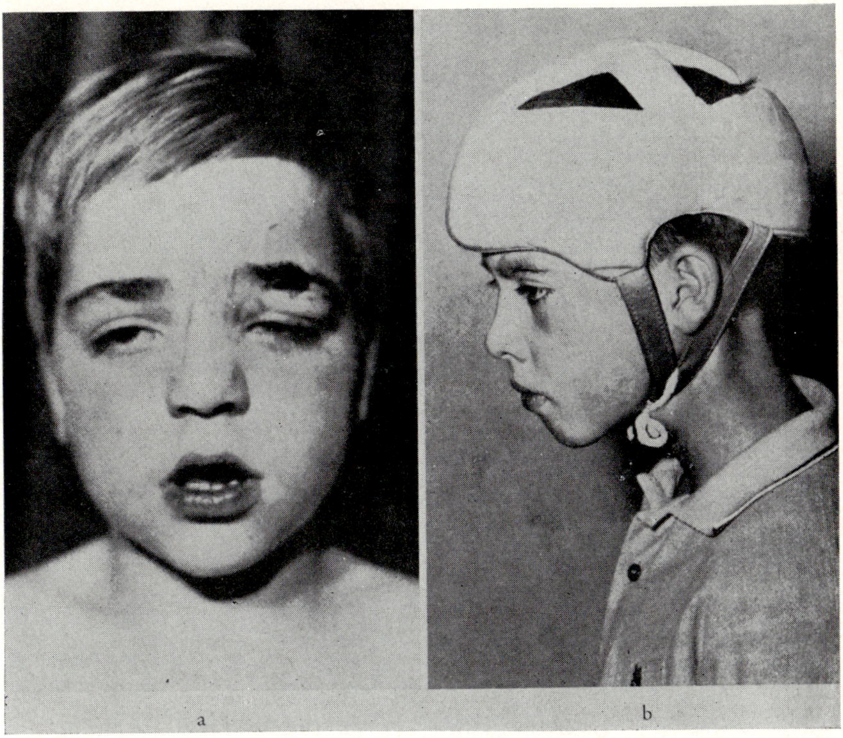

FIGURE 17. (Left) This 6-year-old boy shows facial lacerations caused by numerous sudden falls due to atonic-akinetic attacks. (Right) Protective headgear for children suffering from traumatizing atonic-akinetic seizures. (Reprinted with permission from R. Kruse: Das myoklonisch-astatische Petit mal, Berlin, Springer, 1968.)

academic interest since, in a very small number of cases, intracranial tumors may be detected. At least a brain scan is advisable.

Neurological deficits are detectable in about 20 percent of the children; some of these defects date back into earliest infancy and may fall into the categories of cerebral palsy. Hydrocephalic and microcephalic skull anomalies may be present.

Intellectual deficits or *mental retardation* of all degrees of severity *are the rule;* the only exception is found in patients with onset of the seizure disorder after the age of 10 years. Profound mental retardation is common in cases with very early onset, especially with preceding untreated infantile spasms or even

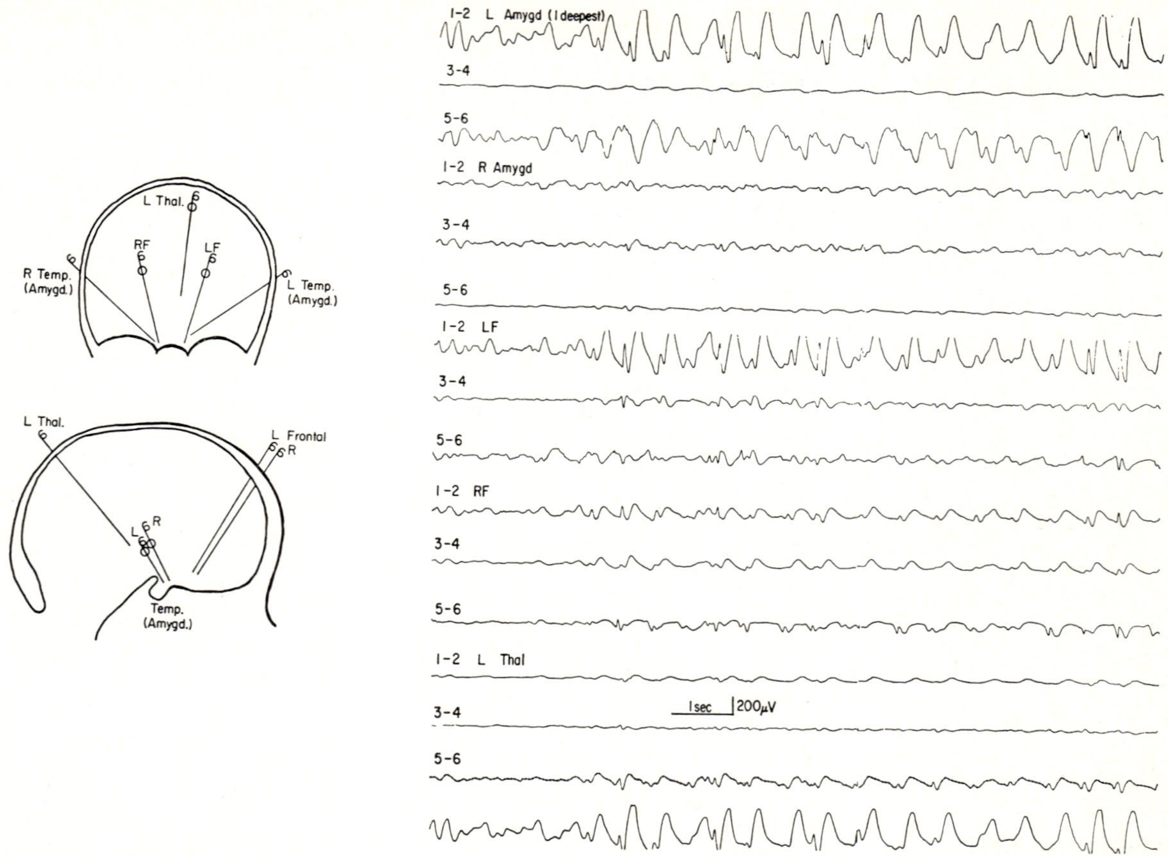

FIGURE 18. Depth EEG in a 15 year old boy (#930129). Severe asphyxia at birth. Lennox-Gastaut syndrome with severe mental retardation. The record shows widespread 1.5-2.5/sec spike-wave activity (the classical EEG feature of the Lennox-Gastaut syndrome.

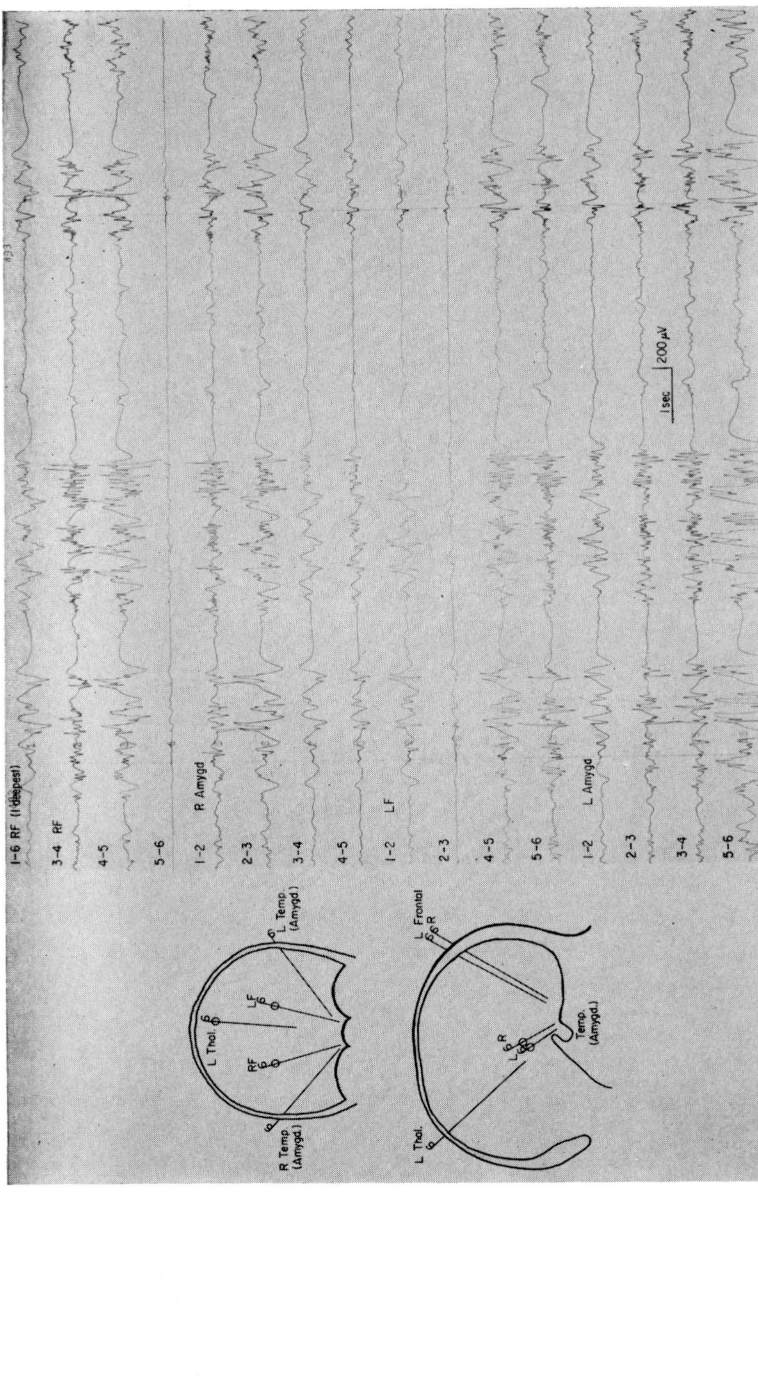

FIGURE 19. The same patient as in Figure 18. Depth EEG. The sleep record shows bilateral-synchronous multiple spikes and runs of rapid spikes.

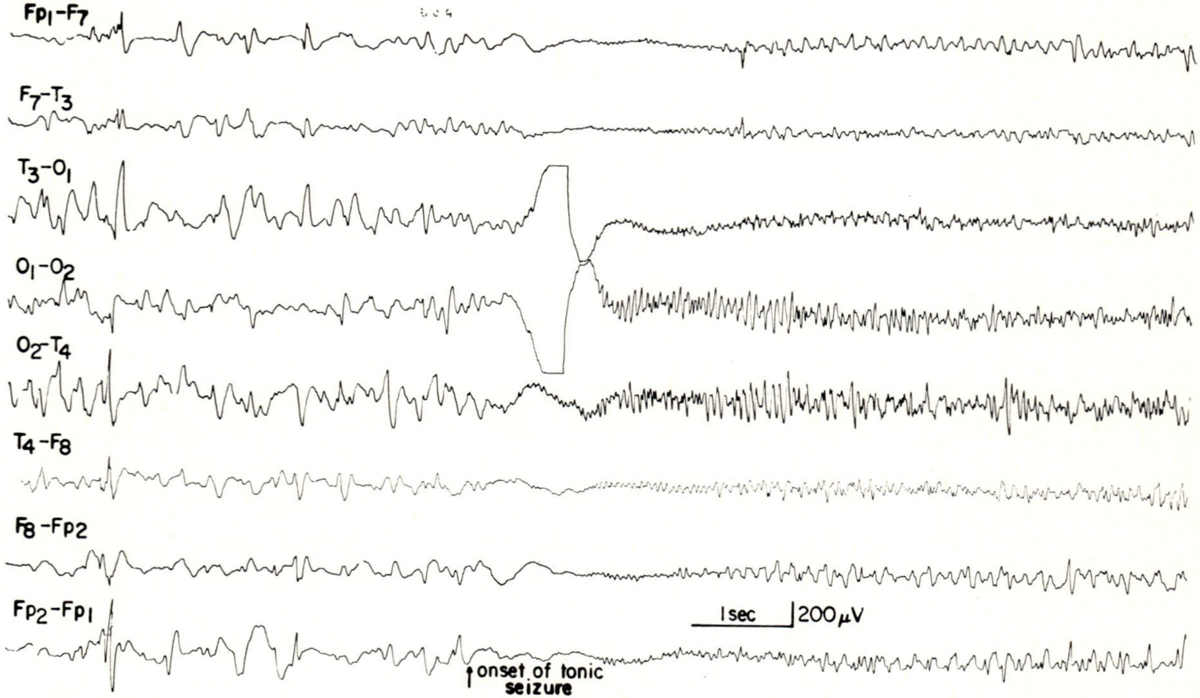

FIGURE 20. Electronecephalogram of a 7-year-old boy, Lennox-Gastaut syndrome. A tonic seizure with stiffening and extension of all four extremities is recorded. Note sudden voltage drop and the following crescendo of sustained rapid spikes.

seizures since birth. *Behavior disorder* with hyperkinetic motility is not very common in association with the mental deficits; in patients with onset after age 10, however, behavioral disturbances may be in the foreground while the mental defects may be negligible.

Like in infantile spasms, *a vast number of etiological conditions may account for this type of convulsive disorder; in the majority* of the cases, however, *the cause will remain undetermined.* Thus, a 3-year-old child with hitherto normal physical and mental development may suddenly have a series of major convulsions without any detectable accompanying disease. From this time on, the child will have frequent violent falling spells (or myoclonic jerks, absences, nocturnal tonic spasms, psychomotor automatisms, etc.) and the intellectual development will slow down. The diametrically opposed case is the baby with neonatal convulsions followed later by hypsarrhythmia with infantile spasms and gradual conversion into the ictal and electrical semeiology of the Lennox-Gastaut syndrome. This child may be hemi- or quadriplegic since earliest infancy and the mental retardation is likely to be profound.

Every type of insult to the brain (infectious, traumatic, anoxic, vascular or metabolic) may give rise to the Lennox-Gastaut syndrome. An additional hereditary component or genetic predisposition to epileptic seizures may be present but its role must not be overrated. In rare instances, a brain tumor may be the cause, either as an independent neoplastic development or in association with tuberous sclerosis.

The *physiopathogenesis* of the Lennox-Gastaut syndrome is obscure. There is no explanation for the "malignant" character of the slow spike wave complex and the atonic akinetic seizures. The frontal lobes might be more involved than other regions but this lies in the realm of speculation (Niedermeyer, 1972).

The incidence of the Lennox-Gastaut syndrome is controversial. In the material of a large medical center with a very active seizure clinic and special interest in seizure surgery, the number of cases is relatively high, even though 2 to 3 percent of the total epileptic material of the center are not exceeded. These values are probably considerably lower in the overall epileptic population, despite the fact that large numbers of children and adolescents with Lennox-Gastaut syndrome are found in institutions for the mentally retarded.

THERAPY. Thus far, the entire armamentarium of anticonvulsants have yielded poor results and the use of hormones (ACTH, steroids) is also futile. *Diazepam* (*Valium*®) has been recommended by Gastaut et al. (1966) and at least transient control or reduction of seizures was noticed. The effect of drugs is not easily assessed because of the extremely capricious changes which may occur in the course of the disorder. Spontaneous cessation of seizures for years may occur but with no concomitant mental improvement; even a "miraculous" case (see Lennox, 1960, and his brilliant case histories) is likely to have seizures in the future. *Ketogenic diet* almost always reduces the number of seizures for several weeks or months; it may even lead to temporary seizure freedom. Desperate parents sometimes ask for *neurosurgical treatment* but in view of the widespread EEG abnormalities, the neurosurgeon will have to resist, in most instances, the parental pressure to operate. *Institutionalization* is very frequently the result of the severe mental defects which may lay an unbearable burden on the life of an otherwise healthy family.

In the management of children with atonic akinetic falling spells, protective head gear (of a football helmet like appearance) will be necessary because of the above mentioned traumatizing nature of the falls.

Should the physician give medication at all? I feel one cannot negate this question, especially because of the psychological impact of total therapeutic passivity on parents and relatives. It may be wise to change medication from time to time, according to the general rules of such changes (see chapter on therapy). A dramatic struggle for a pharmacological enforcement of seizure-freedom has to be strictly avoided; these attempts always lead to drug toxicity and enhancement of mental dullness.

COURSE AND PROGNOSIS. The recalcitrant character of the seizures renders the prognosis extremely gloomy. There is no doubt that the Lennox-Gastaut syndrome carries the worst prognosis among all epileptic conditions. The outlook is not quite as bleak when the seizures start over the age of 10 years since repercussions on the intellectual development may be absent.

Bizarre variations of the seizure frequency are not uncommon and usually not attributable to therapeutic efforts. As it was mentioned before, the seizure disorder gradually changes its character as adulthood is reached. The slow spike-wave complex becomes progressively less distinctive while runs of rapid spikes in the sleep EEG may still linger on. The EEG tends to show more focal spikes and sharp waves over the anterior temporal area and this electrical hallmark of temporal lobe epilepsy corresponds with changes in the ictal symptomatology; psychomotor automatisms move into the foreground. Thus, the Lennox-Gastaut syndrome tends to merge into the pciture of temporal lobe epilepsy by losing its own distinctive features. These mentally deteriorated and usually institutionalized temporal lobe epileptics, however, are often characterized by a fairly specific type of psychomotor automatisms: the "running fits," also called "epilepsia procursiva." The scarcity of good longitudinal studies from infancy into adulthood does not permit authoritative statements in this regard. Therefore, the described trend toward "secondary temporalization" is still debatable.

6) ***Common generalized epilepsy*** (also called "centrencephalic" or "idiopathic")

There has been much controversy about the justification for the establishment of form of *epilepsy "per se"* in which signs of insult to the brain—in the individual history as well as in the neurological and ictal semeiology—are absent. Accordingly, these patients would have seizures merely on the basis of a very strong predisposition to epileptic reactions and this would automatically mean a strong genetic element. The genetic factors in epilepsy, however, are very complex and suggestive of a multiplicity of involved genes.

On the negative side, a history of brain disease or injury automatically disqualifies a given seizure disorder from being listed as common generalized epilepsy; this is also true for the occurrence of neurological signs, mental defects and focal types of seizures which are strongly suggestive of some type of acquired cerebral involvement. On the positive side, one might expect a family history of epilepsy but a genetic component could just as well be a contributory factor in acquired types of convulsive disorder. In common generalized epilepsy, positive family histories are not obtained in the majority of the cases (although a sizeable number of patients—around 10 to 20 percent— do have positive family histories).

The most reasonable and best founded positive diagnostic criteria of common generalized epilepsy lie in a) the *factor of age* (of onset, peak and decline of the seizure disorder), b) the *type of seizures,* and c) the *EEG characteristics.*

The *maximally involved age ranges from 4 to 16 (or 20) years;* there are virtually no seizure manifestations prior to the age of 3 years (except for occasional febrile convulsions in infancy and earliest childhood) and a considerable decrease or gradual disappearance of the seizure is notable in early adulthood; this development is furthered by appropriate treatment.

The most typical seizure in common generalized epilepsy is the classical petit mal absence. The characteristics of petit mal are discussed in Chapter 2. These short-lasting and mild attacks may occur at a frequency of 50 to 100/day or even higher, especially in cases of early onset (around age 4-6 years).

Petit mal absences of later onset—around age 8 to 14 years— are associated with a lesser seizure frequency and their clinical course is slightly different as will be shown later; for these reasons, German authors (Doose, 1964; Janz, 1969) have proposed a distinction between the earlier classical form ("pycnolepsy") and the later form ("juvenile petit mal").

A large number of children with petit mal in childhood will develop grand mal attacks in puberty or prepuberty; the figures lie between 31 percent (Paal, 1957) and 54 percent (Lennox, 1960; Livingston et al., 1965). The grand mal seizures are usually infrequent events and tend to occur in the morning hours and especially after nights of insufficient sleep. The major convulsions may be preceded by *occasional myoclonic jerking* in the morning hours; the flexor muscles of the arms are principally involved.

These jerks and twitches may serve as a stern warning of an imminent grand mal seizure.

There are only three types of seizure compatible with common generalized epilepsy: petit mal, grand mal and myoclonic attacks with bilateral jerking. All of these seizures are based upon bilateral synchronous seizure discharges; focal-cortical elements are alien to this group. A rare special ictal condition is *petit mal status* which occurs in an extremely small number of patients with common generalized epilepsy; a more proper term for this state would be *"ictal stupor"* or *"spike wave stupor"* (Niedermeyer and Khalifeh, 1965) since it is characterized by a stupor-like state lasting hours or days (rather than by a rapid succession of petit mal seizures); it will be discussed in greater detail under the heading of "status epilepticus."

Electroencephalographic findings. Generalized-synchronous seizure discharges and, above all, the 3/sec spike wave complex dominate the picture. While short bursts of these discharges must never be automatically equated with the presence of petit mal seizures, more sustained 3/sec spike-wave bursts of clock-like rhythmicity are the only EEG accompaniment of true petit mal. The subictal and ictal spike wave bursts are easily elicited by hyperventilation in children or adolescents with petit mal. In addition, single and occasional multiple spikes are seen; minor asymmetries may exist but consistent focal accentuation is suspect of additional focal mechanisms and does not fit the picture of common generalized epilepsy. In sleep, spike-wave bursts become less rhythmical and break up into groups of single and multiple spikes. The background activity is usually unremarkable.

All of the electroencephalographic seizure patterns of common generalized epilepsy show a maximum over the frontal midline region. During sleep, these bursts are strongly and consistently associated with arousal responses (K complexes). Some of the patients show marked generalized spiking during intermittent photic stimulation, especially at a rate of 14 to 18 flashes/sec; these bursts may be associated with bilateral myoclonic jerking or even more widespread and prolonged convulsive activity.

Photo-sensitive patients are likely to form a subgroup of common generalized epilepsy with a lesser tendency to develop petit mal, a greater proclivity toward grand mal and myoclonic seizures and predominant 4/sec spike wave-bursts (rather than the 3-3.5/sec frequency) of short duration in the resting EEG and during hyperventilation. Positive family histories of epilepsy are more common in this sub-group (Niedermeyer, 1972).

The *physical findings* are usually normal; major neurological deficits and mental retardation are by definition incompatible with common generalized epilepsy although this epileptic condition could theoretically coincide with completely independent cerebral disease. Behavior disorder is not uncommon and perhaps more often seen in the photo-sensitive sub-group.

The *physiopathogenesis* has been a subject of great controversy. Some investigators have never ceased to abandon the theory of a hidden and clinically undemonstrable focus of epileptogenic character; in this view, one ought to talk in terms such as "cryptogenic" epilepsy (Wilson, 1935). The advent of electroencephalography and the report of generalized-synchronous seizure discharges in petit mal attacks (Gibbs, Davis and Lennox, 1935) prompted the concept of a "common central (midline subcortical) pacemaker" (Jasper and Kershman, 1941); this concept was never shared by Gibbs and his co-workers who considered a cortical origin more likely. The ideas of Jasper and Kershman (1941) were bolstered by the demonstration of non-specific thalamo-cortical pathways instrumental in the "recruiting response" of the cortex and elicited by low frequency electrical stimulation of intralaminar thalamic structures in the cat (Morison and Dempsey, 1942). Furthermore, this theory of a powerful midline structure in thalamic level (in addition to the Jacksonian concept of a "highest level" type of seizures) perfectly fitted Wilder Penfield's ideas concerning the function of consciousness on the basis of extensive cortical and integration within the thalamic level ("centrencephalic system"; Penfield, 1938; Penfield, 1957).

A blend of these theories and experimental findings brought forth the new concept of *centrencephalic epilepsy* (Penfield,

1952; Penfield and Jasper, 1954) typefied by the petit mal seizure and the concomitant generalized-synchronous 3/sec spike-wave pattern. This term became extremely popular among neurologists, epileptologists and electroencephalographers, especially after the demonstration of widespread cortical spike-wave discharge elicited by intralaminar thalamic stimulation in the cat (Jasper and Droogleever Fortuyn, 1947); this was confirmed in further studies (Ingvar, 1955; Pollen et al., 1963). The demonstration of the ascending mesodiencephalic reticular system (Moruzzi and Magoun, 1949), its diffuse connections with the neocortex and its tonic influence on the cortical level in the regulation of consciousness lent further support to the ideas of Penfield and Jasper. Mesencephalic electrical stimulation also produced spike-wave responses in the cat (Weir, 1964) and, in chronic experiments in cats with aluminum oxide midbrain lesions, "spontaneous" spike wave activity was noted (Guerrero-Figueroa et al., 1963).

A sudden freeze of the global motor activity was elicited by electrical stimulation of the mesio-anterior thalamus in unanesthetized animals (Hunter and Jasper, 1949); this "arrest reaction" was subsequently regarded as an animal model of the petit mal attack (Penfield and Jasper, 1954).

In spite of these impressive experimental findings, some investigators did not accept the theory of a centrencephalic pacemaker mechanism in generalized seizure discharges. The significance of the cortex in the production of experimental spike-wave activity was stressed by Starzl et al. (1953); Sager et al. (1959); Okuma et al. (1961); Pradhan and Ajmone Marsan (1963); and Marcus and Watson (1965). Other investigators de-emphasized the role of the thalamus in the generalization of experimentally induced electro convulsions (Jung, 1949) or in the propagation of generalization of epileptic activity from experimental cortical or subcortical foci (Walker and Udvarhelyi, 1965; Udvarhelyi and Walker, 1965). A frontally induced type of arrest reaction was demonstrated by Walker and Morello in the cat (1967).

Depth electroencephalographic data derived from implanted electrodes in human epileptics could hardly provide further evidence for the centrencephalic concept since the cortical level (or limbic and basal ganglia structures) appeared to be substantially or predominantly involved in the generation of generalized-synchronous seizure discharges (Hayne et al., 1949; Williams, 1953; Bickford, 1956; Walker and Marshall, 1964; Angeleri et al., 1964; Bancaud et al., 1965; Rossi et al., 1967; Niedermeyer et al., 1969; Niedermeyer, 1972). In recent years, Gloor (1968, 1969) has emphasized the role of the cortical and the mesencephalic reticular level in the genesis of generalized-synchronous seizure patterns; his concept of "cortico-reticular epilepsy" is based upon his data derived from intracarotid injections of pentylene-tetrazol (Metrazol®) in human epileptics.

The much debated question of thalamic (or subcortical) vs. cortical origin of generalized-synchronous seizure discharges might be irrelevant in human epileptics with common generalized epilepsy. The precipitating mechanisms deserve much greater attention. In recent studies, Niedermeyer (1965, 1966, 1967, 1970, 1972) has studied the *conjunction of generalized seizure discharges and arousal responses* in sleep (Fig. 21). It is felt that *a faulty arousal mechanism* exists in most patients with common generalized epilepsy; the physiological electrical arousal responses of these patients tend to assume epileptic properties. This mechanism has been called "*dyshormia*" (derived from the Greek: "hormaein" for "to incite," "to spur," "to arouse," thus denoting a deviant arousal) and is likely to be due to defective neuronal inhibition on the basis of a neurobiochemical defect.* Even the age determination of common generalized epilepsy could be explained in this manner since the physiological electrical arousal responses (K complexes in the EEG) tend to show a relatively sharp and mildly paroxysmal component, especially at the age between 4 to 16 years. Further details cannot be discussed in this context (see Niedermeyer, 1972).

A primarily photosensitive subgroup of patients with common generalized epilepsy may lack the mechanism of dyshormia; other patients may have both the dyshormic and the photosensitive component (Fig. 22).

The length of this discussion of physiopathogenic mechanisms

* The nature of the presumed neurobiochemical defect could be elucidated by the absence of generalized seizure discharges in REM (rapid eye movement)-

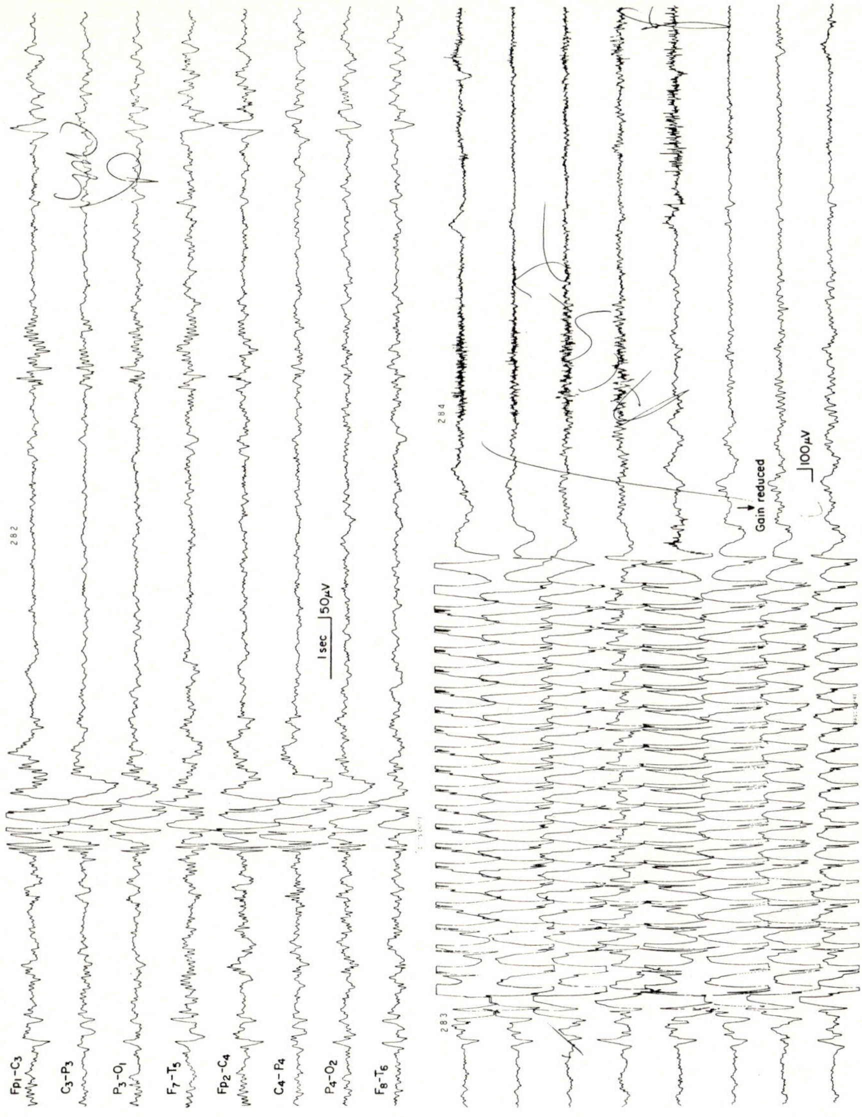

FIGURE 21. Sleep EEG recording of a 15-year-old female patient with petit mal and grand mal (#1452993). The bottom section is the continuation of the upper portion. Note a brief generalized burst of spikes and a few spike-waves in the left half of the upper tracing. This burst is linked with a physiological arousal response (K complex; its trailing slow component is superimposed by spindles). In the lower section, a generalized-synchronous subclinical proxyom of 3/sec spike-wave complex is preceded by the sharp component of a K complex. There is subsequent arousal from sleep. The spike-wave burst is "sandwiched" between the components of the K complexes and thus imbedded in a physiological arousal response.

stages of sleep (Passouant and Cadilhac, 1970) which is thought to be governed by catecholaminergic and cholinergic neuronal systems (Rothballer, 1957; Koella et al., 1960; Jouvet, 1967). The "hypersynchronous" non-REM sleep with production of frequent generalized epilepsy seizure discharges (in common generalized epilepsy) is presumed to be controlled by serotonin-containing neurons in the pontine raphe and preoptic area (acting on midbrain reticular formation) (Jouvet, 1967; Pujol, 1972).

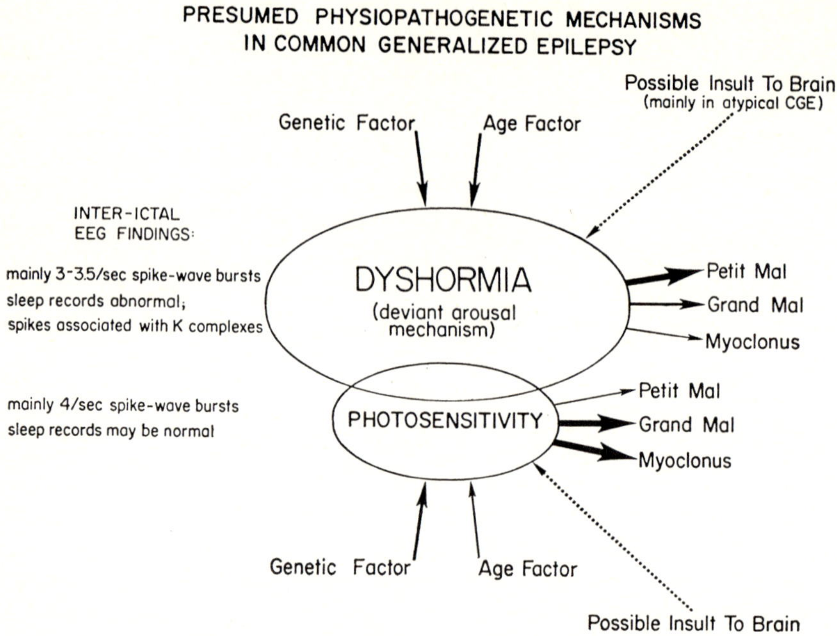

FIGURE 22. Presumed physiopathogenetic mechanisms involved in common generalized epilepsy. The dyshormic and the photosensitive subgroups are shown separately. Note the area of overlap between both subgroups. While age and genetic factor might be equally significant in the dyshormic epileptic, the age factor is probably less important in photosensitivity. Also note the greater propensity to grand mal and myoclonic attacks in the photosensitive subgroup. The interictal electroencephalogram is more likely to show 4/sec (rather than 3 to 3.5/sec) spike-wave complexes in the flicker-sensitive patients with Common generalized epilepsy. Patients with Common generalized epilepsy and 4/sec spike-wave complexes, however, are not necessarily photosensitive.

is inconsistent with the style of this book but the controversy about the origin of generalized seizure discharges attracted so much interest during the past 25 years that one cannot discuss this topic in brevity.

DIFFERENTIAL DIAGNOSIS. Common generalized epilepsy must be separated from other epileptological conditions in which generalized synchronous seizure discharges are also predominant. *Secondary bilateral synchrony* (Jasper, 1949; Tukel and Jasper,

1952) is a term used for generalized seizure patterns due to a primary hemispheric focus which is most likely to be located in the frontal or temporal region. Classical petit mal seizures may occur in such patients who may greatly benefit from the removal of the site of primary focus after the failure of the appropriate anticonvulsive medication (Niedermeyer et al., 1969; Niedermeyer, 1972; see Fig. 4, 7). In rare instances, intracranial tumors may be the cause of the generalized seizure discharges (Ajmone Marsan and Lewis, 1960; Stewart and Dreifuss, 1967). It is very difficult and often impossible to differentiate between primary and secondary bilateral synchrony on EEG evidence alone; some of these cases will remain enigmatic. The remote possibility of a brain tumor cannot be completely dismissed and the physician has to keep a watchful eye on the possible development of intracranial hypertension. There is some reason to presume that epileptics with a hemispheric focus and marked secondary bilateral synchrony are genetically predisposed to the generalization of seizure discharges while the primary cortical focus is the residue of acquired brain disease.

In rare instances, the classical combination of petit mal and grand mal with generalized-synchronous seizure patterns in the EEG may be due to a *lesion in the hypothalamic or mesencephalic level.* Patients with hypothalamic lesions may have endocrine disturbances such as precocious puberty (Hann, 1957; Scherman and Abraham, 1963), cerebral gigantism (Niedermeyer, 1972) or other neuro-endocrine symptoms (Boudin et al., 1954). The differentiation from *metabolic and especially renal disorders* does not present major difficulties; generalized seizure discharges in renal epilepsy are usually less regular (Fig. 23). In some *hypoglycemic states,* however, very well formed spike-wave complexes and occasional occurrence of true petit mal absences may be observed (Niedermeyer, 1972), while more uncharacteristic findings (even absence of spikes) predominant in most patients with hypoglycemic epilepsies (Gastaut et al., 1969).

A typical petit mal and bilateral synchronous seizure patterns have been reported in *cingulate lesions* ("cingulate epilepsy"; Y. Mazars et al., 1966; G. Mazars, 1969, 1970). When the spike-

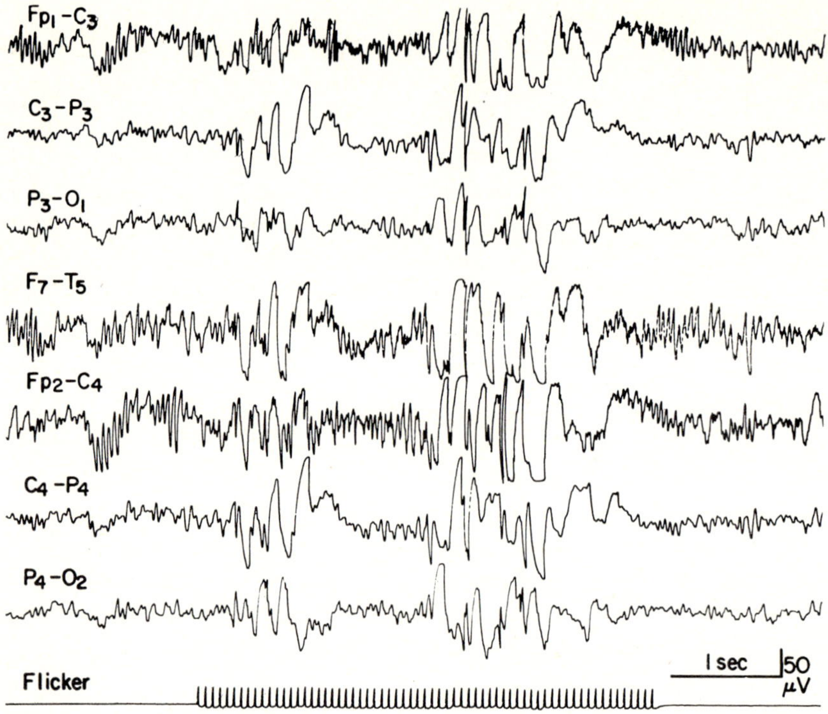

FIGURE 23. Renal epilepsy in a 14-year-old boy (#873407) with nephrosis since age 2 years. Flickering light triggers a generalized irregular spike-wave-burst. He also had spontaneous paroxysmal bursts and rare petit mal-like absences.

wave activity fails to show the slow frequency range (1-2.5/sec) of the *Lennox-Gastaut* syndrome, the electroencephalographic differentiation between this condition and common generalized epilepsy may become difficult; the history, types of seizure and the pattern of mental development will be diagnostically helpful. Generalized seizure discharges in *Essential hereditary myoclonus epilepsy* (*Lafora-Unverricht-Lundberg*) are very irregular and widely mixed with myogenic spikes; the abundance of myoclonic jerking, presence of cerebellar dysmetria and decline of mental function speak heavily in favor of the degenerative myoclonus epilepsy.

THERAPY. *Petit mal* absences usually defy any treatment

based on phenobarbital (or other barbiturates) and/or hydantoines. The introduction of trimethadione (Tridione®) by Lennox (1945) proved to be extremely valuable in the control of *petit mal* absences but a number of undesirable side-effects have made this medication somewhat dangerous. The oxazolidinediones (Tridione and Paradione®) are now more seldom used and have been widely replaced by the succinimides and especially by ethosuximide (Zarontin®). Further details will be given in the chapter dealing with therapy in general. The prevention of future grand mal seizures necessitates additional amounts of phenobarbital or diphenylhydantoin; the amount of 32 mg phenobarbital given in a single dosage at bedtime will be effective in this regard. Patients with grand mal only (or additional myoclonic attacks) respond to the usual phenobarbital diphenylhydantoin treatment.

There is general agreement that *petit mal* absences should be treated as soon as the diagnosis has been established.

Some patients with common generalized epilepsy have certain psychopathic personality traits and take their tablets haphazardly; one of my patients has recently become a drug addict (heroin and some short-acting barbiturates). This is an extremely unusual event in the treatment of epileptics (leaving aside alcohol epilepsy) since most epileptics (and even the temporal lobe epileptics with their own brand of personality disorder) tend to take their tablets almost "religiously."

Hygienic measures will also be discussed under a separate heading; these measures aim specifically at a well regulated sleep-waking-rhythm with a sufficient length of sleep. The violation of this principle might contribute to the emergence of grand mal attacks in teenagers who start *hanging around.* Fatigue in the morning hours seems to enhance the above mentioned mechanism of dyshormia.

Course and prognosis. In most of the cases, the prognosis is bright and the patients become seizure free during the third decade of life. The number of petit mal attacks gradually diminishes during adolescence; these absences may or may not linger on after age 20. If *petit mal* persists into adulthood, the frequency of the attacks is usually very low (around 1/week to 1/month) and the inconspicuous nature of the absences conveys to the patient a feeling of seizure freedom. According to Gibberd (1972), patients who continue having petit mal absences after the age of 20 years may have a rather prolonged course throughout adult life. In practice, however, middle age or elderly patients with true *petit mal* absences are very rarely encountered.

Petit mal absences starting at the age of 10 to 12 years do not respond as well to appropriate treatment as compared with petit mal of earlier onset, especially in the range of 4 to 6 years. This subdivision has been stressed by Kuhlo (1965), Janz (1969) and Doose (1970).

Patients with grand mal only or with some additional myoclonus will not as readily become seizure free (or nearly seizure free) in adulthood. In spite of a sizeable reduction of the seizure frequency, occasional convulsions may occur throughout adult life, often several years apart.

7) *Childhood epilepsies with focal spikes in the electroencephalogram*

Many epileptic children in the age from 3 to 12 years show well defined focal spikes or sharp waves in the EEG. In the majority of these children, the history is unremarkable except for the seizures; there is no suggestion of a previous insult to the brain and the physical findings are mostly normal. The focal spike activity is seen most often over the central region; slightly less common are mid temporal, occipital, parietal and frontal spike foci.

The seizure disorder of these children defies a precise categorization in any of the before mentioned conditions and one could lump these cases together in one group. One has to presume some (clinically and neuroradiologically undemonstrable) moderate cerebral disturbance of obscure etiology.

In the vast majority of these children, the seizures as well as the *focal spikes disappear late in childhood or early in adolescence.* These children *grow out* their seizure disorder. Optimal anticonvulsive medication will be helpful in bringing the epileptic manifestations more quickly under control.

There are certain differences within this group according to the location of the spikes (Gibbs and Gibbs, 1964). Children with occipital spikes are usually in the pre-school age; only 40 percent of them actually have seizures. Children with central and midtemporal spikes have clinical seizure in 50 to 70 percent of the cases; the non-epileptic children tend to have a behavior disorder of the hyperkinetic type. The seizures are predominantly of the grand mal type; some of them have contralateral focal motor seizures, often limited to the face ("Sylvian seizures"; Lombroso, 1967). Children with mid temporal spike foci may also have psychomotor seizures, and they could become candidates for the *mature* adult form of temporal lobe epilepsy with anterior temporal sharp wave foci. Frontal lobe foci are less common; their epileptogenicity is high (around 80%) and the ensuing seizure disorder may become more serious.

Central spikes in children have been the topic of several studies (Y. Gastaut, 1952; Hess, 1958; Isler and Hess, 1960; Blom and Brorson, 1966; Niedermeyer, 1970). These central spikes may show a puzzling relationship to physiological central patterns ("mu-rhythm," Niedermeyer, 1972).

Children with focal spikes and clinical evidence of cerebral palsy with residual motor deficits fall into a different category. Not all of these children have epileptic seizures but the early development of focal spikes has considerable predictive value as the remarkable work of Gibbs and Gibbs (1964; partly based on earlier studies with Perlstein, 1949, 1955) has demonstrated. These authors have broken down cerebral palsy in the usual manner (hemiplegic, di- and quadriplegic, choreoathetoid forms) discussing separately the epileptogenicity and EEG findings of each group.

Children with multifocal spikes (seizure discharges originating independently from more than one region) tend to have more severe and sometimes poorly controllable seizure disorders irrespective of the presence or absence of neurological deficits caused by cerebral palsy. The prognosis, however, is not as bleak as in the Lennox-Gastaut syndrome.

Chapter 5

SPECIAL TYPES OF EPILEPSY ACCORDING TO THE SITE OF THE FOCUS

1) Introductory remarks

THE LOCAL ORIGIN of an epileptic seizure disorder may reveal itself by the focal character of the seizures. Well documented clinical details of a seizure in correlation with electroencephalographic findings as well as the reproduction of ictal phenomena by local cortical stimulation under electrocorticographic control have enormously contributed to a deeper knowledge of epileptology and, moreover, to a better comprehension of cortical functions. None of these observations has rivalled the fundamental contribution of Penfield and his associates.

According to Penfield and Kristiansen (1951), "the initial phenomenon in an epileptic seizure is usually the most important clue to the localization of the original focus of epileptic discharge within the brain. It is also the most reliable guide to the classification of any case of habitual epileptic seizures."

The determination of the focal origin, however, is hampered by various limitations. Many focal epilepsies give rise to grand mal seizures only and even a carefully taken history will not reveal any aura-like manifestations of a focal onset. In other cases, focal seizures are due to a "low threshold area" activated by the epileptic activity of an adjacent (or even distant) primary epileptic focus which may remain clinically silent. Thus, epileptogenic foci just below the Sylvian fissue may give rise to focal motor seizures from the adjoining precentral gyrus, classically starting in the contralateral facial region ("Sylvian seizures"; Lombroso, 1967) or an occipital focus may give rise to distant limbic temporal lobe seizures (Falconer et al., 1962). Of course, the electroencephalogram will be very helpful clarifying such apparent inconsistencies but this method has its imitations. These are only a few examples chosen to demonstrate the frequently arising difficulties in pinpointing the location of a cortical epileptogenic focus.

Let us also recall again the extremely important factor of age since we just have described the limited localizing value of focal spikes in the EEG of epileptic (and often nonepileptic) children. There are fundamental differences between "functional" focal spikes (seen chiefly in childhood) and the focal spikes of truly localizing significance which occur mainly in adults with chronic epilepsies on the basis of a well defined epileptogenic focus with the characteristics of scar formation or other types of pathology (Niedermeyer, 1972). While the former appear to be related to physiological stimuli and sensory input (especially in the case of central spikes; Tassinari, 1968; Niedermeyer, 1970d) the later seem to emerge in an "autochtonous" or "autonomous" manner as the result of changes occurring within the focus with no apparent extrinsic trigger mechanism).

There are infrequent cases of children with *stable* focal spikes due to well defined regional lesions such as porencephaly, microgyria, cortical atrophy or meningocerebral changes in Sturge-Webers' syndrome. Occasionally, such cases of childhood epilepsies will require neurosurgical treatment. These cases are exceptional whereas the majority of children with focal spikes have "unstable" or "functional" foci which are apt to "migrate" (Gibbs, 1958), disappear altogether, change to innocuous patterns (such as the 14 and 6/sec positive spike discharge; Gibbs, 1958) or merge into physiological EEG activities such as mu-rhythm (Niedermeyer, 1970d).

In the following part, we will discuss the "true" and "stable" forms of focal epilepsies.

2) Temporal lobe epilepsy

Seizures arising from the temporal lobe have increasingly

captivated the interest of the neurologist in recent years. These seizure disorders are fairly common in adult life and may reveal the vast variety of temporal lobe and deep limbic functions which, under ictal irritation, may present themselves as bizarre distortions or caricatures of the physiological state.

Psychomotor seizures are the classical ictal manifestation of the temporal lobe. The extremely rich semeiology of these attacks consists chiefly of psychical and motor phenomena; for this reason, the term "Psychomotor seizure" is perfectly appropriate. Autonomic and sensory ictal manifestations also occur; this will be discussed farther below.

Psychomotor seizures may occasionally develop into a grand mal convulsion and some patients with electroencephalographic evidence of a temporal lobe focus may have grand mal only. Petit mal absences, myoclonic attacks, focal motor and other focal seizures are alien to the picture of temporal lobe epilepsy; the only exception is the Lennox-Gastaut syndrome which may encompass all of these seizure types (usually in children with concomitant mental defects).

HISTORICAL REMARKS—THE DISCOVERY OF THE NEUROPHYSIOLOGICAL BASIS. The clinical observations of Falret (1860), Herpin (1867), Samt (1976), Jackson, (1866), Jackson and Beevor (1889) and Jackson and Stewart (1899) outlined the vast domain of epileptic temporal lobe phenomena. The anatomical basis and the relationship of the ictal signs to the temporal lobe was clearly demonstrated by Jackson's autopsy findings. Clinical pathological correlations were based mainly on temporal lobe tumors; ictal and interictal mental changes were stressed in the studies of Knapp (1905, 1918) and Stauder (1935).

The introduction of clinical electroencephalography helped delineate the symptomatology of temporal lobe epilepsy. Gibbs, Gibbs and Lennox (1937) reported ictal rhythmical 4/sec and 6/sec activity in conjunction with psychomotor seizures (a form which subsequently became generally accepted). The ictal EEG findings of psychomotor attacks proved to be more variable and inconsistent than had been recognized by the first describers; a multitude of ictal patterns were listed by Gastaut and Vigouroux

(1958). Gibbs and Gibbs (1947) as well as Gibbs et al. (1948) stressed the importance of anterior temporal spike or sharp wave foci as the most consistent inter-ictal EEG findings in temporal lobe epilepsy; sleep is often necessary to demonstrate these focal discharges (Gibbs and Gibbs, 1947; Niedermeyer and Rocca, 1972) (Fig. 24, 25).

The pathology and neurophysiology of temporal lobe epilepsy was most extensively studied by Penfield and his co-workers (see Penfield and Jasper, 1954). The term "temporal lobe epilepsy" (Jasper, Pertuiset and Flanigin, 1951) originated from this work; this led into terminological confusion when the new morphological term started to supplant the older descriptive term "psychomotor seizures." Of course, both terms are correct and appropriate from different vantage points (Gastaut, 1953). The elements of the psychomotor seizure were reproduced by electrical stimulation of temporal lobe structures in the waking patient; it was shown that the amygdaloid region was most often involved in automatism-type motor responses or confusional-amnestic states, while hallucinatory experiences were most readily elicted by stimulation of the inferior insular region and its neighborhood. Visceral sensorimotor responses and somatic sensations were equally often triggered from amygdaloid and insular regions (Jasper and Rasmussen, 1956; Jasper, 1958). This work obviously deemphasizes the role of the hippocampus which might function more as a powerful propagator rather than an initiator of epileptic activity, probably as a low threshold area picking up and transmitting nearby or distant seizure discharges. In animal experiments, electrical stimulation of the hippocampus produces strong local and propagated distant responses (Green and Shimamoto, 1953; Green and Adey, 1956; Passouant and Cadilhac, 1961; Walker, 1970).

In human epileptic conditions, Jackson's term of "uncinate epilepsy" corresponds with amygdaloid insular seizure manifestations, which, according to Jasper (1958) may also include the entorhinal area and the hippocampus. On the other hand, hallucinatory experiences are thought to be related chiefly to the lateral temporal neocortex (Jasper, 1958).

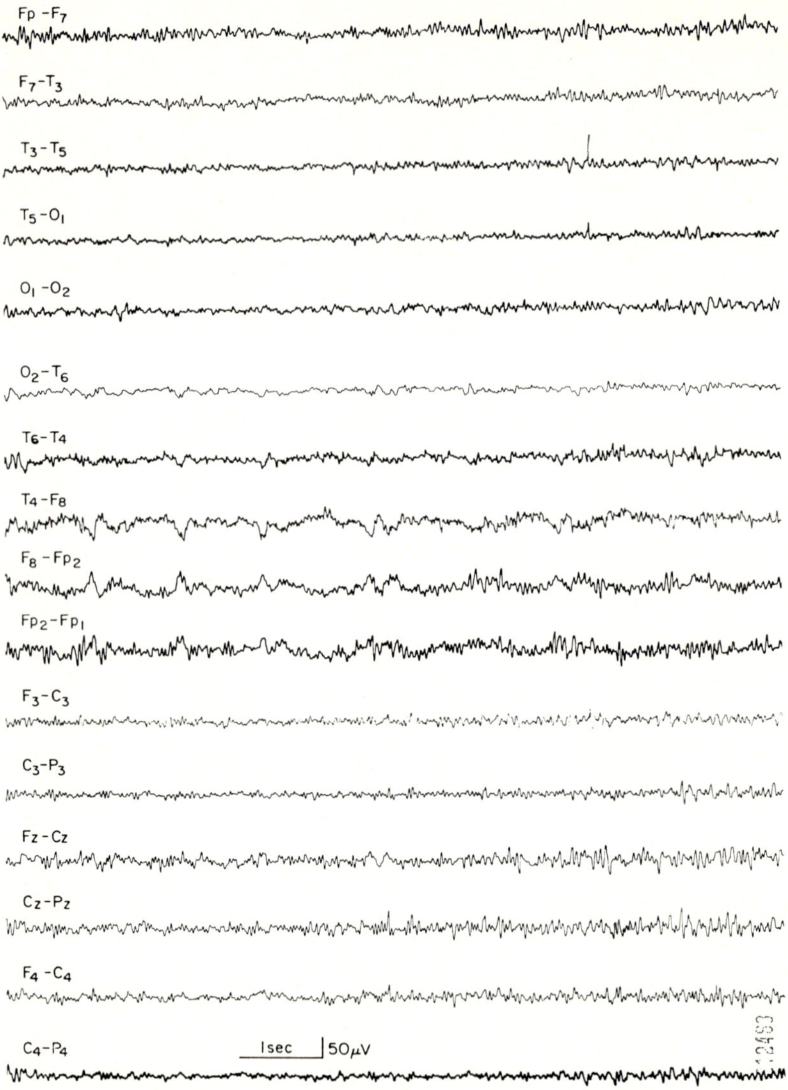

A

FIGURE 24. a) EEG of a 58-year-old male patient with long-standing history of psychomotor seizures. Recurrent sharp waves over right anterior temporal area (electrode F 8, ninth and tenth channel from the top). (Veteran Administration Hospital, Perry Point, Md.; Courtesy of Dr. M. Ereshevich.)

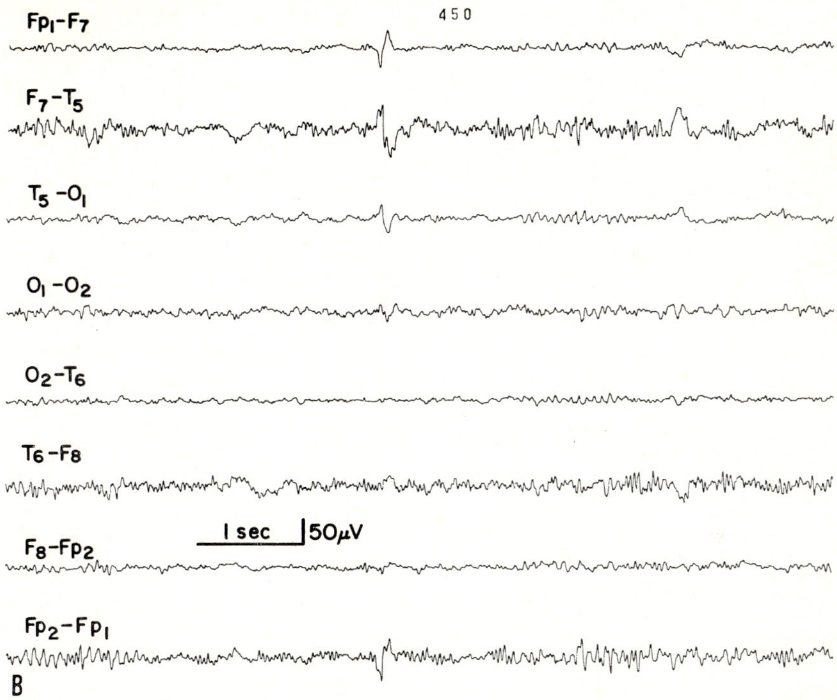

FIGURE 24. b) A left anterior temporal sharp wave focus in the EEG of a 51-year-old woman (#730880) with long standing history of grand mal, psychomotor automatisms as well as chronic schizophrenia with several admissions in a Mental Health State Hospital.

During the past 10 years, the neurophysiological interest in temporal lobe epilepsy seems to have reached a saturation point while psychiatric interest in the psycho cerebral linkages of this condition has steadily gained momentum. Detached from a solid anatomo-physiological basis, misconceptions and unfounded speculations could easily develop. Older theories on the limbic system and emotions (Papez, 1937), limbic system and memory (Kubie, 1953), insights into the Klüver-Bucy syndrome and the bulk of experimental work of MacLean (1955, 1958), Olds (1958) and Delgado (1959), as well as the electrical and biochemical data of Heath and his co-workers (1962) have started an "organic

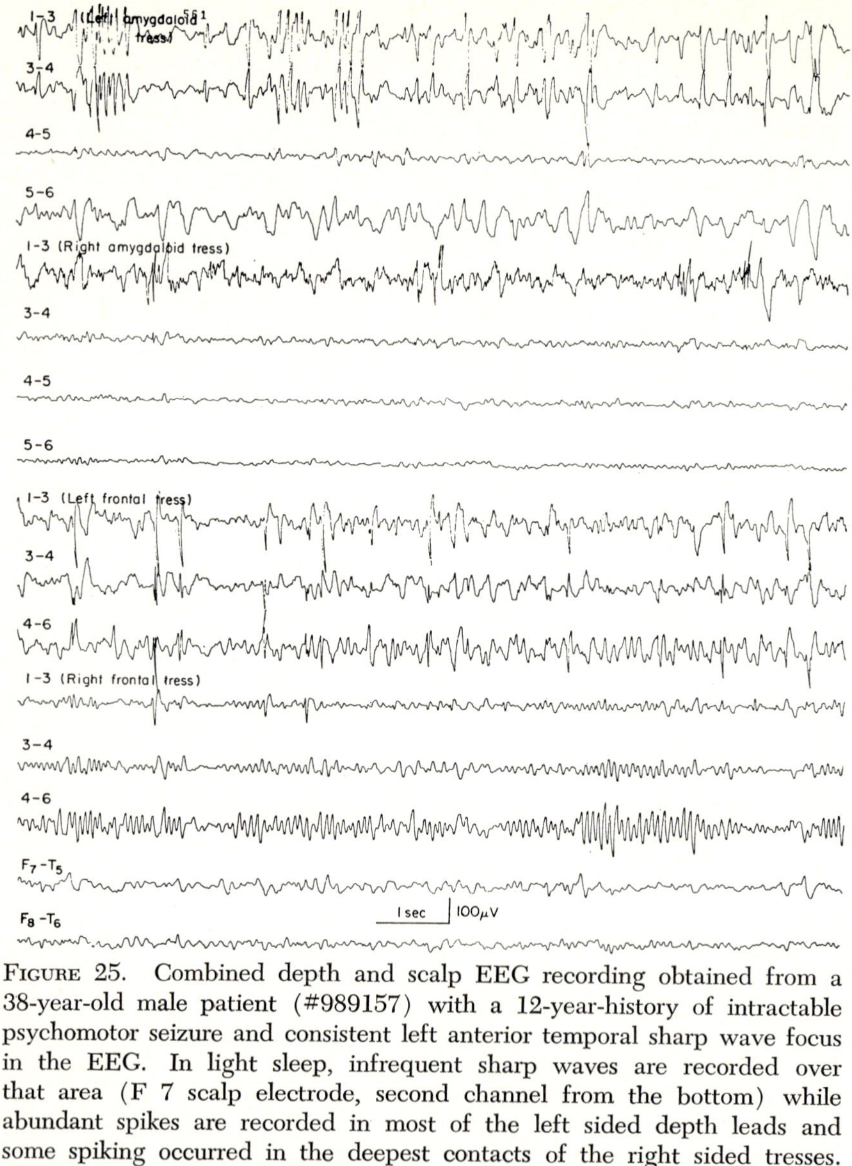

FIGURE 25. Combined depth and scalp EEG recording obtained from a 38-year-old male patient (#989157) with a 12-year-history of intractable psychomotor seizure and consistent left anterior temporal sharp wave focus in the EEG. In light sleep, infrequent sharp waves are recorded over that area (F 7 scalp electrode, second channel from the bottom) while abundant spikes are recorded in most of the left sided depth leads and some spiking occurred in the deepest contacts of the right sided tresses. This tracing is a typical example of the preponderance of spike activity in deep regions (and the relative paucity of seizure discharges in scalp leads). *Localization of depth leads*: *Left amygdaloid tress*: 1 hippocampal gyrus, 2 hippocampal gyrus (inferior border of Ammon's horn), 3 Ammon's horn, 4-6 amygdala. *Right amygdaloid tress*: 1 hippocampal gyrus, 2 Ammon's horn, 3 mid-amygdala, 4 and 5 putamen, 6 claustrum. *Left frontal tress*: 1 and 2 orbital gyrus, 3-6 frontal white matter. *Right frontal tress*: 1 and 2 orbital gyrus, 3-6 frontal white matter.

backlash" in America's Psychiatry. This may lead to shallow theories of the limbic or epileptic basis of psychotic and neurotic conditions as exemplified by the work of Jonas (1965) on "ictal and subictal neurosis."

Ictal symptomatology. The manifestations of psychomotor seizures may be subdivided as follows (after Magnus, 1954):

a) Psychical symptoms
b) Motor phenomena
c) Autonomic symptoms
d) Sensory symptoms

Psychical Phenomena are experienced in an unimpaired but perhaps somewhat modified or trance like waking state. Some of these phenomena are very clear to the patient but he may have great difficulties in describing to others what he experiences (Magnus, 1954). There are feelings "as if everything stopped" or "as if everything occurred in rhythm" and a sense of extreme loneliness or extreme happiness reaching into cosmic, supernatural or divine dimension. Fear and anxiety are often preponderant. The beautiful case reports of Penfield and Jasper (1954), Williams (1956) and Janz (1969) elucidate the complexities of these sensations. Derealization (everything seems strange) and depersonalization with the feeling of a profound intra-personal change may accompany the attacks.

The past present relationship may be suddenly disturbed when the neuronal circuitry of memory mechanisms is altered by the epileptic discharge. Thus, everything may appear extremely familiar to the patient "as though it always had been this way." This "*déjà vu*" experience is a fairly common ictal symptom. It has to be kept in mind, however, that mild *déjà vu* states are often experienced by healthy intelligent and introspective adolescents or young adults; such presumed "neuronal misfiring" may hence occur on a nonepileptic basis, too. The opposite experience, namely extreme strangeness and lack of familiarity ("jamais vu") is less common in psychomotor attacks.

Complex perceptive phenomena fall into the category of psychical seizure manifestations. Such pseudo hallucinations comprise sudden changes of the perceived size of objects which may appear larger (macropsia) or smaller (micropsia, "Liliputian" illusions) in an "Alice-in-Wonderland" like manner.

Vivid reports of such ictal experiences indicate the lack of post-ictal amnesia which otherwise would erase the psychical content of the seizure. Amnesias, however, do occur in seizures manifesting themselves as a *dreamy state* or *twilight state* with no subsequent recollection of ictal experiences.

Psychical manifestations of psychomotor seizures are usually of short duration, mostly less than one minute and sometimes of flash like character with an abrupt experience lasting less than one second. Most of these attacks remain undetected and escape the attention of bystanders because of the only marginal alteration of the outwardly visible state of consciousness. Only admixture of motor phenomena (which may be present in a sizeable number of cases) will betray the patient's epileptic condition.

In childhood, psychomotor attacks, the ictal picture may be dominated by sudden terrifying experiences. The child may suddenly run to the mother searching for protection. Nocturnal terror may also fall into this category but most cases of pavor nocturnus are seen in neurotic children.

Motor phenomena consists chiefly of *automatisms*. Elementary motor activity plays a secondary role but tonic extension of one arm, adversion of the head and occasional brief unilateral clonic twitching may be present.

Psychomotor automatisms are ictal states characterized by complex motor activities detached from volitional control due to the paroxysmal discharge.

Automatisms may be divided as follows:

a) with purposeless movements
- uncoordinated
- coordinated

b) with purposeful movements
- uncoordinated
- coordinated

It is self evident that uncoordinated/purposeless automatic behavior represents the most primitive type and coordinated-purposeful activity the highest type of a psychomotor automatism.

The maladaptive character of the former is very obvious while the higher type may escape detection because of the relatively high level of adaptation. Postural reflex mechanisms remain preserved even in the lowest types and the patient does not fall to the ground in spite of his ictal clumsiness.

A large portion of ictal automatisms is confined to the oral sphere. Such *oral automatisms* include swallowing, lip licking and smacking, grunting, drooling with hypersalivation, mastication with repetitive chewing movements and tasting tongue movements. Sniffing may be a part of an automatism and staring is very common (in contrast to the true intense staring with occasionally bloodshot eyes, as it may occur in psychomotor automatisms, petit mal absences have been often falsely termed "staring spells"; these patients exhibit a blank or vacant expression). According to Magnus (1954), isolated masticatory movements are often seen in the postictal state while rhythmical mastication and other types of automatisms accompany the ictal EEG discharges.

Another large part of psychomotor automatisms is characterized by *picking and searching hand movements,* by *fumbling with clothes,* unbuttoning and buttoning clothing, either in a random manner or more rhythmically executed in a stereotyped fashion. Stereotyped repetition of movements may occur while the patient is working; the seizure then becomes obvious to onlookers because the patient is doing the same thing over and over again. Such repetitive movements occur in a higher level of automatism since some degree of coordination and purposefulness is a prerequisite.

Laughter or giggling may be a manifestation of a psychomotor automatism but such "*gelastic epilepsy*" (Daly and Muller, 1957) may also occur in association with generalized synchronous seizure discharges. According to Gascon and Lombroso (1971), epileptic laughter may originate in various CNS levels but the subserving neuronal circuits are likely to involve limbic structures.

Psychomotor automatisms usually last from 30 seconds to 5 minutes. Automatic behavior of much longer duration (for hours or even days) is very suspect of a psychogenic ("hysterical") dissociative state during which very complex actions may be carried out. This is the category where we have to list most of those well known and often publicized cases as the truck driver who suddenly found himself hundreds of miles away from the place where his memory became blank. This driver had undoubtedly made no mistakes at the steering wheel; he correctly stopped at stop signs or red lights and never made directional errors. In older and mildly arterioclerotic individuals such prolonged amnestic states ("transient global anmesia"; Fisher and Adams, 1964; Steinmetz and Vroom, 1972) with normal outward behavior could be due to transient vascular insufficiency, probably involving the limbic regions (Brain, 1957; Steinmetz and Vroom, 1972) but these cases are rare.

Aggressive acts may be committed in a psychomotor automatism but crime leading to bodily harm hardly ever materializes in the ictal state since the execution of the assault is slow and clumsy. The patient "swings wildly and misses" (Gibbs and Gibbs, 1964) in those rare events of ictal aggression. Sudden rage may be noticed (beautifully documented by Ervin et al., 1969) but one has to keep in mind that hardly any rage attack with criminal assault is committed during a psychomotor seizure. Prolonged post-ictal confusion following a grand mal attack in a deteriorated chronic (mostly institutionalized) epileptic is indeed associated with a relatively high rate of physical assault and occasional fatal outcome but most of these cases fall into a bygone era of epilepsy management. This will be discussed in greater detail in the chapter dealing with psychiatric changes.

In chronic and deteriorated temporal lobe epileptics, "*running fits*" "epilepsia procursiva" are fairly common whereas this type of automatism is very uncommon in socially functioning patients.

Rather infrequent are cases of *speech automatism* in temporal lobe epilepsy. The uttered fragments of phrases or simple perplexity utterances occur in automatisms arising chiefly from the right (nondominant) temporal region or in patients with bilateral temporal lobe foci (Serafetinides and Falconer, 1963). *Ictal speech arrest* or *paroxysmal dysphasia* are due to left sided epileptogenic foci; these cases belong into the category of focal seizures rather than into the more complex set of psychomotor epileptic manifestations.

Autonomic symptoms are frequent concomitant of automatisms; others are more likely to represent an aura-like prelude of a grand mal convulsion due to a primary temporal lobe focus. Such patients may describe an aura of epigastric sensations, either rising or stationary. Hypermotility of the intestinal tract may occur on an ictal or postictal basis. Van Buren's (1963) study of the abdominal aura indicates that abdominal pain is a rather infrequent and short-lasting ictal phenomenon in temporal lobe epilepsy. This is important in view of the overused term of "*abdominal epilepsy*" (Moore, 1945) which label has been inappropriately attached to numerous children and adolescents with attacks of abdominal pain, lasting usually a few hours and, probably in the majority, representing migrainous equivalents.

Other autonomic symptoms include flushing, pallor, cyanosis, brief and innocuous apnea, hyperpnea, dyspnea, goose flesh, sweating and change of the heart rate. These symptoms may constitute isolated seizures but, in general, accompany psychomotor attacks or precede a grand mal seizure.

Sensory symptoms are not readily distinguished from the above mentioned psychical phenomena. Ictal perceptive disturbances comprise all sorts of hallucinations and illusions. The patient is almost always aware of their unreal nature; for this reason, the misperceptions are pseudo hallucinations and illusions.

Best known are *olfactory ictal perceptions* which usually consist of a bad rather than a pleasant odor. Patients with olfactory aura need a particularly careful diagnostic workup since brain tumors are very often the cause of the attacks (more often than in other manifestations of temporal lobe epilepsy). Visual, auditory, gustatory and vestibular sensations are also encountered. The more complex the sensations are (when sceneries are seen instead of elementary visual phenomena) the more likely is the involvement of temporal neuronal networks.

The *epileptic personality* has proved to be one of the most controversial matters of epileptology and will be discussed with the psychiatric aspects of temporal lobe epilepsy in Chapter 11.

The symptomatology of the interval between the seizures may be determined by the basic etiological brain disorder such as a tumor of the temporal lobe which will eventually lead to intracranial hypertension and neurological deficits in addition of the seizures. These cases are omitted from the presentation of inter-ictal signs and symptoms occurring in a residual type of temporal lobe epilepsy (Chapter 11).

ETIOLOGICAL CONSIDERATIONS. NEUROPATHOLOGY. Temporal lobe epilepsy, like all epileptic conditions, is due to a variety of causes. Most frequently encountered are residual epileptogenic foci due to lesions acquired early in life. Perinatal brain damage has been thought to give rise to incisural sclerosis as a consequence of hippocampic herniation ("incisural herniation," Earle, Baldwin and Penfield, 1953). This mechanism, however, does not materialize as frequently as Earle and his co-workers believed (Veith, 1959; Peiffer, 1963).

Most of the residual lesions remain unexplained when the involved area is examined following temporal lobectomy.

Gliosis, mesio-temporal or pararhinal sclerosis are the most common pathological findings. Among the variety of etiologies, repeated, bouts of severe otitis media might have been a rather common cause (Gastaut and Gastaut, 1951) but better control of this condition by means of antibiotics has reduced the incidence of such cerebral complications.

Among acquired lesions of adult life, *intracranial tumors* deserve special attention. Oligodendrogliomas, astrocytomas of all grades and glioblastoma multiforme of the temporal lobe may be the cause. Some low grade astrocytomas may be of very small size and escape detection by neuroradiological studies for many years. The meningeomas of the lateral sphenoid wing may give rise to psychomotor seizures before any neurological deficit or any sign of intracranial hypertension becomes manifest. Large supradiaphragmatic portions of intrasellar tumors and craniopharyngeomas may affect the temporal lobe and give rise to seizures. It must be stressed again that an olfactory type of ictal sensation is particularly likely to be due to neoplastic etiology.

When psychomotor seizures occur in older adults, *cerebrovascular disorder* is the most likely cause. Vascular temporal lobe foci are often limited to the spike activity in the EEG; those with clinical seizures comprise a smaller segment in which grand mal is more common than psychomotor attacks. This will be further elucidated in the discussion of the course of temporal lobe epilepsy (see also Chapter 3 where the variety of etiologies is discussed).

Diagnosis. In the past few years, temporal lobe epilepsy has become an "overdiagnosed" epileptic condition, especially in this country. It seems that the basis for the diagnosis has been overextended. Convincing evidence of classical psychomotor seizures and an anterior temporal spike or sharp wave focus in the interictal EEG tracing provide solid ground for the epileptological diagnosis which, in most cases, has to be followed-up by an etiological diagnostic investigation. The use of diagnostic procedures in epilepsy will be the topic of Chapter 9.

Why have diagnostic presumptions of temporal lobe epilepsy grown so badly out of proportion? The answer lies in the rich ictal semeiology of psychmotor seizures which has struck the fancy of many physicians and especially of numerous psychiatrists. From the occurrence of transcendental experiences in psychomotor attacks, inferences on the experiences of founders of religions have lightheartedly been made. Religious revelations or ecstasies have been equated with temporal lobe epilepsy. All sorts of psychotic and especially schizophrenic hallucinations or delusions have been indiscriminately regarded as manifestations of temporal lobe epilepsy when only a trace of a recurrent attack-like element was found. While psychomotor automatisms may occasionally lead to acts of overt aggression (a very rare event and very unlikely after Rodin, 1972), why not regard all or most of the criminal assaults an ictal discharge of the temporal lobe or its limbic portion? If the scalp EEG remains stubbornly normal, a case of "larval" or "masked" temporal lobe epilepsy with presumed deep seizure discharges is readily construed. The experienced epileptologist has to resist such trends of scientific fashions which, incidentally, have been oddly thriving in courtroom expertises.

The electroencephalographer can easily contribute to the diagnostic mistake. Over the anterior temporal and mid-temporal region, stretches of local slow and moderately sharp activity develop in a large percentage of adults past the age of 50 years

(Fig. 26); a vast majority of these individuals are seizure-free or have minor multiple complaints (failing memory, some dizziness or lightheadedness etc.). This pattern is well known (Strauss et al., 1952; Obrist, 1954; Busse et al., 1956; Kooi et al., 1964) and is likely to denote mild limbic involvement (ischemic Ammon's horn sclerosis). When syncopal attacks and spells of vertigo or acute dizziness occur in such individuals, the presence of some degree of sharp activity in the temporal region may mislead the electroencephalographer to the assumption of a temporal epileptic event. To make matters worse, the epileptic nature of the reported attacks cannot be ruled out either; but this possibility is very small and chances are overwhelming that the patient will benefit from vascular rather than from anticonvulsive treatment. Even indubitable spikes or sharp waves may develop in such cerebrovascular disturbances but their epileptogenicity remains limited. All this must be said to point out the difficulties encountered in the interpretation of these middle-to-old age EEG deviations.

A further diagnostic trap is the mid-temporal spike discharge of childhood which must not be considered as suggestive of temporal lobe epilepsy since the epileptogenicity of this pattern is limited (50 to 70%) and only a few children will later develop temporal lobe epilepsy.

COURSE. THE SIGNIFICANCE OF AGE-DETERMINED FACTORS IN TEMPORAL LOBE EPILEPSY. The very first ictal manifestations of temporal lobe epilepsy in early childhood are often shrouded by enigmatic or equivocal behavioral changes which defy any precise analysis. Elements of automatism are readily misinterpreted at this age; stereo-typed repetition of motor actions, smacking, swallowing, sniffing or grunting may easily escape the attention of the parents. On the other hand, such attacks may be correctly diagnosed as psychomotor seizures but ictal EEG changes may be completely absent as demonstrated on Figure 27. There is good reason to presume that, in childhood, psychomotor attacks may be associated with amygdaloid-hippocampic spiking only.

There is no doubt, however, that psychomotor attacks or temporal lobe epilepsy play a much less important role in child-

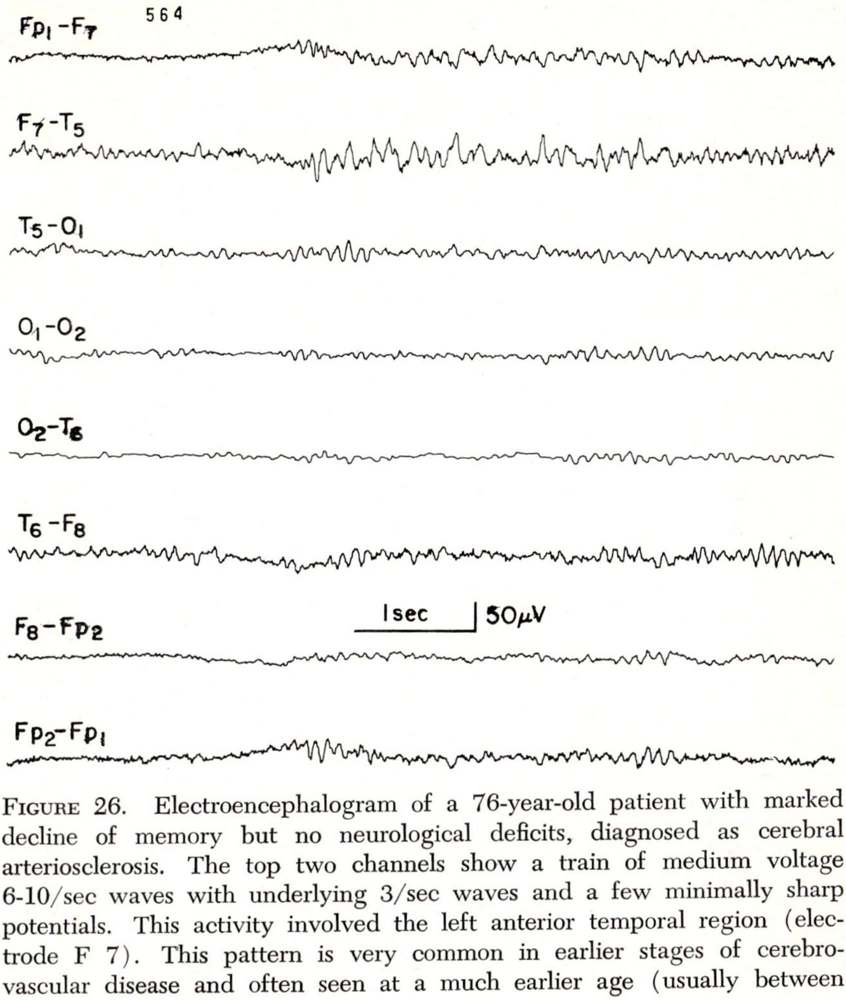

FIGURE 26. Electroencephalogram of a 76-year-old patient with marked decline of memory but no neurological deficits, diagnosed as cerebral arteriosclerosis. The top two channels show a train of medium voltage 6-10/sec waves with underlying 3/sec waves and a few minimally sharp potentials. This activity involved the left anterior temporal region (electrode F 7). This pattern is very common in earlier stages of cerebrovascular disease and often seen at a much earlier age (usually between age 45 and 65 years).

hood than in adult life. The gradually increasing segment of temporal lobe epilepsy with advancing age is paralleled by a gradual "maturation" of the classical inter-ictal anterior temporal EEG abnormalities (Gastaut and Roger, 1955; Gibbs, 1958). Misleading EEG findings are very common in children with temporal lobe epilepsy; diffuse spikes, generalized spike wave bursts, local spikes in other regions (occipital, central), mid-

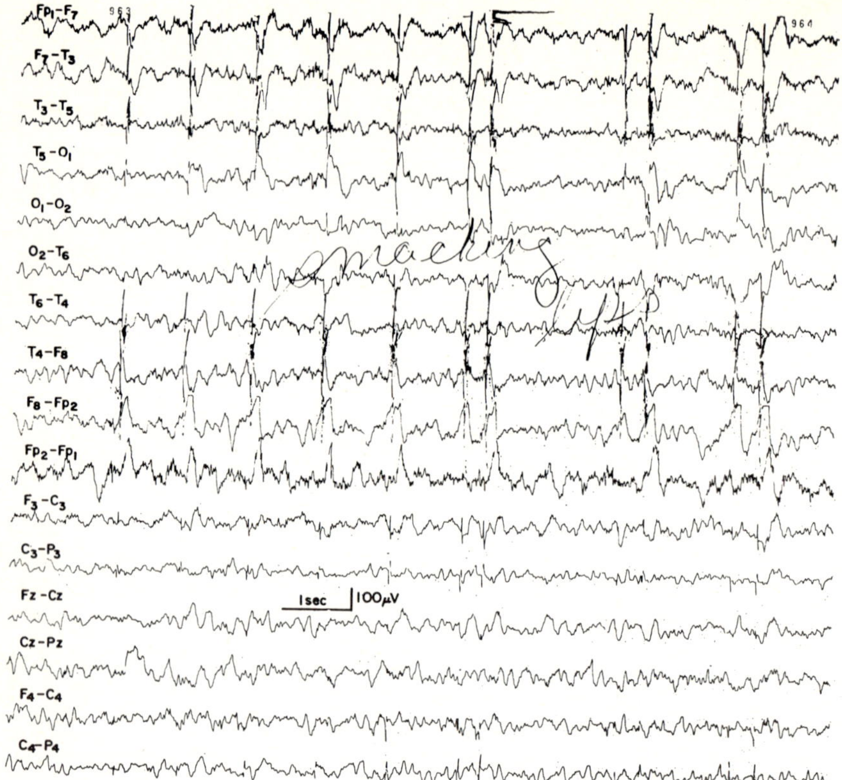

FIGURE 27. EEG of a 4-year-old girl (#1467192) with frequently recurrent attacks of automatic behavior with lip smacking. One of these attacks is recorded in this tracing. All of the large spiky discharges represent muscular artifacts caused by the oral movements; there are no corresponding seizure discharges or frequency changes during the attacks (occasionally, a few inter-ictal left central sharp potentials were noticed). Psychomotor seizures of early childhood may be associated with very atypical or misleading EEG findings. It is presumed that the electrical discharges of these seizures are limited to deep limbic structures.

temporal spikes (only seldom evolving into anterior temporal spikes) and some rather marginal findings may be seen. The increasing incidence of anterior temporal spike or sharp wave foci is beautifully demonstrated in Gibbs' and Gibbs' (1964) synopsis of almost 20,000 cases with paroxysmal EEG changes related to age; the anterior temporal spike focus forms a Gothic steeple standing upside-down on its thin elongated tip (denoting near-absence of this discharge in infancy), gradually widening during adolescence and adulthood with a broad basis in the old age range.

When psychomotor seizures occur in combination with more than one other type of seizure during childhood, chances are high that this case belongs into the category of the Lennox-Gastraut syndrome. During the course of the Lennox-Gastaut syndrome, temporal lobe seizure characteristics tend to become more evident during the third decade of life and, eventually, the patient may lose all the other ictal and electrical characteristics of the Lennox-Gastaut syndrome and will be considered a mentally defective chronic temporal lobe epileptic, usually institutionalized.

This phenomenon of "*secondary temporalization*" was discussed before; it does not pertain to the Lennox-Gastaut syndrome alone and is occasionally seen in cases of Common generalized epilepsy, too. In other words, traits of temporal lobe epilepsy tend to overshadow the other elements of a mixed epileptic condition as age advances. This is even true for some of the psychological and psychiatric personality characteristics of temporal lobe epilepsy which will give some mixed forms a "temporal lobish" flavor (Fig. 28).

While anterior temporal lobe spike and sharp wave activity reaches its highest incidence in old age, psychomotor seizures become less common in the elderly and the overall epileptogenicity of the anterior temporal spike focus falls sharply in aged individuals (mainly arteriosclerotics). We have therefore the paradoxical situation of

a) children with temporal lobe epilepsy (psychomotor seizures) without the typical EEG finding of an anterior temporal focus, and
b) aged individuals with prominent anterior temporal spikes or sharp waves and no clinical evidence of temporal lobe epilepsy (or even no clinical epilepsy whatsoever).

This discrepancy is often encountered.

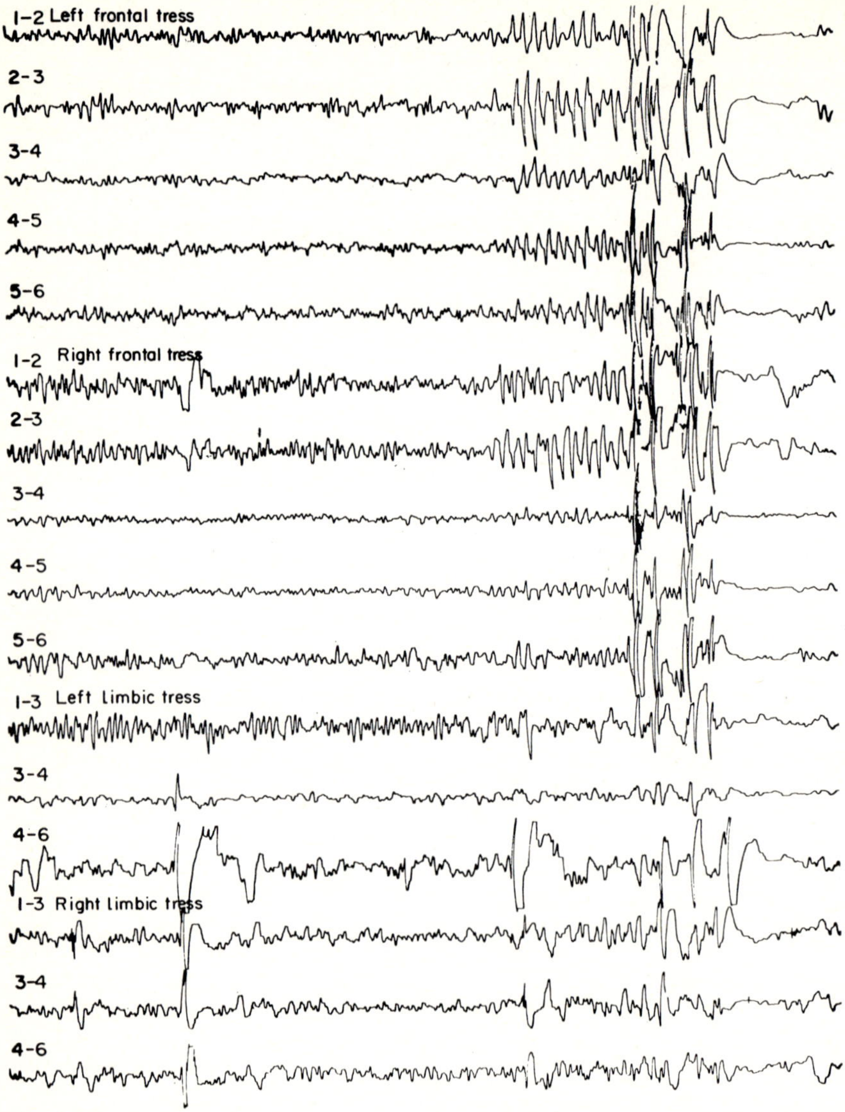

FIGURE 28. Combined scalp and depth EEG recording in a 27-year-old man (#1023687) with Lennox-Gastaut syndrome and seizures (grand mal, adversive, atonic-akinetic) since age of 9 years. During sleep, a burst of bilateral-synchronous rapid spikes is noted in both frontal tresses. There is marked independent spiking in limbic areas and especially in the left Ammon's formation. The independent limbic spike activity is likely to

These incongruencies intimate the *difficulties in the assessment of the incidence of temporal lobe epilepsy.* Among childhood epilepsies, temporal lobe epilepsy (with psychomotor seizures) probably occupies a segment of 1 to 2 percent and certainly less than 5 percent; in adult life, this segment will increase to 5 to 15 percent.

As to the *prognosis,* temporal lobe epilepsy is, in general, a serious type of seizure disorder which may defy anticonvulsive therapy. There are, however, relatively mild cases, too, with good responses to the usual type of anticonvulsants. It is self-evident that these prognostic considerations do not apply to cases of temporal lobe tumors with psychomotor attacks and obvious need for surgical therapy.

THERAPY. Milder cases only respond satisfactorily to appropriate dosages (see Chapter 12) of *diphenylhydantoin* and *primidone,* often used in combination. Primidone, generally known as Mysoline®, is believed to have a specific effect against psychomotor seizures; its combination with phenobarbital is not recommended for pharmacological reasons.

A specific effect against psychomotor attacks has also been ascribed to *methsuximide* (Celontin®) and, during the past decade, to *sulthiame* (Ospolot®, Conadil®) and *carbamazepine* (Tegretol®). Sulthiame is not commercially available in the United States whereas carbamazepine has been, thus far, registered in this country for the sole use in trigeminal neuralgia (tic douloureux) while its effectiveness as an anticonvulsant is still under investigation. This drug prompted very favorable reports from European investigators. Local experiences of

---

reflect the mechanism of secondary temporalization. *Localization of depth leads*: *Left frontal tress*: 1 and 2 gyrus rectus, 3 caudate nucleus, 4 internal capsule, 5 head of the caudate nucleus, 6 white matter. *Right frontal tress*: 1 suprachiasmatic cistern, 2 gyrus rectus, 3 stria terminalis (transition from putamen to caudate nucleus), 4-6 caudate nucleus. *Left limbic tress*: 1 and 2 inferior temporal cortex, 3 inferior amygdala, 4 and 5 inferior hippocampus, 6 posterior Ammon's formation. *Right limbic tress*: 1 inferior temporal cortex, 2 white matter, 3 anterior border of amygdala, 4 inferior posterior amygdala, 5 inferior hippocampus, 6 posterior hippocampus.

Livingston (1972) are encouraging but not overly enthusiastic in view of various side effects (see Chapter 12).

Perhaps the most potent and specific drug for the treatment of psychomotor epilepsy has been *phenacemide* (Phenurone®) but its use has proved to be very hazardous (see Chapter 12) and ought to be restricted to ultimate attempts in desperate cases under most careful supervision.

Surgical therapy has been used in temporal lobe epilepsy more often than in other forms of regional epilepsies. This treatment will be the topic of Chapter 13.

The management of inter ictal personality changes constitutes a major problem. Major tranquilizers of the phenothiazine-group have been used with moderate to good results. More recently, the hormonal therapy (medroxy-progesterone acetate, Provera®) has been recommended by Blumer (1972).

3) *Focal-cortical epilepsies other than temporal*

a) FRONTAL LOBE EPILEPSY. Seizures arising from the convexity of the frontal lobe have a strong tendency to become generalized; prior to the grand mal attack, an aura-like initiating focal phase is often present and helpful in the determination of the local aspect. Epileptogenic frontal lobe foci are much less common than temporal lobe foci (Fegersten and Roger, 1961); craniocerebral laceration might be the most frequent cause.

The work of Penfield and Kristiansen (1951) as well as Penfield and Jasper (1954) has shed more light on the focal seizure patterns of certain frontal regions. The most important seizure types are:

Adversive seizures (turning eyes, head and body, usually to the opposite side)

- *With unconsciousness*: convexity of frontal lobe, chiefly in vicinity of the frontal pole, in middle and superior frontal gyrus, not involving the fronto-orbital region.
- *In a conscious state*: posterior portion of the frontal lobe convexity, neighborhood of the precentral gyrus.

Immediate grand mal with no focal initiation whatsoever, a common event in epilepsies involving the convexity of the frontal lobe.

Autonomic-visceral sensations, usually ascribed to the temporal lobe limbic portion and the insular region, may also occur in frontal lobe limbic (Penfield and Kristiansen, 1951). There is reason to presume that these attacks are due to strong firing into limbic structures. General *bodily sensations* and a *rising epigastric aura* are notable in this regard.

Aphasic and dysphasic seizures as well as *ictal vocalization* may ictally arise from Broca's area (aphasic arrest) or from upper frontal regions neighboring the supplementary motor area.

Ictal thought disturbances and especially *forced thinking,* usually regarded as a temporal lobe phenomenon, may also originate from the convexity of the frontal lobe.

These types of seizures are generally considered representative of frontal lobe epilepsy but this picture, as outlined by the Montreal School, needs some supplementation since the mesial-frontal seizure manifestations due to epileptogenic lesions located within the hemispheric fissure are not included. Most recently, Tharp (1972) has attempted to single out another special type of frontal lobe epilepsy "Orbital frontal seizures" in children.

MESIOFRONTAL EPILEPSY. This term (Niedermeyer and A. E. Walker, 1971) comprises seizures originating from the frontal portion of the interhemispheric fissure and particularly from the supplementary motor region. This type of seizure disorder is not common but deserves special attention for various reasons. It has been frequently neglected or omitted in textbook like presentations of the epilepsies although it presents a difficult problem of diagnosis and therapy.

Mesiofrontal epilepsy is characterized by *tonic seizures* involving predominantly the contralateral limbs and especially the arm which is raised, held stiff in the air with moderate flexion in the elbow joint. Clawing of the hand may also occur. In some cases, both sides are involved. Intense flushing of the face may be noticed. The attacks last about 20 to 40 seconds and end as abruptly as they started; one can hardly detect any clonic component. The patient may fall to the ground but this is due to a gradually developing opisthotonus which shifts the center of gravity in a posterior direction; this is markedly different from the initial fall in a grand mal. Consciousness is profoundly disturbed during the attack but the patient is surprisingly well oriented after the seizure has ended. There is no aura and no warning. The attacks may occur at a rate of 3 to 10/day with a crippling effect on the patient's social life; in some patients, more attacks occur at night during sleep than at daytime. Some patients had grand mal attacks earlier in life but, in the further course, the tonic seizures dominate the picture almost exclusively (Fig. 29).

Mesiofrontal epilepsy is most developed in younger and middle-aged adults. In children and adolescents, this type of seizure disorder is very uncommon but, if it exists, *the tonic attacks may be startle induced.* Sudden unexpected noise is a very effective precipitator.

The literature is very scanty in this area. Foerster and Penfield (1930) reported a posttraumatic case of epilepsy involving the supplementary motor area; the beautiful pictorial documentation of this case has also been presented in the work of Penfield and Jasper (1954). Ajmone Marsan and Ralston (1957) have emphasized a type of seizure attributable to the supplementary motor region; these attacks are characterized by abduction and external rotation of the shoulder and flexion of the shoulder without head turning.

The startle mechanism in association with tonic attacks has been studied by Alajouanine and Gastaut (1958). There is now good evidence that these startle attacks emanate from the supplementary motor area within the mesial portion of the frontal lobe (Bancaud et al., 1967). Most of the patients with startle-induction have a residual hemiparesis (hemiparetic type of cerebral palsy). The underlying pathology in adults with mesiofrontal epilepsy is mainly residual.

The *diagnosis of mesiofrontal epilepsy is particularly difficult due to the frequent absence of EEG abnormalities.* Minute and inconsistent spikes may occasionally occur near the frontal midline; even the ictal EEG may be completely uninformative. Depth EEG studies may also miss the discharge unless a tress of electrodes is inserted into the mesio-frontal region (Fig. 30).

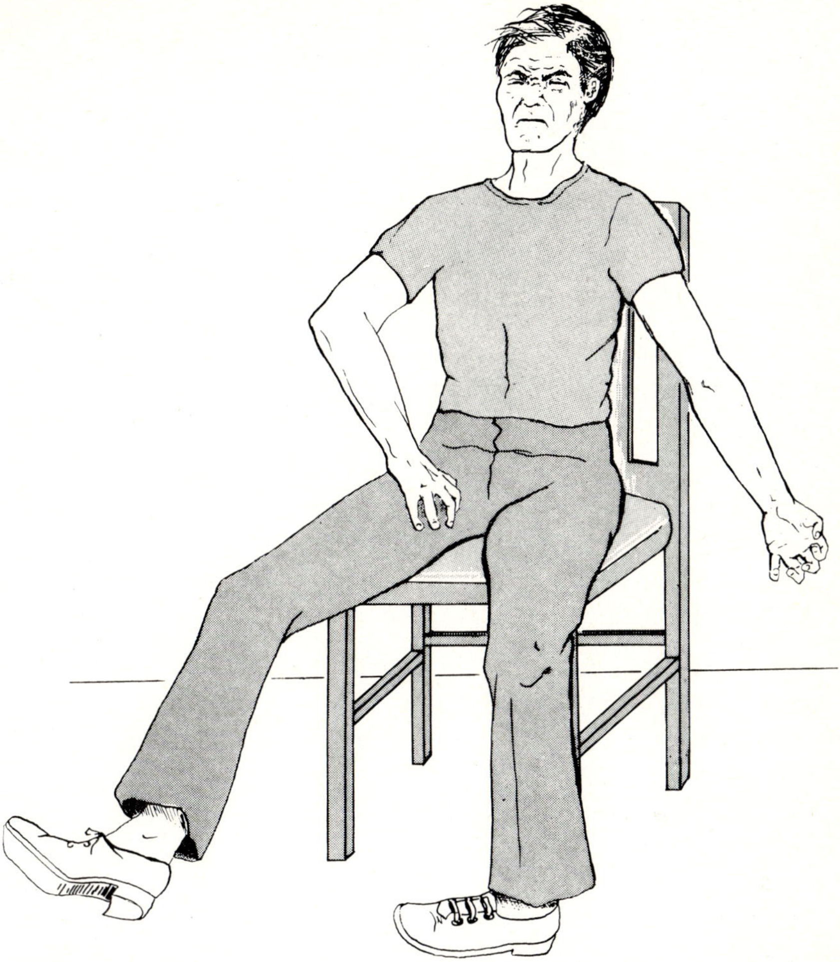

FIGURE 29. Artist's drawing of a tonic seizure occurring in a 48-year-old patient with mesio-frontal epilepsy (#493055) (after the observing physician's sketch). In spite of extreme general tonic rigidity and some retroflexion of the body, the patient did not fall off his chair. The purely tonic attack lasted about one minute; the severely impaired function of consciousness was almost instantly restored after termination of the attack which lasted 50 seconds. (The localization of the focus was confirmed by depth recordings.)

This indicates that there is little or no propagation of the focal inter-ictal discharge.

Cingulate epilepsy encompasses seizures arising from the

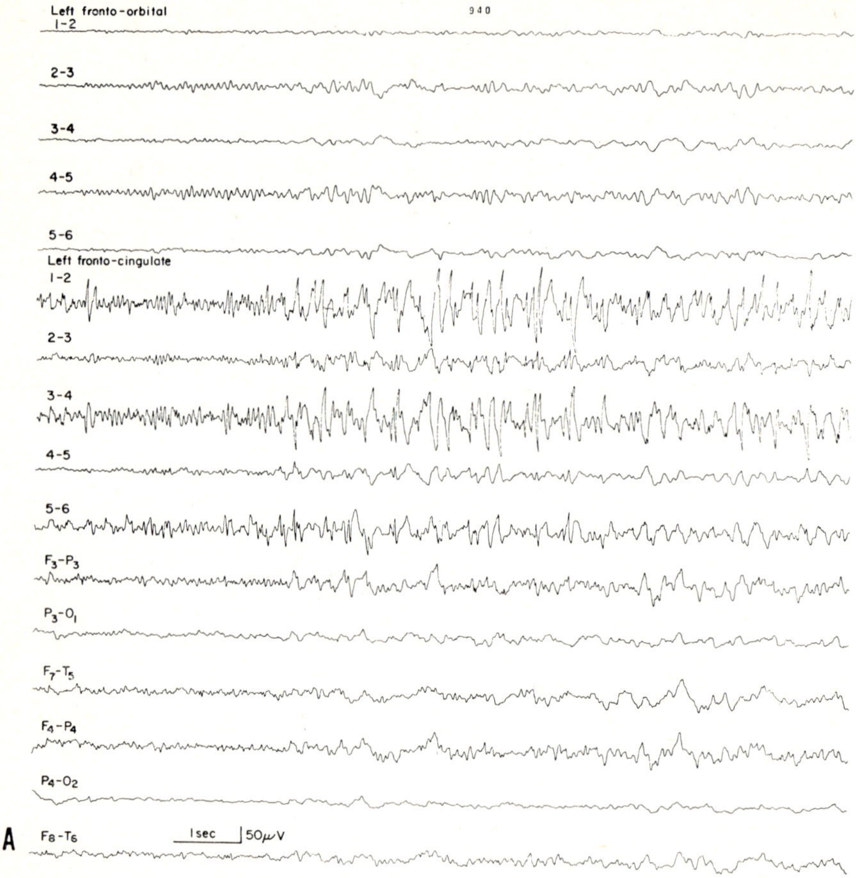

FIGURE 30. a) Combined scalp and depth recording in a 39-year-old female patient with intractable tonic seizures. Mesio-frontal epilepsy). She had scanty and very small left upper frontal spikes in her scalp EEG. Note normal sleep activity with spindles and K complexes in scalp leads and in all contacts of the left fronto-orbital tress whereas almost constantly recurring stretches of repetitive spikes are seen in the fronto-cingulate tress (located slightly above the cingulate gyrus in the lower portion of the supplementary motor area deep in the interhemispheric fissure).

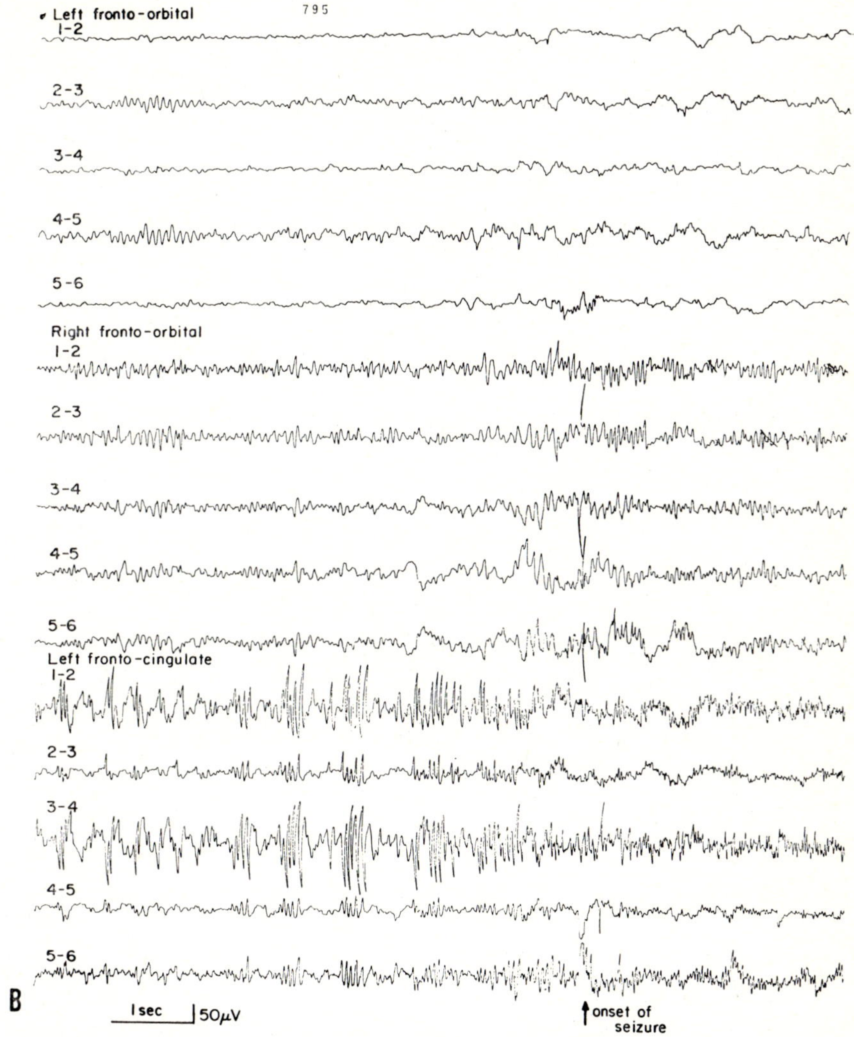

FIGURE 30. b) Onset of a clinical tonic seizure characterized by extension of right (sometimes both) arm and clawing of hand. Rapid spiking in the fronto-cingulate tress is immediately attenuated ("desynchronized") in conjunction with increasing firing rate. Note the almost total lack of participation of the regions explored by the fronto-orbital tresses.

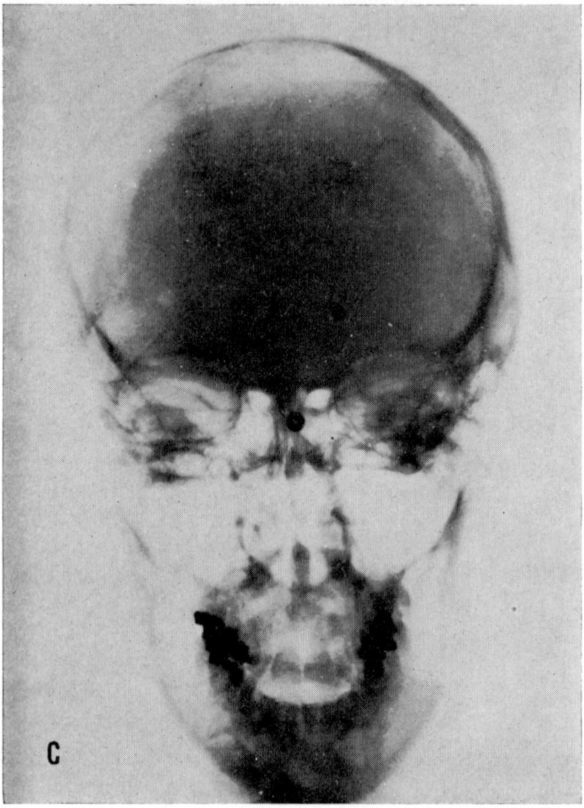

cingulate gyrus and especially from its frontal portion. This poorly understood type of seizure disorder seems to combine elements of mesio-frontal epilepsy (tonic seizures) with petit mal absence like manifestations. Electrically, generalized spike-waves or spike wave like activity has been reported by G. Mazars (1969). Thus, the cingulate gyrus might give rise to considerable spread and even to secondary bilateral synchrony in stark contrast to the spreadless hidden focal seizure discharges of mesio-frontal epilepsy.

This rather lengthy discussion of mesiofrontal epilepsy has been prompted by a vacuum in the literature and the difficulties of diagnostic documentation. The discussion of tonic seizures in Chapter 2 includes a brief review of the differential diagnosis.

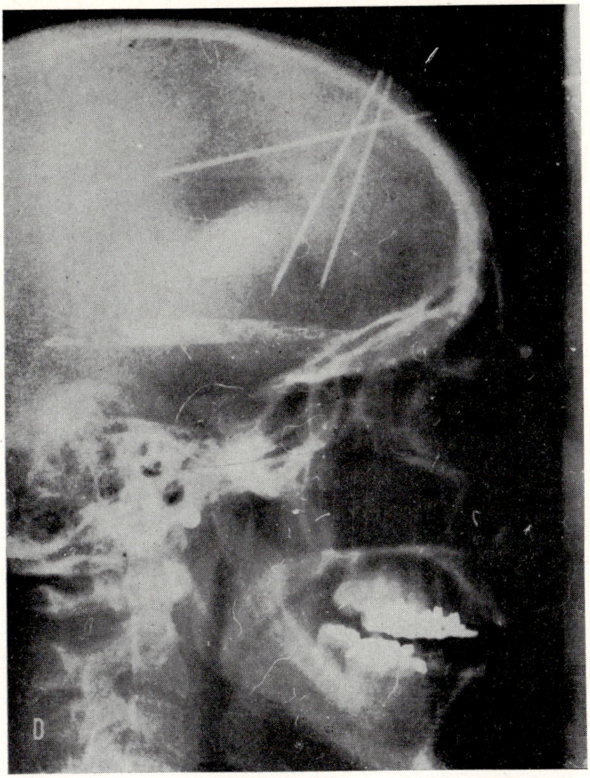

FIGURE 30. c & d) Radiological demonstration of the position of the depth electrodes.

THERAPY. Frontal lobe epilepsy in general will respond fairly well to the combination of diphenylhydantoin and phenobarbital; refractory cases are unlikely to respond to other anticonvulsants and may require neurosurgical treatment. Needless to say, frontal lobe tumors are likely to give rise to seizures; initial grand mal is very common (Hess, 1970) and, according to Janz (1960), grand mal status epilepticus is more often seen in frontal than in other hemispheric lesions.

Mesiofrontal epilepsy represents a therapeutic problem of major proportions and may defy all types on anticonvulsive medication, even in sub-toxic dosages. The long-term effectiveness of neurosurgical removal of the lesion (partial frontal lobectomy) is not well known.

b) FOCAL-MOTOR (ROLANDIC, JACKSONIAN) SEIZURES Clonic twitching of the contralateral extremities (as well as facial and trunkal muscles) is the typical seizure manifestation of a localized discharge within the precentral gyrus. In contrast to frontal and especially mesiofrontal seizures, tonic elements are almost completely overshadowed by the clonic nature of the motor activity.

In accordance with the somato-topic arrangement within the precentral gyrus, the clonic movements are initially limited to one area of the body and tend to spread during the course of the focal-motor attack. Twitching of the left facial muscles and left lingual and pharyngeal muscles may gradually extend to involve the left fingers, hand, elbow and shoulder. It may spread to the left abdominal muscles (which could be by-passed) and eventually to the left lower extremity. In the course of such a *Jacksonian march*, consciousness is almost always preserved. At any stage of the focal motor attack, sudden generalization may supervene and a full blown grand mal will be the pinnacle of this development.

A well-defined local onset of the attack, such as initial left facial twitching, does not necessarily mean that the irritative lesion is located exactly within the facial segment of the precentral gyrus. The threshold for motor responses may differ from area to area (Gelhorn, 1953) and the region of lowest threshold may usher in the clinical attack while the epileptogenic impulses stem from an adjacent lesion. In rare instances, even deep seated lesions are capable of generating focal motor attacks; repeated attacks of contralateral twitching of the masticatory muscles as well as the muscles of the floor of the mouth was reported following a vascular thalamic lesion (Niedermeyer, 1957). In stereotaxic stimulation of the ventral posteromedical nucleus of the thalamus in the human, similar contralateral clonic movements of masticatory, labial and lingual muscles were elicited by Talairach et al. (1949) and Monnier (1955); this could provide an experimental basis for rare cases of "diencephalic Jacksonian epilepsy."

After termination of a focal-motor seizure, there is some

degree of transient weakness in the involved musculature; in children, postictal weakness may reach much greater proportions including *complete postictal hemiplegia* (*Todd's paralysis*). One should note, however, that young children are most prone to have more pronounced *hemiconvulsions* with lesser or greater impairment of consciousness. According to Gastaut et al. (1962), the focal-motor cortex is not primarily involved in the hemiconvulsive attacks of early childhood.

A completely stationary and circumscript type of focal-motor epilepsy has been classically described as a sequel of the Siberian spring-summer-encephalitis with constantly repetitive clonic activity of a limited muscular segment. This type of activity may be sustained for months and years; it is termed *epilepsia partialis continua.* Following the first report of Koshevnikov (1895), Russian authors have frequently discussed the role of the cortical and subcortical levels in the physiopathogenesis of this status like focal motor activity. Such prolonged focal seizure states are very seldom seen outside Siberia with etiologies other than the spring-summer encephalitis. There is reason to presume that one type of epilepsia partialis continua is associated with a completely normal ictal EEG (Niedermeyer, 1954) while other cases occur in conjunction with chronically repetitive spiking over the contralateral motor region (Kugelberg and Widén, 1954). Kristiansen et al. (1971) stressed the subcortical origin of the continuous seizure activity which persisted during temporary blocking of cortical function by craniocerebral cooling (to 15° C) through an extracorporeal carotid shunt.

Among the *causes of focal motor epilepsy,* the possibility of an intracranial tumor must be ruled out with greatest care especially when the seizures start in adulthood. *Parasagittal meningiomas* deserve particular attention in this regard. In these cases, the skull x-ray often shows suspicious bony and vascular changes; the brain scan will confirm the diagnosis with great reliability. It is interesting to note that, in parasagittal meningeomas, the EEG findings are often marginal. The Rolandic area is a difficult place for the EEG diagnosis of local pathology; even the recording of a focal-motor seizure may lack the expected focal spike activity since the epileptic discharge may remain extremely limited. Artifactual muscular overlay is another problem of these ictal tracings.

Among further causes, *arteriovenous malformations* of the centro-parietal regions play a significant role. The first seizures usually occur in adolescence or early adulthood. *Cerebral arteriosclerosis* and *neurosyphilis* deserve special mention among the multitude of possible causes; in tropical countries, parasites must be seriously considered. Traumatic laceration of the Rolandic area may also give rise to a focal motor type of *posttraumatic epilepsy*.

The *factor of age* was mentioned above in connection with the hemiconvulsions of early childhood; these seizures are characterized by impairment of consciousness and a rather mixed pattern of unilateral tonic and clonic motions. Later in childhood, true focal motor seizures with typical clonic movements may occur often limited to the face ("Sylvian seizures"; Lombroso, 1967). These children show midtemporal and central spike discharges in the interval. The vast majority of focal motor seizures occur in adult life.

The *therapy* poses no special problem as far as residual lesions are concerned; both diphenylhydantoin and phenobarbital are effective and often lead to complete seizure freedom. These drugs are of little use, however, in epilepsia partialis continua which, by virtue of its status like nature, is more likely to respond to i.v. diazepam (Valium®)—though only for a limited period of time. The search for a surgically treatable epileptogenic lesion cannot be overstressed.

c) Focal sensory. Parietal lobe epilepsy Paroxysmal *paresthesias of the contralateral half of the body* are the typical seizure manifestation of the *postcentral gyrus*. The paresthesias include a variety of sensations from "pins-and-needles" to "crawling ants." Ictal pain is very unusual but may occur in rare cases. A Jacksonian march like pattern of the attack may materialize.

These seizures represent the sensory counterpart to the above discussed focal-motor seizures; the difficulties of electroencephalographic demonstration are similar and even the etiologies are about the same. In general, however, focal sensory seizures are not as common as focal motor attacks. There are also greater difficulties in the differential diagnosis since there is a variety of peripheral types of recurrent abnormal sensations, especially brachial dysesthesias in association with cervical spyondylosis. Even the referred type of abnormal sensations in the left arm (ulnar portion) occurring in coronary ischemias may mislead the physician.

The *rest of the parietal lobe* does not play a major role in the generation of typical focal seizure patterns. General bodily sensations, brief ("tornado like") episodes of violent vertigo, and occasional epigastric sensations may occur. One of our patients with a well delineated focus close to the inter-hemispheric fissure had attacks of visual illusions (suggestive of oscillopsia) tinnitus and a state of motionlessness or akinesia lasting about 30 seconds (see Fig. 31, 32).

d) Occipital lobe epilepsy. Seizure manifestations arising from the calcarine fissure consist of a wide variety of *elementary visual sensations* such as the perception of gross light (usually brightly colored), a ball of fire or sparks; the sensations may move across the visual field or remain stationary for the duration of the seizure. Blurring of vision, darkness or transient complete blindness are further ictal symptoms. All of these phenomena may constitute an isolated attack or may evolve into a grand mal seizure.

The differentiation from experienced temporal lobe seizures (see above) must be stressed; the temporal ictal illusions and pseudohallucinations are complex. Spread from a primary temporal lobe focus into the occipital region with elementary visual ictal sensations has been reported by Gastaut (1958); hence, occipital lobe seizures occasionally may be of secondary nature.

Attacks of blindness may be accompanied by generalized spike wave activity (Strauss, 1963); these attacks are probably limited to children and adolescents (Fig. 33, 34).

The *differential diagnosis of elementary visual seizures* must include nonepileptic attacks such as the well-known scintillating scotoma of migraine, basilar artery migraine (Bickerstaff, 1961) and various types of cerebrovascular insufficiency affecting the

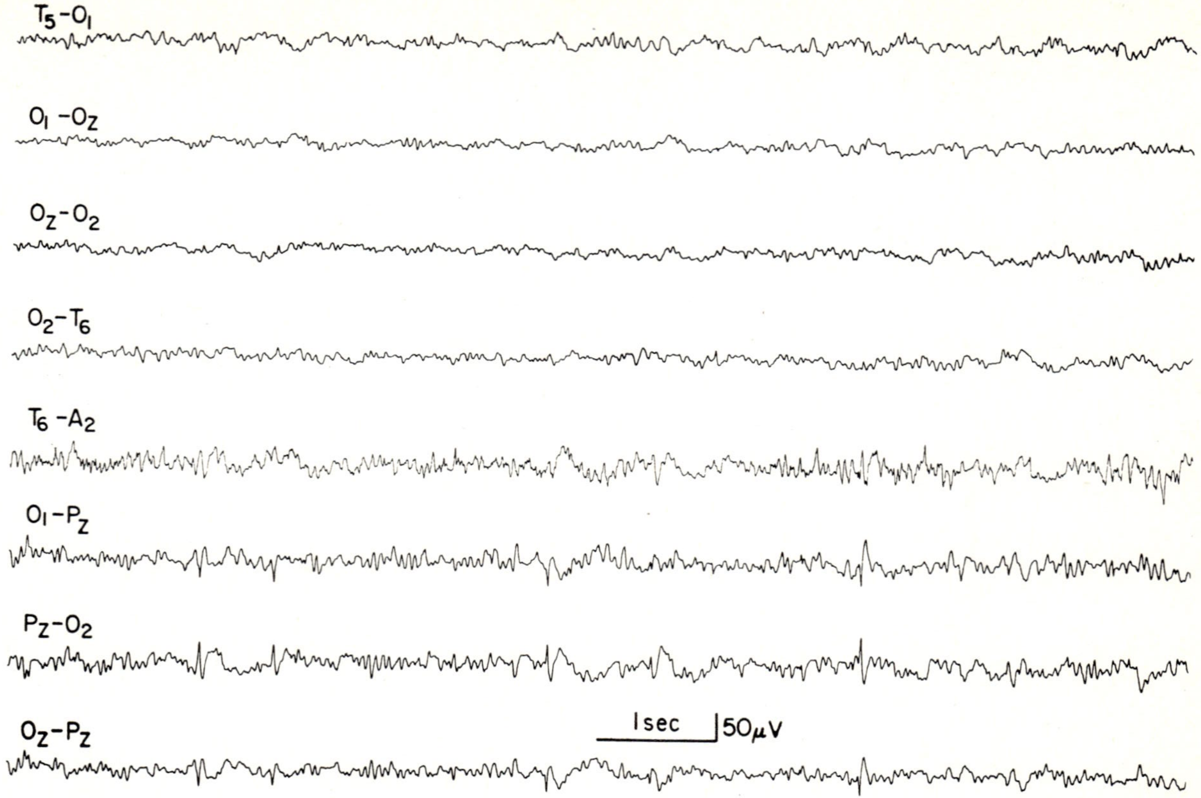

FIGURE 31. EEG of a 23-year old male college student (#1411948) with onset of grand mal at age 20 and frequent attacks consisting of tinnitus, oscillopsia and general akinesis duration of 30 seconds with post-ictal confusion. Note focal spikes over parietal midline region (electrode P z).

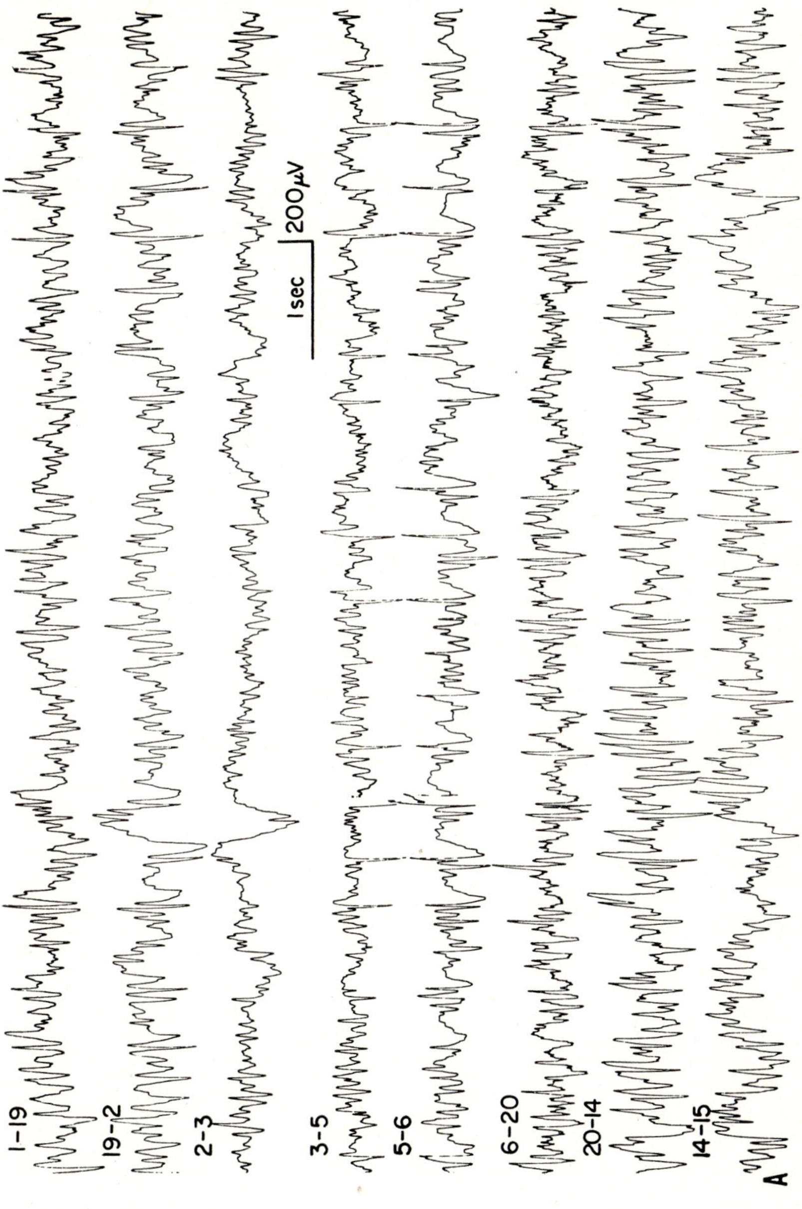

FIGURE 32. a) The same patient; electrocorticogram during surgery in general anesthesia. There is marked focal spiking in electrode #5 which is located in close vicinity to the interhemispheric fissure.

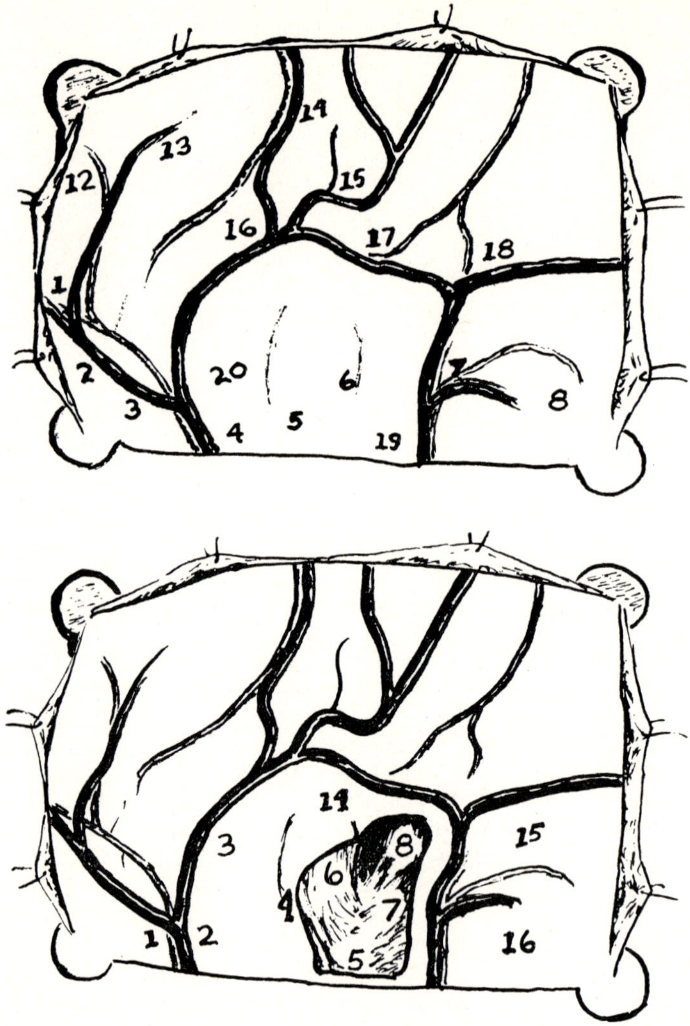

B

FIGURE 32. b) Drawing shows localization of cortical electrodes and surgical excision. The patient's seizure frequency was reduced but no full control was attained in the 1½ year-follow-up-period.

vertebro-basilar system and, more specifically, the posterior cerebral artery (blurring of vision, amaurosis fugax).

Oculoclonic seizures or epileptic nystagmus are due to occipital epileptogenic lesions, usually located outside the

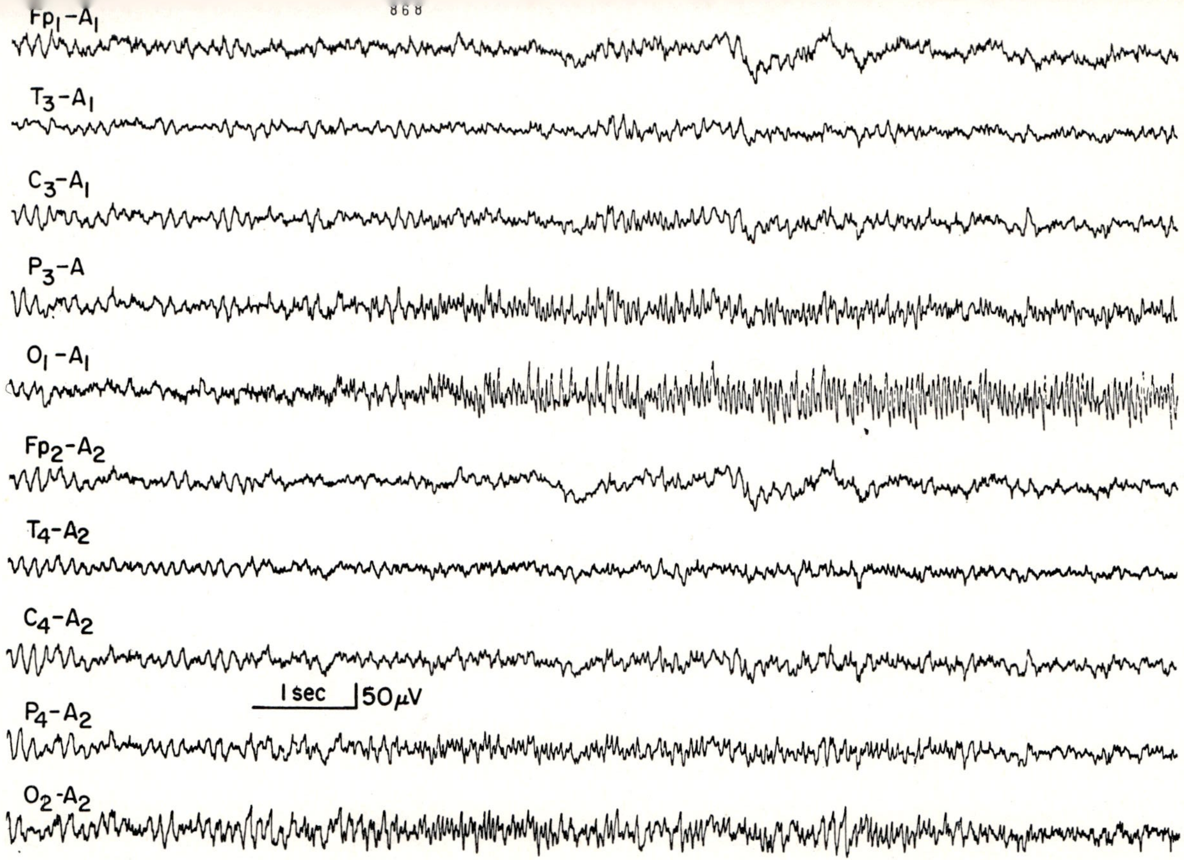

FIGURE 33. The EEG of a 39-year-old female with an onset of occipital lobe epilepsy during her third pregnancy. She experienced flashing red lights, blurring of vision and severe headache during these attacks. Note the left occipital onset and subsequent propagation of rapid spike activity. The patient has become completely seizure-free. (Patient of the Walter Reed General Hospital, Neurological Service, Washington, D.C.; courtesy of Dr. A. D. Huott.)

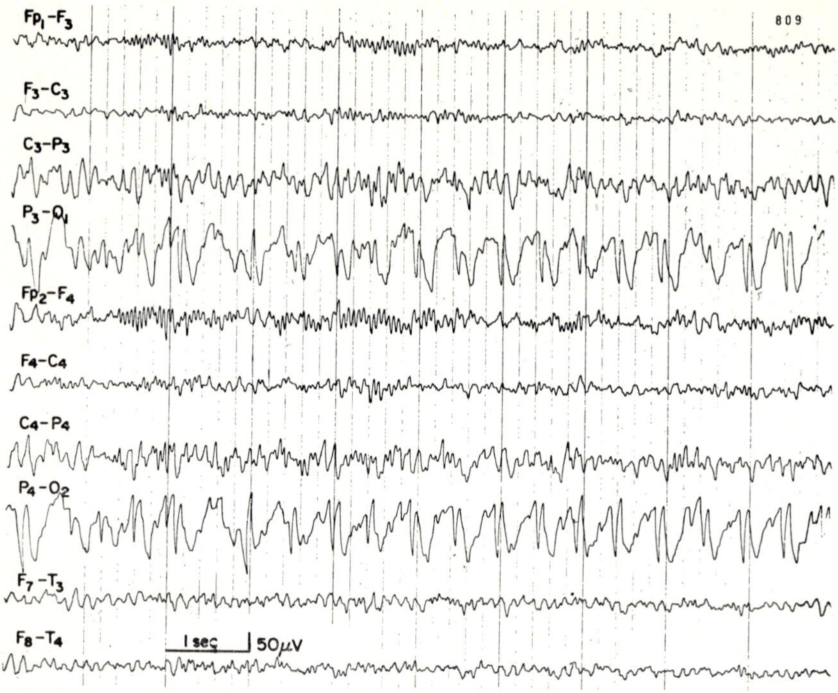

FIGURE 34. The EEG of a 14-year-old boy with episodic loss of vision, mostly associated with the hallucination of one or more female faces. This tracing was obtained during such an episode which lasted almost 9 minutes and was characterized by bilateral occipital spike-wave discharges. Note the basic difference between this bilateral-synchronous mechanism associated with the spike-wave complex) and the typical unilateral focal onset of rapid spiking in Figure 33. (Patient of the Fitzsimons General Hospital, Neurological Service, Denver, Col.; courtesy of Dr. D. S. Madison.)

calcarine fissure. These seizures have been well documented by Gastaut (1960) and White (1971). These attacks of nystagmus-like eye movements may last several minutes and there may be moderate impairment of consciousness.

The etiology of occipital lobe epilepsy is multifold and the elimination of a space occupying lesion is of great importance.

4) Epilepsies of deep (subcortical) origin

Diseases of the *basal ganglia* and the *thalamus* are not associated with epileptic seizures except for very rare cases; one of these possible exceptions was discussed earlier ("diencephalic Jacksonian epilepsy").

Generalized synchronous seizure discharges with classical petit mal or grand mal may develop in patients with *hypothalamic lesions* in association with autonomic-diencephalic and endocrine disturbances (Boudin et al., 1954; Hann, 1957; Scherman and Abraham, 1963; Niedermeyer, 1972) and probably also in rare cases of *mesencephalic lesions*. It has been presumed that such lesions may derange diffuse thalamocortical connections "from below"; the resulting seizures and seizure discharges may imitate the picture of common generalized epilepsy. Diencephalic epilepsy with autonomic manifestations (Penfield, 1929) is a very rare and probably controversial form of seizure.

"Cerebellar fits" denote a time-honored term for *tonic posturing* occurring in *decerebrate states with mesencephalic release-mechanisms*. There is no place for these attacks in modern epileptology. Ischemic factors account for the most prominent form of "cerebellar fits" in posterior fossa tumors (Ingvar and Lundberg, 1961).

Paroxysmal manifestations of the *pontine and oblongata level* are customarily not regarded as epileptic although the basic neuronal disturbance may show unmistakable epileptic traits. Therefore, attacks of *tic douloureux* (trigeminal neuralgia) may represent neuronal discharges of epileptic nature and respond indeed very favorably to certain anticonvulsants. On the other hand, these local discharges never spread into adjacent or interconnected distant areas; this lack of propagation justifies the general opinion of a nonepileptic entity. The glosso-oropharyngeal *myorhythmias* do not belong into the domain of epilepsy.

Spinal epilepsy is thought to consist of *segmental myoclonus* and deserves a place in the semeiology of the spinal cord. Again, the epileptic character remains controversial because of the lack of spread, although neuronal epileptiform activity is likely to be present. The widespread spasms occurring with *systemic administration of strychnine* are based upon marked seizure activity within the spinal reticular formation throughout most levels ("strychnic tetanus," Brémer, 1941). This experimental model of true spinal epilepsy might play a role in human cases of strychnine poisoning and possibly also in infectious tetanus.

5) Unexplained but presumably focal epilepsies in adulthood

A breakdown of an epileptic population into diagnostic-etiological and cerebral-localizing categories shows in a painful and humiliating manner that a large number of cases cannot be placed into any special category. According to Boshes and Gibbs (1972), approximately 25 percent of patients with grand mal seizures (and no other type of seizures) have a completely normal electroencephalogram awake and asleep. Even greater is the number of patients with grand mal attacks of unknown origin and undetermined etiology.

Other patients of this etiologically dubious category show a moderate EEG abnormality known as "small sharp spikes" (Gibbs and Gibbs, 1965) which become evident in drowsiness and sleep (see Table III). These extremely inconspicuous discharges originate from a large area according to the depth studies of Westmoreland and Klass, 1972. With more prolonged sleep recording, widespread small sharp spikes may be replaced by infrequent large anterior temporal sharp waves. There is reason to presume that some of these cases are larval temporal lobe epilepsies with grand mal seizures only and no evidence of psychomotor attacks.

Chapter 6

RARE SPECIAL FORMS OF EPILEPSY (UNUSUAL TRIGGERING MECHANISMS)

1) *Introductory remarks*

In a sizeable number of patients, epileptic seizures occur exclusively in a certain set of conditions such as circadian cycle, menstrual cycle, states of emotionality (often associated with sleep disturbances), sudden withdrawal in a state of chronic alcoholism and others. In much smaller groups of epileptics, the seizures are triggered by one well-defined precipitating factor. One of these factors, sensitivity to flickering light, was discussed as a part of common generalized epilepsy. Startling auditory stimuli are capable of triggering convulsions in infantile lipidosis (Tay-Sachs disease) and tonic attacks in rare cases of mesiofrontal epilepsy; this was also mentioned farther above.

This brief chapter deals with unusual and very intriguing forms of epilepsy. One must concede that these forms of unusual seizure precipitation are rare but, without proper knowledge of their existence, the physician may be inclined to diagnose such attacks as partly or completely psychogenic.

2) *Reading epilepsy*

The precipitation of epileptic convulsions by reading was first reported by Bickford (1954); such cases were subsequently observed by Chavany et al. (1956), H. Stevens (1957), Bingel (1957), Alajouanine et al. (1959), Critchley et al. (1960), Baxter and A. A. Bailey (1961), Lasater (1962), Zlotlov (1964), Shanzer et al. (1965), Gastaut and Tassinari (1966) and Matthews and Wright (1967).

Most of the observers have stressed the role of jerking jaw movements developing in a gradual crescendo while the patient is reading; further continuation of reading will lead to a grand mal attack. The patient is aware of strange laryngeal sensations and the onset of *"jaw clicking"* which plays an important role as a premonitory manifestation according to Bickford et al. (1956). Hypermotility of the jaw with clicking was precisely the main characteristic of a personal unpublished observation. It has been felt that this indicates a peripheral proprioceptive initiation of the attack (Bickford et al., 1956). European authors, however, have laid greater emphasis on focal cerebral factors. In a case of Gastaut and Tassinari (1966), right parietal spiking preceded the generalization of the seizure whereas bilateral-synchronous seizure discharges stood in the foreground in the observations of Bickford et al. (1956).

The patients have only rare attacks; they learn quickly at what point reading has to be discontinued. The proper discontinuation of reading is probably far more effective than treatment with anticonvulsive medication. Some patients, however, have additional spontaneous seizures requiring medication.

The *physiopathogenesesis* of reading epilepsy is still enigmatic since an abnormal spread of proprioceptive input from the jaw musculature or muscles of articulation (due to latent vocal reading) is probably not the only mechanism. Proprioception of the extraocular muscles is a controversial issue. Strictly visual elements (photic stimulation), intellectual concentration, emotional factors deriving from the content of the text and conditioning of a response might be further possible sub-factors (Critchley, 1962; Bickford and Klass, 1969). The role of a genetic element (Matthews and Wright, 1967) and acquired cerebral lesions is poorly understood.

3) *Various types of visually induced epilepsies*

a) Sensitivity to flickering light. The "ordinary" type of photosensitivity (Walter et al., 1946; Gastaut et al. 1948), represents an important segment of common generalized epilepsy (see Chapter 4) but may also occur in other forms of seizure disorder; genetic and structural defects may be inseparably intermingled. Myoclonic bilateral jerking is the most common manifestation; petit mal absences and grand mal attack may also be triggered. The affected age ranges from childhood into the forties and fifties. Although this is the most common of all peripherally induced epilepsies, photosensitivity comprises hardly 1 to 2 percent of the total epileptic population. It must be kept in mind that intermittent stroboscopic stimulation in the EEG laboratory sometimes reveals photosensitivity (which would lead to convulsions unless the activation is discontinued) in patients with no history of epileptic seizures. Some of these individuals have psychiatric problems.

What is easily triggered in the EEG laboratory by the powerful flashes of the strobe lamp (chiefly at rates of 6-20/sec, especially 14-18/sec) occurs under the following natural conditions:

Play of light through foliage of trees, from a brilliant moving object, from waves of the sea.

Rhythmical interruption of light by a row of trees (seen from a moving vehicle) or by the blades of a helicopter (occasional cause of helicopter crashes due to photosensitivity of the pilot).

Some patients are referred for *self-induced seizures;* these are mostly young adults who trigger absence or automatism like brief attacks by rapidly moving their hands in front of their eyes in bright sunshine; some of them derive sexual pleasure from these seizures. These patients are usually not found in the group of common generalized epilepsy, some are mentally retarded and institutionalized.

The *physiopathogenesis* is not fully understood (see Bickford and Klass, 1969). The treatment ranges from simple avoidance of intermittent visual stimuli or elaborate extinction procedures (coupling of visual stimuli with auditory stimuli by means of special hearing aid type eye glasses; Forster et al., 1965) to the usual type of anticonvulsive therapy (especially when spontaneous seizures also occur).

b) PATTERNED VISION SENSITIVITY AND TELEVISION INDUCED

SEIZURES. The very rare epilepsy-inducing effect of *geometrical patterns* must be separated from the nonepileptic activation of lambda waves in the electroencephalogram (Scott, Groethuysen and Bickford, 1967; Bickford and Klass, 1969) caused by viewing half tone patterns. A pattern of vertical black stripes may give rise to generalized synchronous spikes or spike waves with clinical seizures (Bickford and Klass, 1969; Chatrian et al., 1970); horizontal and diagonal stripes are much less epileptogenic.

Seizures induced by watching television are thought to be due to the same mechanism which is involved in patterned vision sensitivity (Bickford and Klass, 1962). Switching channels is probably the most critical situation in this type of photosensitivity. The fact that the average American spends much of his free time in front of the TV screen must be taken into account when the history reveals seizures coincidentally occurring while watching TV. True television induced epilepsy is very rare.

c) SEIZURES INDUCED BY VISUAL EXPLORATION. Gastaut and Tassinari (1966) separate these intrinsically triggered attacks from the photosensitivity to extrinsic visual stimuli. A 4-year-old patient of Gastaut and Tassinari (1966) had myoclonic seizures while looking at a colored scarf. Klass and Daly's (1960) patient had tonic spasms when he was viewing his left hand; the patient of Mitchell et al. (1954), had a "fetish-like" induction of his attack by looking at a safety-pin and was relieved by temporal lobectomy. Additional emotional factors are fairly obvious in such a case.

d) SEIZURES INDUCED BY EYE CLOSURE. These are, in rare instances, observed in patients with a history of petit mal in childhood. The attacks consist of brief absences and slight myoclonus and may persist into adult life.

4) Musicogenic epilepsy

Very few cases of musicogenic epilepsy have been reported since the first observation of Critchley (1937). These seizures are most likely to occur as temporal lobe automatisms rather than as grand mal attacks and are (usually invariably) induced by listening to music and, in some of the cases, exclusively by a special tune (Weber, 1956; Joynt et al., 1962; Titeca, 1965).

These attacks are not consistently reproducible and an additional emotional factor is very likely. Epileptogenic foci within the temporal lobe, especially on the right (non-dominant) side, are the most common substratum of musicogenic seizures.

5) *Startle epilepsy*

Unexpected strong stimuli and especially loud sound may precipitate convulsions in a small number of epileptics. Tonic-clonic convulsions lasting only a few seconds can be elicited in *infantile amaurotic idiocy* (*Tay-Sachs disease*). These attacks are associated with flattening of the EEG (Gastaut and Tassinari, 1966).

Another type of startle epilepsy has been demonstrated by Alajouanine and Gastaut (1958) in young individuals with the hemiplegic form of cerebral palsy. The sudden noise produces a tonic spasm of the paretic extremities, either without any electrical epileptic discharges ("startle synkinesia"), or with a vertex spike followed by EEG desynchronization ("startle epilepsy"). Depth EEG studies performed in an intractable case of startle epilepsy with residual hemiparesis revealed a focus involving the supplementary motor region within the frontal lobe (Bancaud et al., 1967), and the patient greatly benefitted from the removal of the affected region.

According to Gastaut and Tassinari (1966), diazepam (Valium) is more effective than other drugs in the treatment of startle epilepsy.

Epileptic seizures induced by intermittent auditory stimuli (as a counterpart of flicker sensitivity) are virtually nonexistent in the human but play a major role in rodents.

6) *Tapping epilepsy*

Somatosensory stimuli may produce myoclonic phenomena of undisputed epileptic character. Widespread body jerks noticed during examination of the deep tendon reflexes may lead to the detection of a case of tapping sensitivity; this was first demonstrated by Dawson (1947), and an extremely small number of similar cases has been reported since.

7) Arithmetic-induced epilepsy

Calculation as a triggering mechanism of epileptic seizures has been reported by Ingvar and Nyman (1962).

8) Movement induced epilepsy

This seizure precipitating mechanism has been noted in connection with paroxysmal choreoathetosis (H. Stevens, 1965; Perez-Borja et al., 1967) and tonic seizures (Burger et al., 1972).

9) "Reflex epilepsy"

This term is seldom used in American and Western European medicine whereas numerous investigators in Eastern European countries would probably list most of the above mentioned modes of peripherally elicted seizures in the category of reflex epilepsy.

This concept is based upon experimental observations of Brown-Séquard (1950), Amantea (1920), Clementi (1929) and Speransky (1935); it proved to fit well with Pavlovian ideas on higher central nervous system activities and had profound repercussions on the thoughts of neurological scientists in Eastern Europe.

It is a matter of semantics as to whether one categorizes peripherally induced epilepsies as reflex epilepsies; the term "reflex" obviously has a different and more restricted connotation in the Sherringtonian world of thoughts when compared with the Pavlovian conception.

Peripheral irritation and subsequent central bombardment may certainly lead to neuronal epileptic responses but this is probably confined to cases of failing inhibitory mechanisms either due to structural lesions or biochemical deficiencies. Thus, one could explain reports of a peripheral cutaneous scar leading to epileptic manifestations ceasing after its removal. Scollo-Lavizzari and Hess (1967) reported focal-motor attacks in a 41-year-old patient triggered by touching the right arm and associated with left centroparietal spiking). Gastaut and Tassinari (1966), used the term "vegetative reflex epilepsy" for a 9-year-old child in whom major convulsions were consistently elicited by administration of a cold water enema or the injection of prostigmine with its well known effect of vagal intestinal hypermotility. Multiple spikes accompanied the development of abdominal discomfort which preceded the grand mal attack. The child had a history of severe measles encephalitis; this fact again stresses the existence of a cerebral lesion in peripherally induced seizures.

Dubious are old reports of epileptic seizures caused by intestinal infestation with ascaris lumbricoides and seizure-freedom after antihelminthic cure. One could invoke a very strong allergic mechanism (see allergic epilepsy, Chapter 3), but even this appears to be far fetched.

Abundant literature concerning the controversial problem of reflex epilepsy is found in the proceedings of the International Symposium on Reflex Mechanisms in the Genesis of Epilepsy, Liblice, Czechoslovakia, 1960 (Epilepsia, Amsterdam, 1962).

Chapter 7

STATUS EPILEPTICUS

1) *Introductory remarks*

STATUS EPILEPTICUS IS A state of prolonged or continuous seizure activity or a state of recurrent seizures in rapid succession with no recovery or consciousness between the attacks. It is not simply a sequence or cluster of seizures. A real status epilepticus lasts more than 12 hours once the initial treatment has failed to abort the series of attacks and duration over several days is not uncommon. Focal as well as generalized types of seizures may meet the criteria of a status. Unabated clonic twitching of a muscular segment in epilepsia partialis continua (see Chapters 2 and 5) may go on for years without major impairment of the patient's general health whereas a grand mal status may be fatal after 48 to 72 hours of uncontrolled convulsions.

There has always been a tendency to use the term status epilepticus in an excessively generous manner. Clusters of convulsions, especially in neonates and infants (Aicardi and Chevrie, 1970), are very common and some epileptics have their grand mal seizures in clusters only, especially females in the premenstrual stage. What could sound like a purely academic terminological distinction, becomes a matter of pragmatic value when reports are presented concerning treatment and efficacy of certain anticonvulsive drugs in status epilepticus. Clusters of grand mal usually will stop without any special treatment whereas the successful active termination of grand mal status may be extremely difficult. It will be shown in the following presentation that true status epilepticus is a rare condition.

2) *Grand mal status epilepticus*

Any patient with grand mal seizures could theoretically develop a status; the rarity of such an event indicates that the brain is endowed with potent inhibitory and seizure terminating mechanisms capable of preventing a following seizure before recovery of cerebral function has materialized clinically and electrically (see also Chapter 1 on inhibitory and seizure-terminating mechanisms).

These seizure terminating mechanisms apparently fail in status epilepticus. Three factors may contribute to such a failure: abrupt discontinuation of anticonvulsive medication (especially in the case of phenobarbital), gastrointestinal disturbances of drug absorption and intercurrent infectious diseases (Hunter, 1959).

Status epilepticus may develop in patients with a well defined epileptogenic focus (most often in frontal region according to Janz, 1960) as well as in primarily generalized epilepsies. There are also cases of status with no previous history of seizures. Undiagnosed brain tumors may occasionally lead to the fatal end by means of a grand mal status epilepticus. Modern advances in the treatment of seizure disorders have reduced the incidence of status epilepticus.

The severity of a true status grand mal cannot be overrated. Such a patient is usually admitted in a major neurological department after one or more days of futile attempts to stop the seizures in a smaller hospital. He is in a *profound coma* during and between the attacks but, at this point, there is no evidence of alarming brain stem signs. *Hyperthermia* is usually present, often exceeding 103° F or 39°C, mostly without apparent cause and presumed to be of hypothalamic origin. Sometimes it may be due to pulmonary congestion or frank pneumonia with associated electrolyte problems. Blood leucocytosis may exist with no evidence of infection; albuminuria is also common and of rather enigmatic genesis.

In this state of coma and instability of central automic

functions, *one major convulsion follows another in intervals of a few minutes* so that even a careful observer may lose track in the precise seizure count. The tonic-clonic sequence essentially remains preserved although slight modifications may develop; the usual length of a grand mal ranging from 60 to 90 seconds may be slightly shortened; seizures lasting less than 40 seconds can hardly be listed as grand mal any longer.

Once the status has run out of control to this degree, chances are very slim that further administration of anticonvulsants will succeed. At this stage, therapy must concentrate on adequate oxygenation.

Electroencephalographic studies of status epilepticus grand mal are surprisingly scanty. The ictal EEG is almost completely obscured by artifacts unless the patient is curarized under artificial respiration. The fascinating finding is the *lack of the post ictal silence* or flattening which is the rule after a single grand mal; it usually lasts somewhat less than one minute and is followed by very irregular slow activity which rather quickly becomes less slow on its way to normalization and clinical awakening during the next few minutes. In status grand mal, however, the last clonic jerks are immediately followed by a slow irregular inter-ictal tracing from which another seizure takes its origin very soon. The lack of the period of post ictal silence has been interpreted as suggestive for the *breakdown of an inhibitory seizure terminating* system or mechanism (Niedermeyer, 1959, 1960; Madison and Niedermeyer, 1972) (Fig. 35, 36).

When the seizures stop after successful intensive care unit treatment with artificial respiration, coma may still persist for one or a few more days; this partly depends on the blood level of barbiturates. After awakening from coma, the patient remains mentally dull and slow, and exhibits marked cerebellar signs which gradually subside over the following few weeks.

The *physiopathogenesis* of grand mal status epilepticus might be determined by the following sequence of events: The first cluster of major convulsions might damage the seizure terminating system which may be partly biochemical but is greatly dependent on cerebellar structures (Dow, 1965). The

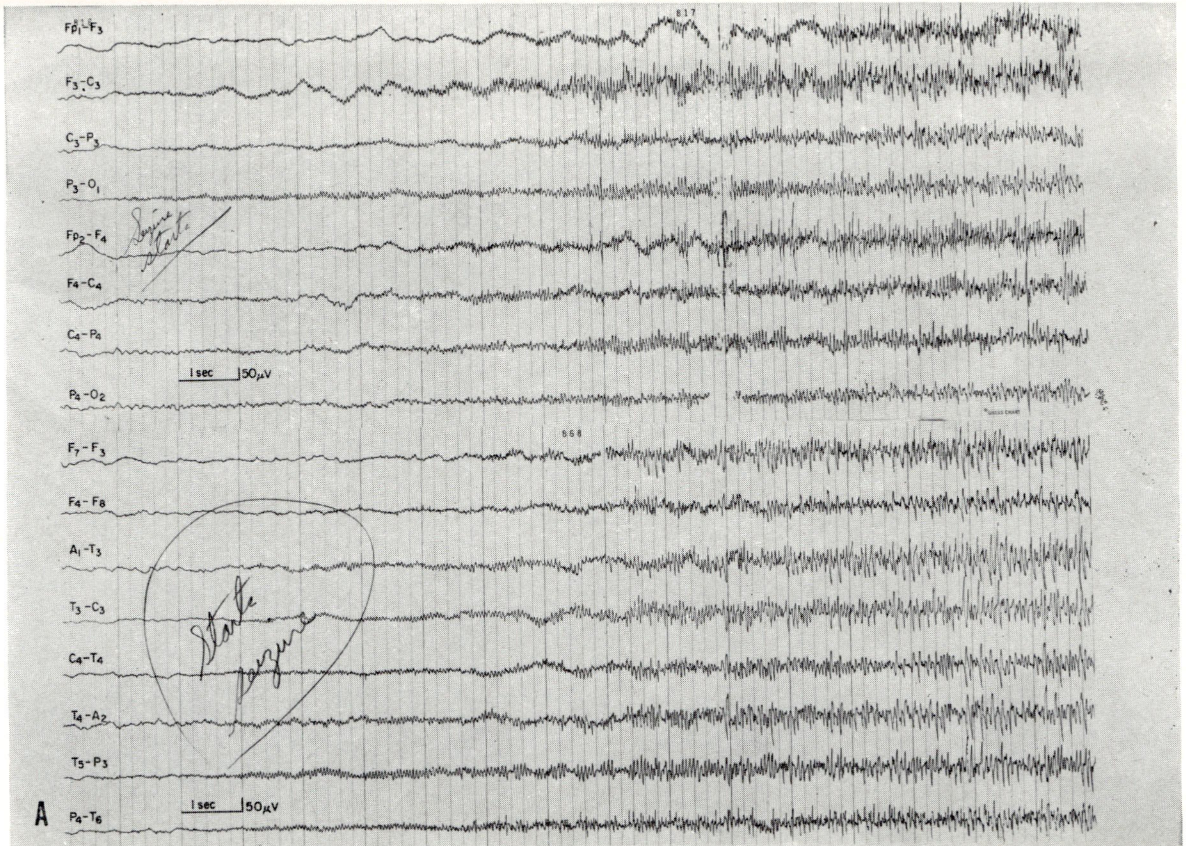

FIGURE 35. EEG recordings obtained in a 20-year-old female patient with severe status epilepticus grand mal in a state of curarization and artificial respiration. The cause of the status was obscure; the patient was no known epileptic and probably had an acute or subacute transient brain disease. (Patient of Fitzsimons General Hospital, Neurological Service; courtesy of Dr. D. S. Madison.) a) Both the upper and the lower 8 channels show the onset of two different grand mal seizures in the course of the status. In both instances, the seizure is initiated by left parietal repetitive spiking with subsequent spread and generalization within 3-4 seconds.

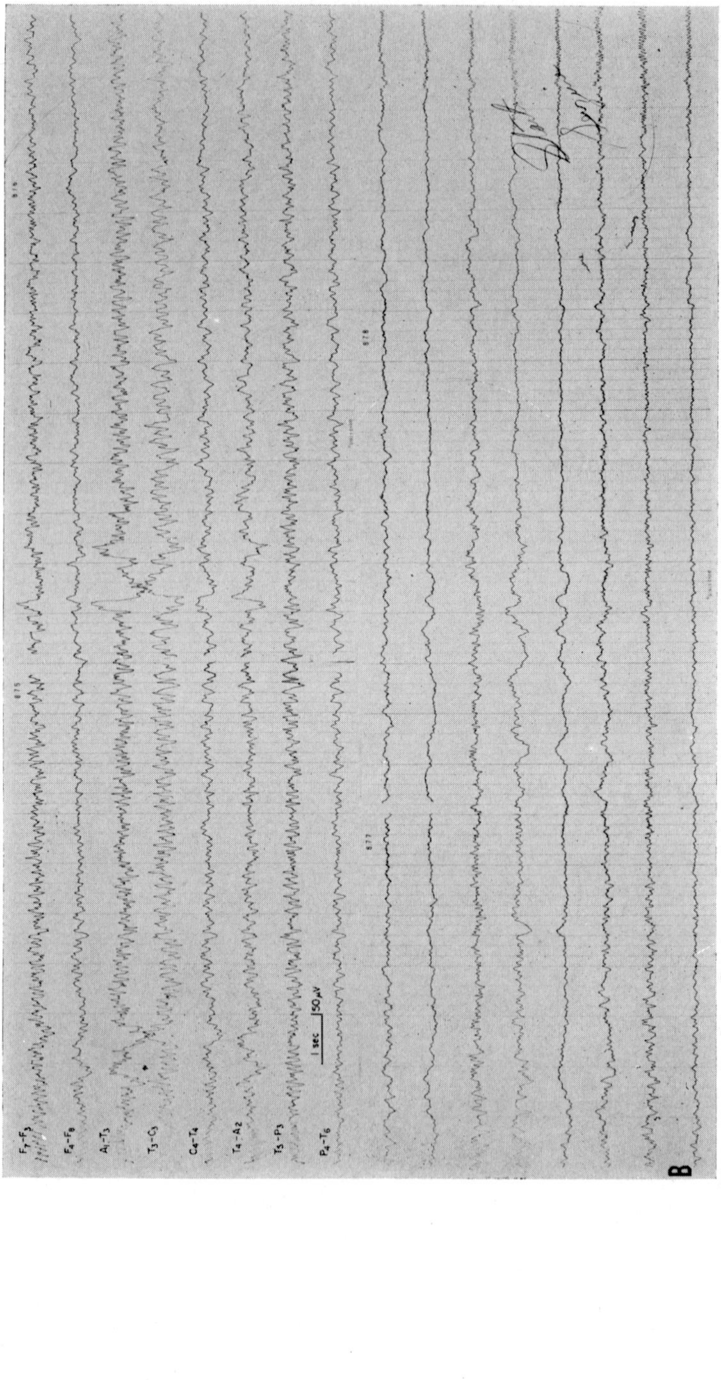

FIGURE 35. b) The bottom part is the continuation of the upper part. It shows the final stage and the termination of a grand mal seizure during the same episode of status. Note the general decrescendo of seizure activity the lack of abrupt termination (compare with Fig. 3), the gradual transition into poorly defined activity of moderate voltage, the total lack of postictal silence (or near-flatness) and the onset of the next seizure (right lower corner). The patient eventually recovered after vigorous treatment.

sensitivity of Purkinje cells to hypoxia is well established and ictal hypoxia (Scholz, 1951) may start the vicious circle. Persistent coma, hypoventilation and the countless attacks further contribute to the complete breakdown of the inhibitory mechanisms; oxygenation may reverse this development when started at a point before irreversible neuronal damage has occurred. All of these statements form a working hypothesis which explains satisfactorily the lack of electrical silence in the EEG, and the response to artificial respiration (Fig. 36).

Therapy. During the first day of seemingly uncontrollable major convulsions, the use of *i.v. diazepam* (*Valium*) is the drug of choice, preferably in combination with i.m. phenobarbital. The first injection of 10 mg may be ineffective and will have to be repeated several times; chances are fairly high that, after a total of 40 to 60 mg, the status will be brought under control. Phenobarbital i.m. in dosages from 100 to 500 mg will only succeed in simple "clusters of seizures" and not in true grand mal status; nevertheless, it is a useful adjunctive treatment in addition to diazepam. Great emphasis must be laid on the slow injection of diazepam (Valium); a rate of 5 mg/minute must not be exceeded in order to avoid respiratory depression or arrest. Other derivatives of benzodiazepine have proved to be more potent than diazepam (Gastaut, 1970) but are not registered in this country.

The parenteral use of *paraldehyde* may also be effective in the earlier stages of status epilepticus. The i.v. administration of 1 to 3 ml (slowly injected over a period of 2 to 3 minutes) is preferable to the i.m. injection of 5 to 10 ml; deep and correct intragluteal injection can avoid subsequent tissue necrosis. The rectal route may also be used.

Unreliable is the effectiveness of parenteral diphenylhydantoin which has been given i.v. in dosages up to 1000 mg. Trimethadione has been recommended in cases of primarily generalized epilepsies with grand mal status but its effectiveness is doubtful. The use of general anesthesia with ultra-short acting barbiturates may be helpful on the first day.

The emphasis on respiration, clearing of airways and cerebral

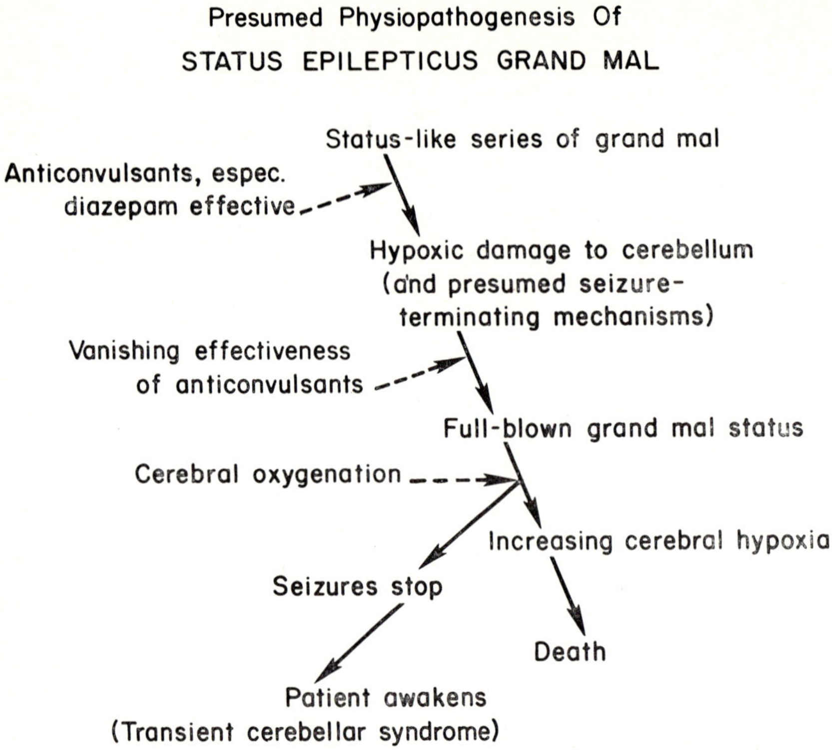

FIGURE 36. Scheme of presumed physiopathogenetic mechanisms of status epilepticus grand mal.

oxygenation implies intensive-care-type treatment. This permits ample use of muscle relaxants such as curare and succinyl choline which help to avoid cardiocirculatory exhaustion by suppression of the muscular effects of the convulsions. The composition of i.v. fluids and the use of antibiotics depends on the individual nature of the case; metabolic and respiratory acidosis may have to be treated specifically.

When the cause of seizures and length of seizure disorder are unknown, it is wise to study the possibility of a brain tumor as the cause; unfortunately, X-ray studies and brain scan cannot be done while frequent convulsions occur. *In children a severe status epilepticus-like condition is very likely to indicate active acute brain disease such as encephalitis or intracranial venous thrombosis.*

New methods of treatment and especially the introduction of diazepam (as treatment for the first day) and artificial respiration have helped to further reduce the incidence of grand mal status and, respectively, to diminish the frightfully high mortality of 50 or more percent. Avoidance of abrupt discontinuation of anticonvulsants and more appropriate methods of changing from one anticonvulsant to another have also done their share in lessening the incidence of this dreadful condition.

3) *Petit mal status* (*Ictal stupor, Spike wave stupor*)

The term *petit mal status* was introduced by Lennox (1945) and is still somewhat controversial. This term would imply a state of petit mal lapses occurring in rapid succession and this is obviously not correct in most of these cases. It could also be used in order to denote one or more unusually prolonged petit mal attack. There is no doubt, however, that most cases reported as petit mal status represent twilight states lasting hours or, more often, a few days. The behavior is stuporous with very slow mentation but the patient's contact with his environment is not suspended and the impairment of consciousness is hence by far lighter than in a typical petit mal absence. In a report on six cases with a review of the literature, Niedermeyer and Khalifeh (1965) have suggested terms such as "ictal stupor" or "spike wave stupor" instead of *petit mal* status.

Petit mal status is a rare condition but not quite as rare as the severe, life threatening type of grand mal status. It occurs at various ages, probably not before the age of 2 years but from then on into middle and even older adulthood. These patients may have

a) a history of classical *petit mal* (with or without occasional grand mal) in the frame of common generalized epilepsy,
b) an isolated condition with no occurrence of any other type of seizure, probably also in the context of common generalized epilepsy, or
c) an early or later manifestation of the Lennox-Gastaut syndrome, with a variety of other seizures and mental deficits.

Such a patient is suddenly found in a stuporous state, able to keep his eyes open or take food; he may answer some questions (usually after repeated questioning only) very slowly and in a slurred speech. His behavior appears strange but no complex automatisms are usually noted. Subtle myoclonic twitching is very common, usually in the facial musculature. At the height of the episode, one or more grand mal convulsions may occur.

This state ceases as abruptly as it has appeared, usually after 1 to 2 days. Throughout this state, the EEG shows prolonged (but usually not continuous) generalized-synchronous spike-wave discharges, mostly 3 to 4 sec in common generalized epilepsy and somewhat slower in the Lennox-Gastaut syndrome (Fig. 37). With increasing age, an admixture of fast spiky activity may be noted (Gumnit et al., 1965). Complete normalization of the EEG may occur immediately with the cessation of the twilight state. Some patients have but one petit mal status in their life.

From the viewpoint of *differential diagnosis,* virtually continuous generalized slow spike-wave activity may be seen in children with advanced Lennox-Gastaut syndrome but this alone must never be regarded as evidence of petit mal status unless clinical stupor exists. Temporal lobe status, acute psychosis and hysteria must be ruled out.

There is no real need for *therapeutic measures* since the duration of the attack is unlikely to be shortened with the possible exception of the earliest stage when diazepam (Valium) might be capable of terminating the status.

4) *Temporal lobe (psychomotor) status*

Some cases of temporal lobe epilepsy may have prolonged and repetitive psychomotor automatisms for hours or even days. This condition is very rare (Cossa and Martin, 1949; Scott and Masland, 1953) and it is doubtful as to whether this type of status can be shortened by therapeutic measure. According to Lugaresi et al (1971), there is no known case of prolonged automatism with typical concomitant EEG activity.

5) *Adversive, focal-motor and other types of status epilepticus*

A prolonged, status like sequence of adversive seizures is not very uncommon; the patient may lapse into deep coma and the condition may remotely resemble a modified grand mal status

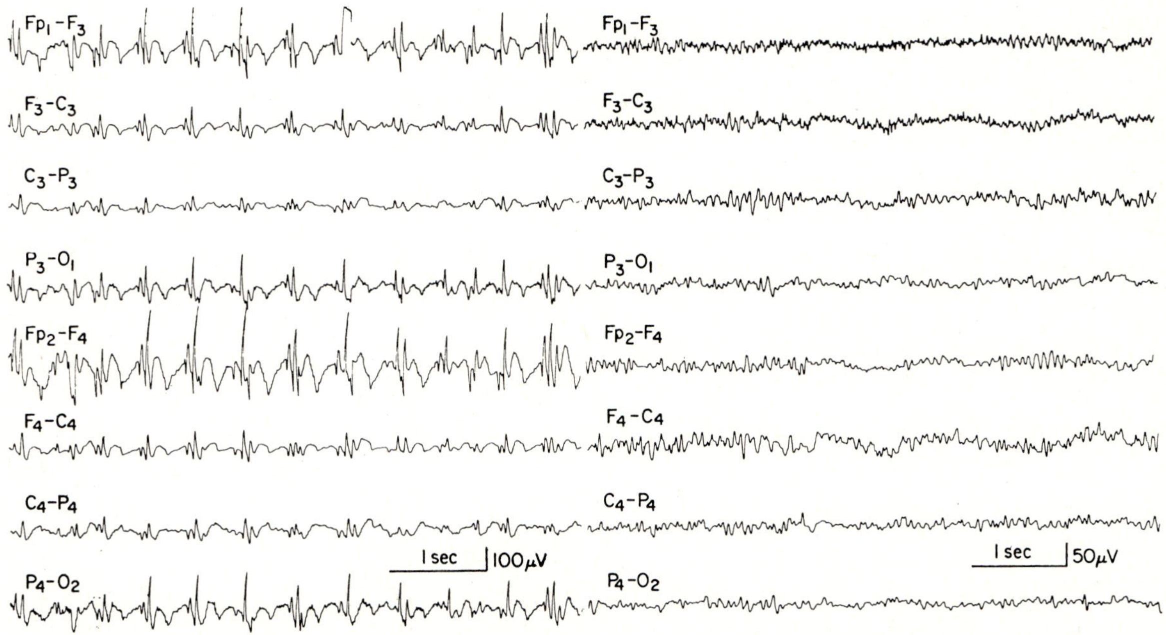

FIGURE 37. *Petit mal* status (ictal stupor, spike-wave stupor) in a 47-year-old male patient (#112434). History of petit mal since age 6 and grand mal since age 15. *Left tracing*: Note rhythmical generalized-rhythmical generalized-synchronous spikes during status. *Right tracing*: The same patient during the same recording session after Diazepam (Valium®) 10 mg i.v. total disappearance of spike activity and diffuse drug-induced fast activity.

epilepticus without reaching the severity of the latter. Diazepam i.v. in the early stage and intensive care type treatment in the case of persistence of seizures and coma are indicated.

The status form of focal motor seizures is *epilepsia partialis continua* and was mentioned in Chapter 5.

A status like repetition of other forms of focal seizures is possible but does not play any particular role in practical clinical medicine.

Chapter 8

"BORDERLAND OF EPILEPSY"

1) Introductory remarks

THIS TERM HAS been introduced by Gowers (1907) and encompasses a variety of recurrent attacks of various nature and origin. Electroencephalographic evidence has proved convincingly that a) absences termed "*pycnolepsy*" (Friedmann, 1906; Sauer, 1916) are nothing but classical *petit mal* seizures, and b) attacks of narcolepsy (irresistible sleep attacks) and the entire *complex of narcolepsy-cataplexy-sleep paralysis can be separated from epileptic manifestations.*

Unfortunately, other types of attacks were not as readily defined by the EEG as epileptic or non-epileptic entities. There is still a good deal of controversy about these forms of seizure or spell. The following paragraphs will show that the term "borderland of epilepsy" ought to be used with caution and restraint. The modern trend of overexpanding the realm of epilepsy has been discussed farther above with regard to temporal lobe epilepsy and recurrent behavioral changes; this tendency has also become obvious in numerous recent studies dealing with the following types of attack.

2) Migraine

In typical cases, migrainous attacks are initiated by visual disturbances lasting about 5 to 20 minutes and consisting of scintillating scotoma, teichopsia (visual field defects of the "fortification spectra" type) or homonymous hemianopsia. This first stage of the attack has been attributed to focal intracerebral vasoconstriction whereas the subsequent stage of mostly unilateral headaches with accompanying severe nausea and vomiting has been thought to be due to an abnormal degree of extracranial vasodilation (Wolff, 1948). These classical attacks usually start in early adolescence and recur throughout adult life. Hereditary predisposition to migraine is a well established fact.

Classical migraine is a very common ictal syndrome; the incidence of migraine is considerably enlarged by the addition of atypical cases, usually characterized by absence of the initiating stage of visual disturbance ("ordinary migraine," Graham, 1955).

The *physiopathogenesis* of migraine is still poorly understood. A genetic component is indubitably present. It has been presumed that the migraine attack might be precipitated by a fall in the plasma serotonin level (Anthony et al., 1967). Such a metabolic disturbance, however, could be due to a primary CNS dysfunction (Pearce, 1969).

Ictal EEG studies have shown normal findings in the vast majority of the cases during both the initiating stage of vasoconstriction (scotomata etc.) and the following stage with predominant headaches and nausea (Heyck, 1956; Gibbs and Gibbs, 1964). Focal delta activity during the scotoma phase was noted by Engel et al. (1947). In a small percentage of the cases, migrainous attacks *may be associated with transient hemiplegia* (complicated migraine, "migraine accompagnée"); such severe attacks may be *accompanied by unilateral slow* (theta and delta) *activity* in the EEG (Heyck, 1956; Rosenbaum, 1960; Bradshaw and Parsons, 1965; Heron, 1966). These temporary EEG changes are readily understood when one considers that the presumed migrainous intracerebral vasospasm might be associated with cerebral edema or infarction (Whitty, 1953) which could lead to permanent cerebral tissue damage (Schumacher and Wolff, 1941). *Inter-ictal EEG findings* are normal in the majority of the cases (Gibbs and Gibbs, 1964). Some patients, however, have consistently abnormal EEG findings with paroxysmal characteristics. Weil (1952) separated *"dysrhythmic migraine"* with marked EEG abnormalities and lack of response to ergotamines (but good response to anticonvulsants) from typical migraine. This view has been supported by the data of Kooi et al. (1965) who feel that patients with migraine and abnormal paroxysmal EEG records constitute a heterogeneous group with "coincidental convulsive diathesis" as an important causative factor. Some degree of photosensitivity with slow and spiky discharges in the EEG during intermittent photic stimulation has been noticed by Heyck (1958). Migrainous individuals often show a wide range of photic driving to varying flicker frequencies (even above the 20/sec flash rate); this "H response" was noted by Golla and Winter (1959). This could indicate an *enhanced excitability of the central visual system* in migraine (and especially in patients with the classical initiating ophthalmic phase).

Epileptic elements are completely absent in a large percentage of a migrainous population; other patients may have a mild paroxysmal component as evidenced by EEG abnormalities. Extremely few patients have an undeniable linkage with epilepsy. Their attacks may start with typical scintillating scotoma (sometimes preceded by a sudden sensation of ravenous hunger) but are followed by loss of consciousness and a typical grand mal which must be carefully distinguished from the more common event of a syncopal attack. Thereafter, the patient may even have headaches with nausea and vomiting for several hours with subsequent normalization. These patients have normal neurological and neuroradiological findings; anticonvulsive therapy is unable to suppress the infrequent seizures but the addition of a long-term ergotamine (Hydergin®) may be helpful (usually two or three sublingual tablets daily).

The possibility of *symptomatic migraine* due to arteriovenous malformations, brain tumor or other cerebral disorders must be taken into account in the clinical evaluation of migrainous individuals; this is particularly important in cases with a negative family history. In such patients, additional epileptic seizures could occur as a further manifestation of the cerebral lesion.

Nothing is gained, however, when the entire complex of migraine is considered "borderland of epilepsy." This has been clearly expressed in the work of Barolin (1966) who feels that migraine and epilepsy are essentially different entities. A linkage of both disorders is limited to a minority. The view has been expressed that hypersensitivity to tyramine could precipitate both migrainous and epileptic attacks (Scott et al., 1972). In spite of such possible jointly shared biochemical mechanisms, one must not forget that migraine is one of the most common neurological disorders and that a migrainous population will show very little overlap with an epileptic population.

3) ***Paroxysmal abdominal pain***

Brief episodes of intense abdominal pain may occur as a manifestation of temporal lobe epilepsy, but these epileptic manifestations are rare as Van Buren (1963) has shown in his study of ictal abdominal-visceral phenomena. Walker and Marshall (1964) observed ictal spiking in the right pallidum during such short attacks in a temporal lobe epileptic with implanted depth electrodes.

As was stated earlier, the term "abdominal epilepsy" (Moore, 1945) has been greatly overused. This term has been applied to attacks of abdominal pain in children, often associated with nausea, lasting for hours and sometimes longer than one day. In earlier days, useless appendectomies were performed in many of these children. One has to agree with Pond (1963) when he points out that ". . . to assign an epileptic basis to the latter (referring to paroxysmal abdominal pain) because of the symptomatic resemblance, is as irrational as ascribing an epileptic basis to habit spasm, merely because the movements resemble myoclonic jerks and the motor cortex is presumably involved in both phenomena."

There is good reason to presume that most of these rather long lasting attacks of abdominal pain are early manifestations of migraine which will reveal itself during adolescence with its classical symptomatology. The electroencephalographer will occasionally notice marked diffuse slowing in the tracing at the height of the attack; this is evidently due to ketosis and other metabolic changes secondary to vomiting (Vahlquist and Nylander, 1954).

A reduction of the frequency of these attacks by anticonvulsants and especially by diphenylhydantoin does not prove the epileptic nature of the attack; most of the anticonvulsants have farther reaching effects and are able to dampen heightened neuronal excitability in general. It is often surprising that some pediatricians use the term "abdominal epilepsy" so generously despite the fact that the notion of epilepsy could have a frightening effect on the parents and all this in the face of inadequate evidence of epilepsy.

4) Attacks of vertigo and dizziness

Sensations of vertigo, dizziness or giddiness may occur as an aura like prelude of major convulsions but isolated attacks of epileptic vertigo are rare (Niedermeyer and Hinchcliffe, 1965). Real epileptic vertigo is very short lasting and extremely severe; a major convulsion may follow immediately (Barac, 1968).

Attacks of vertigo and dizziness are, in the vast majority, secondary to labyrinthine, vestibular and nerve and pontine involvement; frequently recurrent short attacks are the rule in cases of vertebro-basilar artery insufficiency while severe bouts of vertigo will last for hours or days in Menière's disease. The circulatory nature of orthostatic dizziness is obvious.

Chapter 9

THE USE OF DIAGNOSTIC PROCEDURES IN EPILEPTIC PATIENTS

1) Introductory remarks

THE DIAGNOSTIC EVALUATION of a patient presenting with a history of seizures has to deal with the following principal questions:

a) *Are the reported attacks of epileptic or nonepileptic nature?*
b) If the epileptic character is well established, *is there any evidence of a focal origin?*
c) *What is the cause of the epileptic seizures?*

The first question implies considerations regarding the differential diagnosis between various types of attacks; this will be further discussed in the following chapter and the preceding discussion of the so-called borderland of epilepsy (Chapter 8) provides further information for the reader.

The second question implies the localizing value of focal epileptic seizures (see Chapter 5) and falls into the domain of cerebral localization in clinical Neurology.

The third question is a nosological or etiological one. The physician has to be aware of the fact that epileptic manifestations are abnormal cerebral reactions due to a large number of diseases or insults to brain tissue. This is the very first statement of this book; it must act like a "*Leitmotiv*" in all of the physician's diagnostic considerations.

Unfortunately, the second and the third question often remain unanswered. Small residual scars may be the result of a seemingly trivial and forgotten brain insulting event in the patient's early history; a genetic predisposition may be present in an undetectable manner. The answer to the first question may initially elude careful history taking but a series of clinical tests (with or without actual seizure observation) will eventually clarify the issue in the vast majority of the cases.

The type and sequence of ancillary clinical diagnostic procedures are the topic of this chapter. Certain basic rules can be recommended but no rigid diagnostic scheme can be given. The human element must be taken into account; the patient's anxieties or his indifference are important factors in determining the course of the clinical evaluation.

A thorough history, general physical and neurological examination are the foundation of the clinical workup. Even a very careful examination will often prove to be normal. In addition to classical neurological signs, one has also to search for subtle "degenerative stigmas" such as a high palate, hypo- or aplasias of certain muscles, anomalies of fingers and toes, not to speak of obvious birth defects such as hare lip and cleft palate. Authoritative articles of the early part of this century have laid much emphasis on the degenerative element (Hartmann and diGaspero, 1914 and many others); our present knowledge of birth defects, genetic syndromes and chromosomal aberrations has taught us that such disturbances occasionally may be associated with epileptogenic brain defects (McKusick, 1966).

In addition to the information derived from his clinical examination, the physician will need diagnostic laboratory methods which will be discussed in the following.

2) *Electroencephalography*

The capability of recording paroxysmal discharges in the inter seizure interval is one of the greatest assets of electroencephalography. This method is completely based upon functional electrical phenomena and their deviations; such functional or "dyfunctional" events are the basis of epileptic manifestations (in opposition to morphological changes such as shifts of cerebral parenchyma or occlusion of cerebral vessels). While the EEG will always be somewhat hampered in the precise diagnosis of cerebral lesions by virtue of its functional character, the same drawback turns into an enormous advantage when one deals with the diagnosis of epileptic seizures. For this reason, the *EEG evaluation is a necessity in the diagnostic workup of a patient with a history of seizures.* In this domain, electroencephalography has taken a position almost comparable to that of the chest X-ray in lung disease.

This implies that a requisition for an electroencephalogram will be the first step in the diagnostic laboratory evaluation. There are notable exceptions, of course. A middle aged patient with one recent grand mal, a history of headaches for the past few weeks, slight recent loss of mental acuity and the objective finding of papilledema may have a glioblastoma or astrocytoma; then a brain scan is certainly more urgently indicated than an EEG. Acute epileptic conditions in toxic metabolic disorders such as acute renal failure, may require a series of other tests first, although an EEG may be very worthwhile.

In academic medicine, the costs of a diagnostic test are often underrated and, in neurological disorders, EEG's are frequently requested "for completeness sake"; the same is true for other diagnostic tests. Of course, this attitude has to be castigated.

The EEG does not represent any further stress for the patient; it is a completely painless test. This is particularly important in infantile convulsions and in epileptic manifestations of frail individuals.

The EEG evaluation aims at the same set of questions presented farther above in the introduction to this chapter. A satisfactory answer to all three of these questions (epileptic vs. nonepileptic seizures, focal origin, etiology) can only seldom be given. Occasionally, no answer can be found even in the apparently most simple of all questions, namely the distinction between epilepsy and hysterical attacks in certain patients. Mild paroxysmal EEG abnormalities are not unusual in patients with hysteria. As to the seizures themselves, both grand mal and a stormy hysterical sequence of motions are most likely to be obscured by muscular artifacts in the tracing.

It is very difficult to find the correct answer to a pragmatist's question concerning precise percentages of right and wrong answers or false negative and false positive EEG findings in an epileptic population. According to Bickford (1963), a normal EEG excludes epilepsy in 70 percent without activation and in 90 percent with activation. These figures have to be taken with the grain of salt. The epileptic sample can be enormously "manipulated." One could adopt the view that infants or children with febrile convulsions are not epileptics; this is clinically correct in the overwhelming majority but wrong in terms of abnormal physiology (which is epileptic in nature). Thus, the largest segment of individuals with epileptic manifestations may either be included or excluded. The same is true for alcoholics with withdrawal seizures who form another large segment of epileptics in the slum areas of big cities. Both of these segments are characterized by normal interval EEG tracings in the vast majority; the negativity of these findings is certainly a diagnostically valuable contribution of the EEG and no drawback. This list of examples could be further extended.

A complete EEG record contains *activations such as photic stimulation* (aiming at the detection of flicker sensitive epileptics) *and hyperventilation* (aiming chiefly at the detection of classical petit mal but also at the demonstration of generalized seizure discharges in a broader sense and an occasional activation of an otherwise silent focus). *Sleep,* either spontaneous or induced by oral administration of appropriate dosages of Chloral Hydrate or Secobarbital, is no real activation but it gives a wider spectrum of physiological states for the EEG evaluation. Sleep recordings are valuable in most forms of epilepsy but particularly in temporal lobe epilepsy. In infants, there is a greater difficulty in securing readable waking record and many infantile tracings are limited to sleep.

Telemetric EEG recording for prolonged periods has yielded important insight into the circadian distribution of clinical and subclinical ictal activity. This technique has been used by J. Stevens and co-workers (1971) as well as by Geier (1971) but remains limited to special research centers.

Neuropharmacological activations with pentylenetetrazol

(Metrazol) or ethyl-methyl-glutarimid (Megimid®) are of rather limited value since generalized bursts of spikes or spike-waves are normal responses (although elicited with varying thresholds in different individuals). Both drugs, however, are capable of occasionally triggering seizure discharges from an otherwise silent epileptogenic focus. *Hypoglycemia* can enhance generalized seizure patterns. *Sudden withdrawal of chronic anticonvulsive therapy* for 24 to 48 hours prior to the scheduled EEG will clearly improve the electroencephalographer's chance of finding electrical seizure activity. This practice is widely used but cannot be recommended. Leaving aside the chance of provoking the return of long controlled convulsions and the remote chance of a status epilepticus, the EEG findings are chemically manipulated since the element of a *withdrawal rebound* of epileptic activity exists; this pertains chiefly to phenobarbital. The slow metabolism of phenobarbital will not lead to a severe withdrawal syndrome as is the rule with chronic intake of short acting barbiturates in addicts. I personally feel that it is better to evaluate the present state of electrical activity in a well controlled epileptic rather than to improve the "batting average" of obtaining positive EEG findings at the expense of the patient's feeling of safety and security. *Sleep deprivation* (staying awake all night prior to the EEG scheduled for the morning hours) leads to a build-up of already existing EEG abnormalities but endangers especially patients with common generalized epilepsy for whom a well regulated waking-sleeping cycle is an important matter (see Chapter 14). He may be already post ictal when he comes to the laboratory.

The insertion of *special electrodes* may be helpful in the assessment of buried and poorly accessible foci in temporal lobe epileptics. *Nasopharyngeal electrodes* are easily introduced but often marred by artifacts; these electrodes may pick up seizure discharges from the basal portions of the temporal lobe. *Sphenoidal electrodes* are inserted from anterior or from lateral (below the zygoma) approaches with no particular difficulties and may yield excellent recording from an area located in closest proximity of the tip of the temporal lobe.

The insertion of *depth electrodes* is a neurosurgical procedure carried out in the operating room under X-ray control with or without stereotaxic devices. These electrodes are implanted mainly into temporal and frontal regions; the approach has to take into consideration the anatomy of major vessels. Such implants are performed for a duration of 1 to 2 weeks or longer; daily recordings are carried out. *This method is strictly limited to candidates for seizure surgery* (see Chapter 13). About 10 percent of the patients are likely to develop complications, usually minor intracranial bleeding or infection. Major complications, however, are not too rare and even fatal outcome has been observed.

3) *Brain scan*

The evaluation of the craniocerebral uptake of radioactive substances is an excellent test for the detection of a presumed intracranial lesion. Most brain tumors are demonstrable by this method; hemispheric meningiomas (not seldom an Achilles-heel of EEG diagnosis) are almost always localized. Particularly impressive is the demonstration of brain abscesses.

For these reasons, a brain scan ought to be requested in all those patients in whom an intracranial tumor could be reasonably presumed as the cause of the seizures. This is particularly true for adults with recent onset of seizures and especially those with focal attacks or an aura like focal initiation of grand mal. This test is expensive and probably unnecessary in the large majority of childhood epilepsies. The type of radioactive material as well as special technical aspects of the brain scan cannot be discussed here. A *dynamic brain scan* is particularly valuable in cases of a presumed vascular disturbance such as an arterio-venous malformation.

EEG, brain scan and an additional skull X-ray may be regarded as the most commonly used series of ambulatory tests in the work up of an epileptic adult.

4) *Echoencephalography*

This quickly performed diagnostic method is extremely useful in cases of acute epilepsy and in general, in all cases of seizure with suggestion of a space occupying process.

5) *Cranial arteriography (angiography)*

The visualization of the intracranial vessels by intracarotid (intravertebral or right brachial artery) injection of radio-opaque material provides an excellent demonstration of vascular anomalies as well as shifts of the vascular tree caused by space occupying lesions (tumors, abscesses, subdural hematomas). This test requires hospitalization of the patient and presents certain risks for the patient.

Therefore, the arteriogram should be requested in the special diagnostic pursuit of epileptogenic vascular lesions (arterio-venous malformations in particular) and space occupying processes (usually after a positive or equivocal result of the brain scan).

6) *Pneumoencephalography*

The filling of the cerebral ventricles and the subarachnoid space with air or gases following the withdrawal of CSF is presently not as frequently used as in earlier years. In the diagnosis of epilepsies, this method may demonstrate residual cerebral damage such as local or widespread cortical atrophies or small local atrophies involving limbic structures enlarging the inferior horn of the lateral ventricle. Porencephalic lesions are also well demonstrated and likely to escape other methods of neuroradiological diagnosis.

In space occupying lesions, the arteriogram is generally preferred over the air studies; sudden changes of the CSF dynamics may rapidly lead to cerebral complications thus dimming the prognostic outlook.

7) *Reasons for requesting (and not requesting) neuroradiological diagnostic methods in epileptic patients*

The diagnostic evaluation of the epileptic must be reasonably thorough but not compulsive. One has to keep in mind that space occupying lesions and arterio-venous malformations are not among the most common causes of epilepsy while, on the other hand, the failure to diagnose such lesions at an earlier stage may be a tragic mistake.

Following the advent of the brain scan, this dilemma has eased considerably; a negative brain scan will give some peace of mind to the patient as well as the physician. In adults with a history of epileptic seizures since early childhood, brain scan and neuroradiological methods are usually of academic rather than pragmatic value. Infants or small children with febrile convulsions and a normal EEG usually do not need further diagnostic workup. Children with petit mal absences and typical EEG abnormalities need a brain scan and neuroradiological studies only when the seizures remain recalcitrant for some time.

The elimination of active intracranial lesions is not the only goal of the diagnostic workup. In infants, a large number of metabolic and toxic conditions must be ruled out in an internal pediatric workup. Even the possibility of an *inborn error of metabolism* (lipidosis, phenylketonuria and others) must be considered. Later in life and especially during adulthood, grand mal attacks may be the *first manifestation of a systemic lupus erythematosus.* The cerebral microangiopathy of lupus erythematosus will gradually bring forth other neurological complications such as cerebrovascular accidents, delirium or psychosis. Early demonstration of LE-cells and accompanying renal changes are diagnostically helpful.

These are only a few examples stressing the fact that epileptic manifestations cut across a large segment of medicine. Specialized seizure clinics are most welcome but their physicians must always be aware of lingering diagnostic problems in a substantial number of patients in whom epilepsy is a sign of ongoing or progressive disease and not simply a residue of a bygone period of life.

Chapter 10

DIFFERENTIAL DIAGNOSIS: EPILEPTIC VS. NON-EPILEPTIC ATTACKS

1) *Introductory remarks*

THE ABOVE DISCUSSED "borderland of epilepsy" (Chapter 8) raises differential diagnostic questions with respect to attacks which have been thought to be somewhat related to the epilepsies. The differentiation from other clearly nonepileptic spells is the subject of this chapter.

Acute transient loss of consciousness or sudden behavioral changes of nonepileptic character are most commonly caused by

a) circulatory disturbances giving rise to acute cerebral ischemia,
b) sudden changes of blood chemistry, and
c) psychogenic alterations.

Naturally, our considerations exclude all of the prolonged states of altered consciousness and are limited to short lasting attacks which may closely or remotely resemble a major convulsion or other types of epileptic seizures.

2) *Syncopal attacks*

Syncope denotes a sudden and brief loss of consciousness due to a discrete episode of generalized cerebral ischemia; it is thus a manifestation of acute generalized insufficiency of the cerebral circulation (Naquet and Vigouroux, 1972). A considerable number of clinical conditions or well-defined diseases may lead to syncopal attacks and a variety of pathophysiological mechanisms may bring forth such transient cerebral ischemia. The classification of Engel (1962) elucidates the extent of conditions and mechanisms leading to syncope;

a) Syncope with peripheral circulatory inadequacy
   - Vasodepressor syncope
   - Postural hypotension

b) Syncope with cardiac disorders
   - Heart block (Adams-Stokes syndrome)
   - Paroxysmal tachycardia
   - Coronary insufficiency and myocardial infarction
   - Aortic stenosis and insufficiency
   - Congenital heart disease

c) Syncope with respiratory and pulmonary disorders
   - Hyperventilation
   - Breathholding
   - Laryngeal syncope
   - Cough syncope
   - Sneezing
   - Valsalva
   - Pulmonary hypertension, pulmonary embolism

d) Syncope with cerebrovascular disorders
   - chiefly due to vertebro-basilar artery insufficiency

e) Fainting of primary psychic origin
   - Conversion hysteria
   - Acute stress
   - Neuroses and psychoses

The *vasodepressor type of syncope* has also been termed *vasovagal* because of prominent vagotonic mechanisms. Venipuncture, the sight of blood, minor injuries or the receipt of frightening news are some of the triggering factors. Muscle weakness, epigastric discomfort, sweating, nausea, restlessness, facial pallor, sighing, respiration and yawning are the earliest symptoms (Engel, 1962). This may proceed to lightheadedness, blurring of vision and to sudden loss of consciousness with muscular hypotonia and falling to the ground. In attacks exceeding 15 to 20 seconds duration, irregular clonic movements are likely to occur (Engel, 1962) According to Naquet and Vigouroux (1972), however, a special type of *convulsive syncope* is characterized by a tonic spasm occurring 2 to 3 seconds after the faint. The spasm is usually followed, by one or two generalized jerks. This convulsive type of syncope is more likely to occur in attacks with transient asystolia.

Gastaut and his co-workers (Gastaut and Gastaut, 1957; Gastaut, 1958; Naquet and Bostem, 1964) have stressed the non-epileptic character of syncopal attacks with convulsive movements. The studies of Hann and Franke (1953), Low et al. (1955), Broser (1958) and Durst and Krump (1959) have also shed more light on this subject.

A combined vasodepressor orthostatic type of syncope may occur in male patients during nocturnal urination; these attacks have been termed *micturition syncope* (Gastaut and Gastaut, 1956; Eberhart and Morgan, 1960; Lyle et al., 1961; Lukash et al., 1964; Donker et al., 1972). These patients are otherwise in good health like many other sufferers from vasovagal attacks.

Special vasodepressor mechanisms are involved in the *syncope associated with hypersensitivity of the carotid sinus* in which a cardio-inhibitory component leads to asystolia (Ferris, 1935; Weiss et al., 1936). Elderly and quite obviously severely arteriosclerotic patients are occasionally referred for an EEG because of "frequent minor epileptic attacks" or, even worse, *petit mal;* EKG monitoring with the electroencephalogram showing good evidence of subclinical or clinical *Adams-Stokes attacks.* Both carotid sinus hypersensitivity and Adams-Stokes attacks may present themselves as convulsive syncope.

In *congential heart disease,* syncopal attacks are common but epileptic seizures may also occur (Tyler and Clark, 1958; Kalyanaraman et al., 1968). Syncope, breathholding spells and also true grand mal convulsions may occur in children with *familial dysautonomia* (*Riley-Day's disease*) (Niedermeyer et al., 1967).

Breathholding spells are related to the syncopal attacks and frequently observed in older infants and small children. Emotional stress and crying provokes these attacks which have been divided into pale and cyanotic types (Lombroso and Lerman, 1967; Gastaut, 1968). The precise underlying pathophysiological mechanisms are complex and not fully understood. These children have almost always normal EEG tracings in the interval. Livingston (1972) has been impressed with the high incidence of familial occurrence. Pathophysiologically poorly understood are "*apneic seizures*" of infancy (Hooshmand, 1972) with a possible epileptic mechanism and a therapeutic response to atropine.

3) Attacks caused by sudden changes of blood chemistry

a) HYPOGLYCEMIA. The symptomatology of the hypoglycemic attack is characterized by sweating, jitteriness, tremulousness, nervousness, irritability, imperative hunger, mental fatigue, muscular weakness and, less commonly, headaches, nausea and vomiting. The clinical symptoms and signs are the same regardless of the underlying cause (Fajans and Thorn, 1966). According to these authors, hypoglycemias are classified as follows:

Organic hypoglycemia
- Pancreatic islet cell tumor, functioning
- Non-pancreatic tumors associated with hypoglycemia
- Anterior pituitary hypofunction
- Adrenocortical hypofunction
- Acquired extensive liver disease

Hypoglycemia due to specific hepatic enzyme defects
- Glycogen storage disease
- Hereditary fructose intolerance
- Galactosemia
- Familial fructose and galactose intolerance

Functional hypoglycemia
- Reactive functional (postprandial hypoglycemia)
- Reactive secondary to mild diabetes
- Alimentary hypoglycemia (after gastroenterostomy, subtotal gastrectomy)
- "Idiopathic hypoglycemia" of infancy and childhood
- Alcoholism and poor nutrition

Exogenous hypoglycemia (due to insulin or sulfonylurea compounds)
- Iatrogenic
- Factitious

Hypoglycemia may secondarily trigger a grand mal attack if the biochemical alteration is potent enough to lower the level of consciousness to a semicomatose state. The time honored Sakel-cure of schizophrenia with daily induction of insulin coma for several weeks provided abundant evidence for frequently intervening grand mal seizures in hypoglycemia (in otherwise non-epileptic individuals).

b) TETANIC ATTACKS. A low calcium blood level gives rise to increasing central and peripheral nervous system excitability. Tetany with typical carpopedal spasm may be caused by hypocalcemic states but may also occur in normocalcemic individuals with psychosomatic problems such as hyperventilation syndrome. The carpopedal spasm is probably a completely peripheral neuromuscular phenomenon triggered by hypocalcemic and/or alkalotic states. Epileptic seizures of the grand mal type may develop on the basis of severe hypocalcemia (see also Chapter 3).

c) OTHER HUMORAL CHANGES. In its early stages, the carcinoid syndrome with excess serotonin leads to short lasting attacks which gradually change into an almost permanent state. Bright red flushing starting in the face and neck, wheezing, tachycardia, colicky abdominal pain and diarrhea are the most common symptoms which bear some resemblance to the rare visceral manifestations of temporal lobe epilepsy.

4) Psychogenic seizures

a) MAJOR HYSTERICAL ATTACKS. A wild, disorderly sequence of tonic and clonic movements culminating in an impressive arching of the back used to be a rather frequent event in the 19th century when these attacks became the object of detailed descriptions. Occurring chiefly in females (exclusively in women according to archaic views), these spells have been psychodynamically interpreted as a conversion of repressed affect and sexual drive into a display of stormy motor activity with strong histrionic overtones. Victorian women used to be the most common victims of such hurricanes of emotion.

The classical hysterical attack with its rapidly changing scenery can be easily distinguished from a grand mal attack or a psychomotor automatism. But, alas, not all hysterical attacks are classical and problems of differential diagnosis are frequently encountered (Liske and Forster, 1964). The real difficulties start when one deals with a patient who has unequivocal evidence of epilepsy and additional hysterical manifestations. The *combination of epilepsy and hysteria* has been recently studied by Rabe (1970) on the basis of 41 observations and is thought to be not merely coincidental. The extensive study of Rosen and Walker (1963) on the use of hypnosis in patients with epileptic and hysterical seizures has stressed the difficulties of separating both groups. One could speculate that a poorly defined factor of "neuronal hyperexcitability" could favor both an epileptic condition and the lowered impulse control in hysteria.

It would be erroneous to assume that the "new freedom" of our days has radically eliminated hysterical attacks. This indicates that the socio-cultural aspect alone cannot account for the occurrence of hysteria. A more recent *combination of hysterical attacks and large dosages (or toxic levels) of anticonvulsive medication* has been reported by Niedermeyer et al (1970). Common daily stresses under slight drug-induced mental obtundation may lead to frustrational reactions and hysterical attacks. If not properly diagnosed, a vicious circle is inevitable when an increasing number of attacks is produced by an increasing amount of medication.

b) Other types of psychogenic spells. In addition to classical hysteria, neurotic mechanisms may subconsciously express themselves in a wide variety of ictal pictures. *Fainting, shaking and trembling,* mutism or complete *hysterical stupor* must be singled out as the most common types of reaction.

Hysterical stupor has to be diagnostically separated from ictal stupor (*petit mal status*) which is associated with constantly recurrent generalized seizure discharges in the EEG. Intravenous sodium amytal may terminate a psychogenic stupor with a strong emotional abreaction consisting of a tearful disclosure of the traumatizing event. Authentic post epileptic stupor may be followed by agitation and dangerous aggressiveness; this will be discussed in Chapter 11. The EEG is of little help in the post-convulsive stupor since low voltage tracings prevail and seizure discharges are mostly absent. The acute schizophrenic-catatonic stupor may also abruptly change into acute agitation.

Both post convulsive and catatonic stupor have become rare events in the past decade.

Psychogenic tremor has been observed chiefly in the male and especially in the stationary type of trench warfare in World War I.

5) Faked epileptic seizures

Malingering and the artful imitation of grand mal, focal motor and other epileptic seizures pose occasional problems of differential diagnosis and are more often encountered in times of war.

The most logical diagnostic approach appears to be electroencephalography, but one has to recall that a normal EEG does not rule out the presence of an epileptic seizure disorder. Activation tests such as pentylene-tetrazol (Metrazol) i.v. cannot clarify the issue. Certain neurological "tricks" and a solid psychological workup may be very helpful. The use of Erben's maneuvers (Erben, 1930) during a well played post-ictal coma may clearly demonstrate that the state of flaccid paralysis is no paralysis at all. A normal complexion (instead of initial pallor changing to cyanosis), presence of pupillary and deep tendon reflexes (usually suppressed in a grand mal) are suspect. An "ictal" EEG record is not easily obtained and may be just as artifact-obscured as a real ictal grand mal tracing (Fig. 38). Immediate quick post-ictal placement of a few electrodes and demonstration of a perfectly normal waking record after a seizure of supposedly grand mal character (within a few minutes after the attack) could help to provide evidence of the factitious nature. Well played focal motor attacks with Jacksonian march (which can be easily taught) cannot be clarified by EEG evidence and will necessitate a sequence of neuroradiological examinations unless a psychological or psychiatric workup reveals the phony character of the seizures.

Less skilled malingerers actively resist with squeezing when one tries to open the eyes in the postictal period. Active squeezing, however, frequently occurs in hysteria and other psychogenic attacks.

One has to keep in mind that malingering is a consciously and

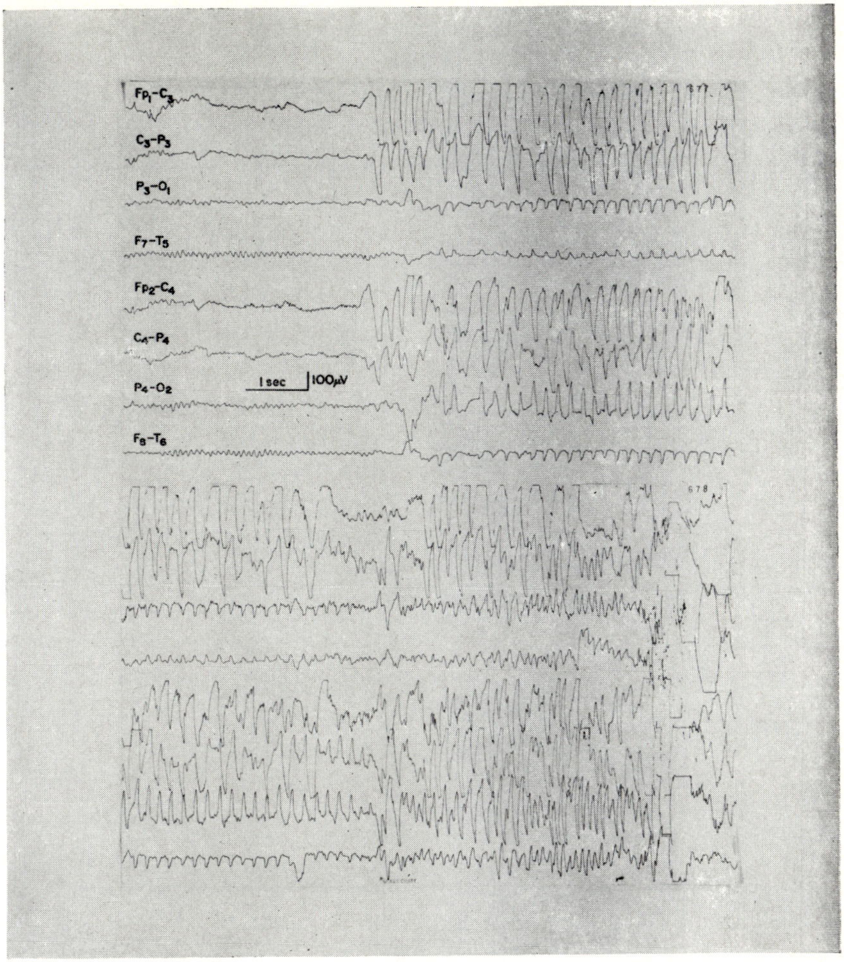

FIGURE 38. Factitious (faked) major convulsion with predominant clonic motor activity. This "attack" was willfully performed by one of our EEG technicians (a 22-year-old female with considerable histrionic talents). Note "pre-ictal" stretch with posterior alpha rhythm. All of the dramatic EEG changes are artifactual and due to movements.

hysteria a subconsciously controlled state. There is certainly a gray zone between both conditions; this bordering area is usually filled with individuals struggling for a compensation. This struggle may lead to a combination of conscious factitious and subconscious-neurotic elements. A final compensation payment of a lump sum often miraculously cures the ailment.

CHAPTER 11

PSYCHIATRIC IMPLICATIONS OF EPILEPSY

1) Introductory remarks

THE READER OF most of the European standard textbooks of psychiatry will find therein a chapter on epilepsy. The psychiatric aspects of the epilepsies were strongly emphasized and the psychiatrist dealt with epileptological problems more often than the neurologist. The reasons for this linkage of the epilepsies with psychiatry are multifold. The epilepsies were still veiled by a nebulous mysticism even in the mind of the otherwise scientifically oriented physician of the early twentieth century. Epilepsy was thought to be an incurable disease progressing into a state of dementia on a road marked by psychotic episodes. Generalizations used to be made from the severe forms to the entire domain since milder forms were not recognized as such or kept secret by the patient's family.

Moreover, the principles of anticonvulsive treament were not as widely known and anticonvulsants with little sleep-inducing side effects were still unknown. The clarification of the neurophysiological substratum of epileptic activity by means of electroencephalography started with the beginning of the middle third of this century.

This was the time of combined neuropsychiatric departments at major medical centers in many countries. The diagnostic workup of a presumed epileptic usually started in the psychiatric service where around the clock observation was possible. Everything was geared to the observation of a spontaneous seizure and the description by the witnessing attendant (frequently a poorly trained and inept person for this task) since the physician could hardly arrive in time. In general, that generation of neuropsychiatrists placed the greatest emphasis on the distinction between a grand mal and a psychogenic seizure. The symptomatology of psychomotor automatisms was already known to a few keen observers but most of this knowledge was buried in old journals and little use could be made of terms like "psychical equivalents."

My own neuropsychiatric training falls into the last segment of that period. This gave me the opportunity to witness the start of an impressive liberation of the epileptic. This favorable development has by-passed only a small minority of hopelessly intractable cases.

Ironically, after the gradual detachment of the epilepsies from psychiatry and the full recognition of neurological etiologies and neurophysiological substrata, psychiatry has recently made an active move in the direction of epileptology. This statement is made, of course, with some reservations since there is a considerable pluralism of psychiatric schools. The section of Chapter 5 dealing with temporal lobe epilepsy briefly discussed these recent developments. Some psychiatrists are seeking a reorientation along modern neurophysiological lines and have discovered temporal lobe epilepsy as a fascinating model bridging soma and mind. Others consider temporal lobe epilepsy and the limbic system the key for the understanding of violent crime. These recent trends and developments could become detrimental to Epileptology. Sober clinical and basic research must be the guideline instead of the presently "fashionable" indulgence in over simplified models of limbic neuronal circuitry.

The psychiatric aspects of epilepsy are best dealt with by a subdivision into ictal, post ictal and inter ictal psychical manifestations. Ictal events and personality traits should be separated; the former can lead to actions which are "out of character" and alien to the patient's mental and emotional makeup. There still remains the nagging question as to whether supposedly interictal events, such as an outburst of rage in an adolescent teased by his peers, are due to epileptic neuronal activity. Common sense must find the answer. There have always been irritable and thin skinned but essentially healthy individuals with a mildly lowered threshold of impulse control; hence, one does not have to conjure an epileptic mechanism for trivial and understandable human responses. If such an outburst, however, consists of senselessly beating, severely injuring or even killing a physically much weaker schoolmate, a serious impulse control problem is evident. Again, the question arises as to whether the brutal beating occurred during a seizure, i.e. in a state of a complete neurophysiological breakdown of inhibitory cerebral functions. Even in this case, an ictal event is very unlikely. It is often forgotten that most epileptics are brain-damaged to a smaller or larger extent. Irritability may be a prominent feature in an originally placid male adult who had a car accident with cerebral contusion a few years earlier. Let us assume that he never had seizures and that his EEG shows some residual local slowing but no seizure discharges whatsoever. This example indicates that *the underlying cerebral impairment may strongly determine a person's impulse control regardless of the presence or absence of epileptic seizures.*

Another often forgotten factor pertains to the *anticonvulsive therapy and its neuropharmacological effects.* In children, phenobarbital is notorious for the enormous degree of irritability which renders hyperkinetic children more restless than ever. This effect may occasionally exist in adults.

2) *Ictal psychical manifestations*

Changes of consciousness range from mild or moderate impairment (in petit mal, psychomotor seizures, certain adversive and other focal attacks) to the profound coma of the grand mal and have been the topic of preceding chapters. *Complex automatic behavior* and *experienced psychical phenomena* are almost entirely limited to the domain of temporal epilepsy (Chapter 5). Another important manifestation of abnormal ictal behavior falls into the category of *petit mal status* (or *ictal stupor*) presented in detail in Chapter 7.

The above description of temporal lobe epilepsy shows that

ictal aggression is an extremely rare event. The clumsiness of such an attack can hardly be exaggerated and physical damage is very seldom inflicted.

A rather violent ictal response in temporal lobe epileptics may be seen when pentylenetetrazol (Metrazol) is effectively used for the clinical electrical documentation of a seizure. Such responses are rare since this drug may be either ineffective or produce misleading responses such as generalized spike waves, immediate grand mal or a tonic type of attack attributed to the supplementary motor area (Ajmone, Marsan and Ralston, 1958). A *Metrazol-triggered psychomotor seizure, however, may be associated with some rage* necessitating restraining of the patient. This could be due to the most unpleasant experiences (e.g. sensations of imminent death) of the patient in the stage preceding the attack.

3) *Post-ictal manifestations*

The clinical and electrical recovery from a single grand mal convulsion usually occurs within 5 to 15 minutes; a post-convulsive sleep may ensue for a few hours. The restoration of cerebral activity may be delayed for hours and days in some cases; this prolongation of the post ictal state has become a very rare event in our days. *The post convulsive delirium has been the hallmark of a chronic and severely deteriorated epileptic;* better treatment has reduced the number of these patients who are mostly found in institutions for epileptics or chronic mental cases. In originally nonepileptic psychotics, repeated electrically-induced convulsions (electroshock treatment) may eventually lead to a post convulsive delirium.

This delirious state is characterized by dramatic outbursts of agitation with frequently repetitive acts of extremely violent aggression. Psychiatric attendants used to fear these aggressive acts far more than all other types of agitation occurring in catatonia, post traumatic syndromes, alcoholism and drug addiction. Punches are delivered with lightening like speed, well aimed and extremely effective (to make matters worse, most of these patients are strong male adults). A heavy object, if in reach, will be used for crushing and not infrequently fatal blows.

The underlying mechanism for this behavior lies in a *partial post-ictal recovery with persistent breakdown of higher cortical systems of inhibitory function.* The outbursts may occur intermittently while the patient was just quietly talking to the attendant or physician. Sudden pupillary dilatation is immediately followed by sitting up, jumping out of bed and deliverance of punches. There is reason to presume that the patient has sudden *threatening hallucinatory misperceptions* which makes him believe that he is being attacked.

When EEG studies can be carried out in this state, the record shows a rather ill-defined low voltage character with no categorical abnormalities and with notable absence of spikes. Anticonvulsants and strong sedatives or major tranquilizers are of little help and may make things worse. In psychiatric institutions, the termination of the post ictal delirium has sometimes been attempted by means of artificially induced convulsions (electroshock) with occasional success. The duration of 1 to 2 weeks is probably the time limit for postconvulsive delirium. In most cases, it is advisable to weather the storm by keeping the patient physically restrained without the use of larger amounts of anticonvulsants, hypnotics or tranquilizers.

Other manifestations of a post convulsive state may include exhibitionism or sexual aggression and are therefore of considerable medico-legal interest. It must be pointed out again that delirious or psychotic post convulsive states are uncommon. The expert physician in the courtroom must provide convincing evidence when he contends that an alleged crime was committed in a post ictal episode.

4) Inter-ictal psychical and behavioral changes

a) The "epileptic personality." The concept of specifically epileptic personality traits was strongly proposed by leading German psychiatric schools, especially prior to World War II. Sluggish mental processes affecting thoughts more than speech ("The epileptic thinks slower than he speaks"; Lange, 1936), perseverance in thought, speech and affect, lack of flexibility, adaptability and creativity as well as marked circumstantiality, pedantry and selfrighteousness were considered prominent features of the epileptic personality. Other authors, however, placed greater emphasis upon antisocial traits and the quick-tempered character of "the epileptic." According to Bumke (1942), these rather specific mental changes were indicative of "idiopathic" ("genuine") epilepsy whereas gradual non-specific mental deterioration and dementia would occur in both idiopathic and symptomatic forms of epilepsy.

This view was strongly opposed by psychodynamically oriented psychiatrists who felt that all of the above mentioned mental and behavioral changes were secondary responses of the patient to his disorder and the discriminating attitude of Society.

b) The role of the temporal lobe in the determination of epileptic personality changes. It has become evident that the slow, persevering and circumstantial epileptic is more likely to suffer from an acquired (rather than idiopathic) type of epilepsy and that the temporal lobe is mostly involved in such patients. Stauder (1936) associated the "enechetic" type of personality with processes of the temporal lobe (even prior to the use of the EEG); Gibbs, Gibbs and Fuster (1948) and also Gastaut (1953) provided EEG evidence for the linkage of personality changes and temporal lobe epilepsy. The "enechetic" or "viscous" type, however, was not the only one encountered in temporal lobe epilepsy since excessively impulsive and also schizoid or even frank schizophrenic patients were found in the sample.

We will discuss separately these different changes which have been associated with temporal lobe epilepsy.

c) The "slow" type of personality and temporal lobe epilepsy. Psychopathology has coined various terms for the sluggish, persevering, and circumstantial epileptic:

"glischroid" (Minkowska, 1923),
"enechetic" (Stauder, 1936),
"ixothymic," "ixoid" or "ixophrenic" (Strömgren, 1936),
"viscous" (Kretschmer, 1956).

These terms denote that the natural free flow of thought and affect is impeded and supplanted by stickiness or adhesiveness which is quite different from the apathetic emptiness seen in other rather non-specific cerebral syndromes.

This type of personality develops gradually and represents a mental change rather than a combination of true personality traits. Its association with pedantry renders history-taking a difficult task; the patient continuously sticks to trivial details which he describes with irritating accuracy while the physician is desperately pressing for essential information. His self-righteousness may be associated with an oily sanctimonious attitude paired with missionary zeal; such noisy and shallow religiousness, however, is less often seen in these days.

The "slow" type is the most commonly encountered type of personality change in temporal lobe epilepsy; this is in accordance with the findings of Gastaut (1953) and Bingley (1958) who also found minority subgroups of other personality types in this seizure disorder.

d) The irritable and aggressive type. The "hyperactive" type has been described by Gastaut et al. (1955) who considered "accelerated but imprecise" intellectual processes to be a major feature in this subgroup. This group would correspond with the antisocial and quick-tempered epileptic of the earlier literature. Serafetinides (1970) has linked aggressive behavior with dominant hemisphere involvement and hence with speech and memory impairment in temporal lobe epileptics.

The impulse control is insufficient in the aggressive subgroup and criminal acts may occur but are not particularly common. It was pointed out farther above that violent behavior in epileptics and especially in temporal lobe epileptics is most likely to be an inter ictal event; it is extremely seldom an act committed during seizures but it may occur (though very rarely in our days) in a very severe and dangerous form in the course of a prolonged post-ictal state.

The fallacy of equating aggressive behavior with temporal lobe epilepsy has been pointed out by Rodin (1972) on the basis of large samples of aggression prone individuals and temporal lobe epileptics (Fig. 39).

e) The schizoid and schizophrenic type. Schizoid per-

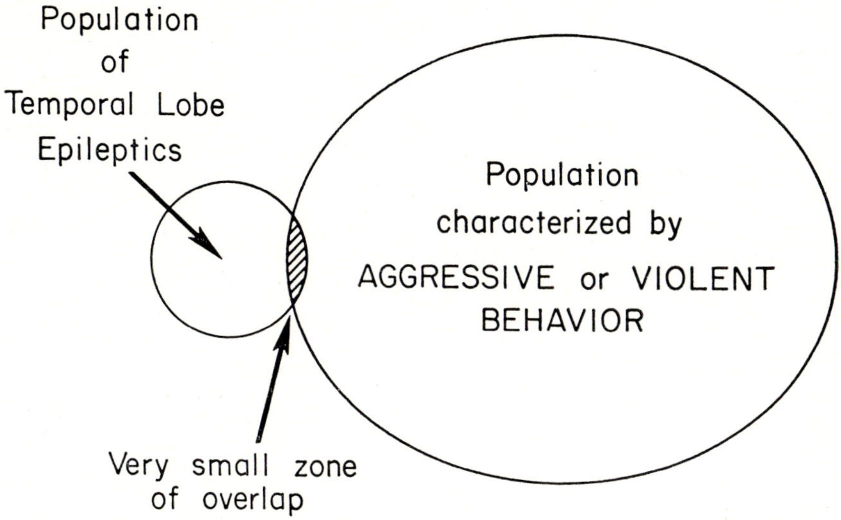

FIGURE 39. Schematic comparison of a basically "aggressive" population and a population of patients with temporal lobe epilepsy. Note the very small zone of overlap. This drawing could be bolstered by the data of Rodin (1972), which are even more restrictive (practically permitting no overlap whatsoever).

sonality traits have been frequently observed in patients with temporal lobe epilepsy (Gibbs and Gibbs, 1952; Hill, 1953; Ervin et al., 1955; Landolt, 1955; Rodin et al., 1957; Dongier, 1959/60; 1960, 1963; Flor-Henry, 1969). Some patients develop chronic schizophrenic psychotic states with paranoid hallucinatory symptomatology undistinguishable from "ordinary" schizophrenia. Attempts to demonstrate a basic temporal lobe (or limbic) disease in all forms of schizophrenia have failed to yield any convincing results. As a matter of fact, schizophrenia has remained an enigmatic disorder of ill-defined nosological outlines.

The occurrence of schizophrenia in temporal lobe epileptics cannot be explained on the basis of mere coincidence. In some patients, the psychosis tends to improve when the seizures are particularly frequent. This inverse relationship may lead to a seesaw like change from *predominant epileptic manifestations to a preponderance of the psychosis and vice versa.* Usually, these patients appear to be much better off when they suffer from frequent seizures; their affect is adequate and thought processes unimpeded by misperceptions and delusions. These seesaw like changes may occur in spontaneous rhythmicity, especially in patients recalcitrant to anticonvulsive medications; in other patients, a sharp increase of medication or starting a new anticonvulsant may bring forth temporary seizure-freedom at the price of a psychotic flare up.

Most of these patients find themselves in institutions for mental cases or chronic epileptics. Not all of these patients are temporal lobe epileptics and not all of the psychotic states are of schizophrenic character. The seesaw relationship can be seen in the EEG which may change rather abruptly from severe epileptic abnormalities to complete normalcy, with the swing toward temporary seizure-freedom and activiated psychosis ("forced normalization"; Landolt, 1955). This was further substantiated by Dongier (1959/60) and Flor-Henry (1969).

Surgical treatment with temporal lobectomy may have very beneficial effect on the seizure disorder whereas the co-existing schizophrenic psychosis tends to persist (Serafetinides and Falconer, 1962).

f) Nonschizophrenic psychotic states. Confusional states, twilight like interictal episodes and manic depressive manifestations are presumed to be more common in epilepsies with generalized seizure discharges rather than in temporal lobe epilepsy (Dongier, 1959/60; Flor-Henry, 1969). This is a comparatively small group and such samples can be studied effectively only in institutions. According to Bruens (1971), only 16 percent of the psychotic-epileptic material are not confined to the temporal lobe (from the EEG viewpoint).

A statistical analysis by Flor-Henry (1969) could shed some light on the laterality of temporal lobe foci and the type of psychosis. According to this investigator, epileptic involvement of the dominant temporal lobe is more likely to be associated with schizophrenic disturbances whereas the affection of the nondominant temporal lobe is more likely to be accompanied by manic-depressive changes.

g) FUGUES AND PORIOMANIA. Episodes of aimless wandering or apparently well organized travelling by car or public means of transportation may be carried out in a state of amnesia; this has been often attributed to epilepsy. Most of these attacks occur in nonepileptic persons and are most often due to dissociative states based on subconscious neurotic or hysterical mechanisms. Some of the episodes have been observed in epileptics but the ictal nature of such events is very doubtful. This has been pointed out in the discussion of temporal lobe epilepsy (Chapter 5).

h) SEXUAL DISTURBANCES. Global hyposexuality is a very common finding in temporal lobe epilepsy and occurs in the vast majority of these patients (Gastaut and Collomb, 1954; Gastaut, 1958; Blumer and Walker, 1967). The global character of the defect implies that there is loss of libido as well as potency; the frigidity of female patients reaches the degree of total sexual "anesthesia."

This finding stands in stark contrast to states of hypersexuality reported in other, nonepileptic temporal lobe diseases such as temporal lobe tumors (Van Reeth et al., 1958). Destructive processes of the temporal lobe in man has been conceived as analogous to the *Klüver-Bucy syndrome*, produced in monkeys by bilateral temporal lobectomy. These animals became extremely hypersexual after the experimental ablation; this was associated with docility, gross memory deficits for visual perceived signals (psychic blindness), marked oral tendencies and hypermetamorphosis (an excessive tendency to take notice of all stimuli in sight).

There is reason to presume that the irritable, mentally sluggish and hyposexual temporal lobe epileptic represents a diametrically opposed picture and one could further argue that the irritative epileptogenic involvement of the temporal lobe inverses the Klüver-Bucy syndrome which is based upon bilateral ablation or destruction of the temporal lobes. Hyposexuality may greatly improve with successful seizure control due to medication or temporal lobectomy.

i) SYNOPSIS. There is no evidence that an "epileptic personality" exists. Personality changes attributed to epilepsy in general are mostly confined to temporal lobe epilepsy. Some of these mental and behavioral changes can be understood in the light of experimental data obtained in studies of the limbic portion of the temporal lobe.

Irritability and hyposexuality are the most common behavioral deviations in temporal lobe epilepsy; the former may lead to acts of aggression due to interictal impulse control problems; we have stressed before the rarity of ictal aggression. In smaller subgroups of temporal lobe epileptics, difficulties of impulse control stand clearly in the foreground while another subgroup is characterized by schizoid changes or clear cut schizophrenic psychosis. Nonschizophrenic psychotic states are even less common and are seen either in epileptics outside the temporal lobe group or occasionally in temporal lobe epilepsy with involvement of the non-dominant side.

Chapter 12

ANTICONVULSIVE TREATMENT

1) Historical introductory remarks

THE MODERN ERA of anticonvulsive therapy began in 1857 with Locock's incidental observation of the seizure-reducing effect of *potassium bromide*. This effect was confirmed in Clouston's study (1868); further details have been presented by Tower (1960). Toxic effects became obvious in 4 of Clouston's 29 patients, when the daily dosage was gradually increased to an amount of 150 grains (9.6 gm). Grand mal and focal seizures were most responsive to this treatment.

Perhaps the most important step forward was made in 1912 when Loewe, Juliusburger and Impens independently introduced *phenobarbital* into therapy; in the same year, Hauptmann made the first clinical observation of the excellent anticonvulsive effect of this drug in epileptic patients. Again, grand mal, focal motor and other focal attacks derived the greatest benefit from this drug which gradually supplanted potassium bromide because of greater effectiveness and safety. Its side effects proved to be essentially harmless but its hypnotic component induced variable degrees of drowsiness and sleepiness. *Petit mal* and psychomotor seizures showed little or no response to the drug.

After 20 years of stagnation, attempts aiming at a non-hypnotic anticonvulsant resulted in the introduction of *mephobarbital* in Germany (Prominal®, marketed in this country as Mebaral®, 1935). Its anticonvulsive effect was somewhat similar to phenobarbital but in spite of its reduced hypnotic properties, this drug never found general acclaim. Further investigative work concentrated on the *hydantoines.* One derivative was already used in Germany during the thirties (Nirvanol®) for the treatment of Sydenham's chorea. *Diphenylhydantoin* was synthetized 1908 by Biltz; its anticonvulsive effect was described by Merritt and Putnam (1938) and the drug subsequently was marketed as Dilantin®. Its range of action is similar in many respects to phenobarbital with predominant effectiveness against grand mal and focal cortical seizures although, in a broader sense, some of its action might even exceed the limits of epilepsy due to more global effects on excitable membranes.

With the introduction of diphenylhydantoin, the search for an anticonvulsant with minimal or negligible hypnotic side effects had come to an end. In the foreground of further experimental studies stood the investigation of drugs with special therapeutic action on petit mal and psychomotor seizures.

These efforts prompted the introduction of *oxazolidinediones,* which proved to be specifically effective against *petit mal* absence. *Trimethadione* was synthetized by Spielman (1944); its anticonvulsive effect was demonstrated by Lennox (1945), Perlstein and Andelman (1946) as well as Richards and Everett (1946). The impressive narrow-range efficacy of the drug (virtually limited to classical petit mal) was marred by a particularly high incidence of undesirable side-effects with dangerous toxicity to the bone marrow. Among subsequently studied further derivatives of the diones, *paramethadione* (Paradione) proved to have the same anti-*petit mal*-effect as trimethadione with slightly less toxicity. Studies of other potential specific drugs for petit mal absences were carried out with *succinimides by* Miller et al. (1951, 1953) in the Parke-Davis laboratories and Zimmerman (1951) demonstrated favorable clinical results *phensuximide* (Milontin®) and *methsuximide* (Celontin) were subsequently introduced but their effectiveness in petit mal was eventually superseded by *ethosuximide* (Zarontin) after the first clinical reports of Vossen (1958) as well as Zimmerman and Burgemeister (1958). Because of lesser toxicity, ethosuximide has widely supplanted the oxazolidinediones in the treatment of *petit mal.*

During the same period, potentially effective substances against psychomotor seizures were under investigation. *Phenacemide* (Phenurone) was introduced by Gibbs, Everett and Richards (1949) and found to be effective in patients with temporal lobe automatisms unresponsive to other anticonvulsants. This potent drug, however, is seldom used in these days because of serious toxicity. *Primidone* (Mysoline), a desoxybarbiturate, was synthetized by Bogue and Carrington (1949) and reported as an effective anticonvulsant by Handley and Stewart (1952). Although closely related (and, as we will see later, metabolically partially broken down) to phenobarbital, its clinical effect has been thought to include psychomotor seizures. Such an additional special action against psychomotor seizures was also ascribed to the above mentioned methsuximide (Celontin).

Further anticonvulsants were studied in view of a possible specific effect on psychomotor seizures in temporal lobe epilepsy. *Sulthiame* (marketed as Ospolot in Germany) a derivative of the sulfonamides, was first thought to be a potent anticonvulsive drug in the treatment of various types of seizures and especially temporal lobe epilepsy (Engelmeier, 1960; Flügel et al., 1960; Raffauf, 1960) but such favorable initial reports could not be confirmed in further investigations (Fenton et al., 1964; Gordon, 1964). This drug has not been marketed in the United States.

Carbamazepine (Tegretol) was developed in the Geigy laboratories concurrently with studies of antihistaminic drugs which prompted the introduction of imipramin (Tofranil®) as an antidepressant psychopharmacon. Blom (1962) reported good results in the treatment of trigeminal neuralgia (*tic douloureux*) with carbamazepine; its antiepileptic action was reported following clinical trials by Bonduelle et al. (1962), Lorgé (1963), Müller (1963), Pakesch (1963), Tchicaloff and Pennetti (1963), Jongmans (1964) and Hagen and Richter (1964). This drug has found wide acclaim as the most effective medication for temporal lobe epilepsy. In spite of very good results obtained by Livingston et al. (1967), carbamazepine is available in the United States only for the treatment of trigeminal neuralgia and not for anticonvulsive purposes.

This historical review of modern antiepileptic drug therapy must be supplemented with a few words on drugs with a secondary anticonvulsive effect of limited range. Some of these *adjunctive anticonvulsants* have yielded very remarkable results when appropriately used.

The treatment of infantile spasms (hypsarhrhythmia) is practically dependent on the favorable action of such adjunctive antiepileptic drugs. The introduction of *ACTH* for the treatment of infantile spasms by Sorel and Dusaucy-Bauloye (1958) represents a milestone in epileptology. Its remarkable effect may also be obtained by *corticosteroids.*

Diazepam (Valium), a benzodiazepine, has advanced from a tranquilizer to an anticonvulsive drug of limited but well delineated range; its excellent effect in status epilepticus (Naquet et al., 1965) and especially in early stages of a status was pointed out in Chapter 7. It was also shown (Chapter 4) that some effectiveness has been ascribed to this drug in the treatment of seizures occurring in the extremely recalcitrant Lennox-Gastaut syndrome (Gastaut et al., 1966). *Nitrazepam* (Mogadon) is another benzodiazepine and has been widely used in the treatment of infantile spasms. In spite of encouraging reports of Liske and Forster (1963) and several other investigators, this drug has not been marketed in the United States.

We will bypass in this review the use of various other adjuncts of anticonvulsive treatment such as dehydrating agents and sympatho-mimetic energizers which will be discussed farther below.

In general, these historical data show that a certain plateau has been reached after a fifteen year period, from the late thirties to the early fifties, characterized by exciting advances in the field. The pace has definitely slowed down since. It is also somewhat embarrassing for America's Epileptology to see that the momentum in the field has completely shifted to the European countries. This has occurred in spite of the fact that perhaps the most active group of investigators in the pharmacology of anticonvulsants are carrying out their work in Salt Lake City, Utah, under the leadership of L. S. Goodman and D. Woodbury. This discrepancy is obviously due to bureaucratic chains; a heavy and partly necessary burden in these days of over indulgence in drugs and in view of our recent knowledge of unexpected long-range effects of new medications.

2) *Barbiturates*

Barbiturates are compounded of malonyl (Form 1), urea (Form 2) forming barbiturate (Form 3) which represents barbiturate with 3 radicals R_1, R_2 and R_3. The differences

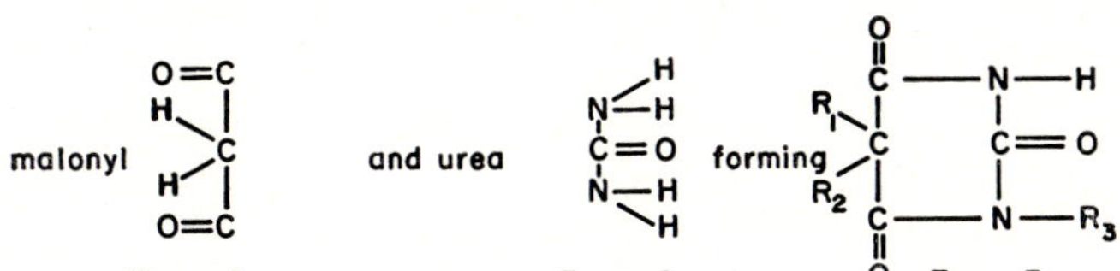

Form. 1 Form. 2 Form. 3

between the three barbiturates with anticonvulsive action (phenobarbital, mephobarbital and metharbital) are based on the following different radicals (after Bush and Sanders-Bush, 1972):

	R_1	R_2	R_3
N-methyl-phenobarbital	C_6H_5	C_2H_5	CH_3
Phenobarbital	C_6H_5	C_2H_5	H
(Mephobarbital, Mebaral®)			
N-methyl-barbital	C_2H_5	C_2H_5	CH_3
(Metharbital, Gemonil©)			

Phenobarbital

(Form 4).

Since its introduction (1912), phenobarbital has been one of the most widely used anticonvulsants. It is probably the safest of all anticonvulsants and it is inexpensive. Its anticonvulsive action is directed chiefly against grand mal and focal seizures; it is moderately helpful in the treatment of psychomotor seizures

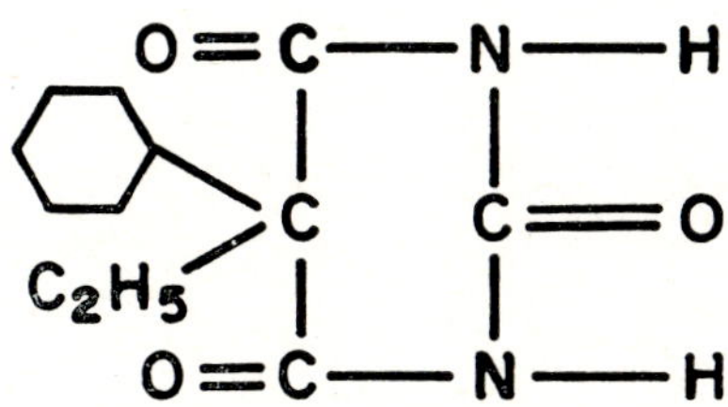

Form. 4

and of little or just temporary use in the therapy of *petit mal.*

The anticonvulsive action of phenobarbital is thought to be "multiple and non-selective" (D. Woodbury, 1969) and may primarily affect the neural synapse (Schmidt and Wilder, 1968). Its *absorption* in the gastro-intestinal tract is slow; maximal serum levels are reached after 10 to 12 hours; maximal brain concentration occurs after 10 to 15 hours (Domek et al., 1960).

Phenobarbital is slowly metabolized and slowly excreted in the urine. The drug disappears at a rate of 11 to 27 percent per day; the corresponding range of half-life is 53 to 140 hours (Maynert, 1972). The metabolic breakdown occurs in the liver largely by oxidation of the ethyl- and phenyl-radicals. About 30 percent of phenobarbital is excreted unchanged in the urine.

The dosage of phenobarbital lies in the range of 1 to 3 mg/kg/day. The most common starting dosage for adults is approximately 100 mg (usually 32 mg three times daily). A daily total of 300 mg should not be exceeded. The degree of drug-induced somnolence shows fairly marked inter individuals variations and may serve as a guide line in the determination of the long range dosage. According to Svensmark and Buchthal (1963), there is a low concentration of the drug in fat tissue; this has to be taken into account when phenobarbital is administered to obese individuals.

Initial amounts for children vary from 30 to 60 mg/day; newborns and infants receive amounts ranging from 15 to 30 mg. Livingston (1972) advocates the tablet form rather than the liquid form (phenobarbital elixir) which is more expensive.

The *intramuscular route* using soluble salts of phenobarbital is safe; *intravenous administration* does not offer any advantages (for instance in status epilepticus) and may lead to undesirable effects.

Therapeutic *levels of serum concentration* lie between 1 to 4 mg/100 ml (10-40 mcg/ml) with a safe average range of 1 to 2 mg/100 ml. According to Svensmark and Buchthal (1964), these levels are usually obtained after 2 to 3 weeks with a daily intake of 1 to 2 mg/kg. Toxicity develops with a serum concentration of more than 5 mg/100 ml but this is subject to inter-individual variations.

Side effects of long-term use are "minimal when one considers the prevalence of its use" (Livingston, 1972). Drowsiness is by far the most common untoward reaction which may necessitate a change of therapy. The wisdom of counteracting somnolence by the administration of amphetamines or Ritalin® is dubious since harmful interactions could develop. *Hyperactivity and irritability* is a very common reaction to phenobarbital in children. Skin rashes of urticarial or morbilliform character are rare. In a very rare *phenobarbital sensitivity-syndrome* (McGeachy and Bloomer, 1953), true idiosyncrasy to the drug causes high fever, mental confusion and toxic damage to various organs. A seldom discussed side-effect is impotence in the male. Such patients may come to the doctor's office angrily asking for another medication but concealing the cause of their dismay; they are very grateful for the physician's understanding. These cases require change of medication.

Phenobarbital toxicity leads to increasing lethargy associated with irritability. Slurred speech, gait incoordination and nystagmus are the most common neurological signs. The electroencephalogram shows considerable admixture of fast activity, mostly in the range of 18 to 25 sec. *Acute poisoning* cannot be discussed in the frame of this book; it has to be dealt with in the intensive care unit. It is very important to keep in mind that the elimination of phenobarbital from tissues is enhanced by alkalosis and especially by the administration of sodium bicarbonate.

Acute withdrawal of phenobarbital in long-term treatment leads to an increase of EEG abnormalities and may give rise to a flare-up of clinical seizures or even status epilepticus. Such an increase of seizure activity is not very common because of the slow rate of metabolism and elimination.

Supply

(after Livingston, 1972)

Phenobarbital Tablets—16 mg.
Phenobarbital Tablets—32 mg.
Phenobarbital Tablets—65 mg.
Phenobarbital Tablets—100 mg.

Phenobarbital Elixir, U.S.P.—20 mg/5 cc (teaspoonful)
Phenobarbital Sodium Sterile Powder—Ampul—120 mg in propylene glycol
Barba-Niacin Tablets—a combination of phenobarbital ½ gr and niacin ¼ gr—scored tablet
Barba-Niacin Forte Tablets—a combination of phenobarbital 1½ gr and niacin ¾ gr—scored tablet
Eskabarb Spansule Capsules—65 mg phenobarbital
Eskabarb Spansule Capsules—97 mg phenobarbital
Luminal Elixir—20 mg phenobarbital/5 cc (teaspoonful)
Luminal Ovoids—16 mg phenobarbital—yellow
Luminal Ovoids—32 mg phenobarbital—light green
Luminal Ovoids—100 mg phenobarbital—dark green
Luminal Sodium Hypodermic Tablets—60 mg phenobarbital sodium
Luminal Sodium Ampul—Powder—130 mg
Luminal Sodium Ampul—Powder—320 mg
Luminal Sodium Solution for Injection—1 cc Ampuls—130 mg—in a special vehicle
Luminal Sodium Solution for Injection—2 cc Ampuls—320 mg—in a special vehicle
Luminal Sodium Solution for Injection—10 cc Vials—160 mg/cc—in a special vehicle
Stental Extentabs—48.6 mg phenobarbital—light pink, coated extended action tablet

Mephobarbital

(Form 5)

Mephobarbital (Mebaral) is less sedative than phenobarbital but is also considered less potent as an anticonvulsant. Major differences between both drugs cannot be expected since the methyl group is removed in the liver. According to Toman (1965), ". . . Mephobarbital is, for all practical purposes an expensive form of phenobarbital."

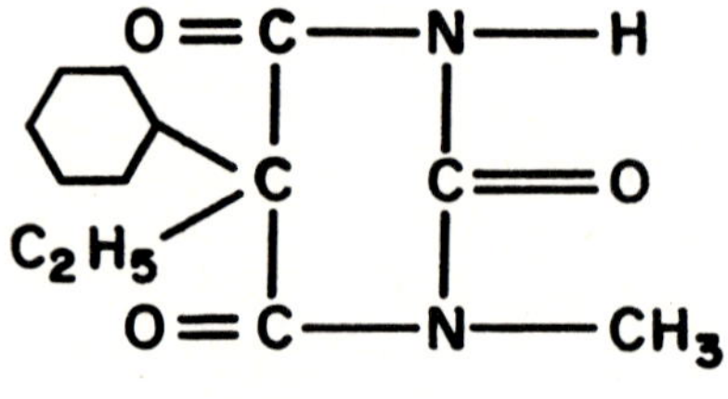

Form. 5

The *dosage* is about twice as high as the amounts of phenobarbital usually prescribed. Daily dosages in adults lie in the range from 200 mg to 600 mg. Mephobarbital is a safe drug; undesirable side-effects are even less common than in the treatment with phenobarbital since drowsiness plays a much lesser role. Livingston (1972) marvels about the very low barbiturate serum levels in patients receiving mephobarbital and hints that the metabolism might be more complex than has been thought.

This drug is not in wide use and its general acclaim is not enthusiastic.

Supply

(after Livingston, 1972)

Mebaral Tablets—32 mg—white tablet
Mebaral Tablets—50 mg—white tablet
Mebaral Tablets—100 mg—white tablet
Mebaral Tablets—200 mg—white tablet
Mebroin Tablets—a combination of Mebaral 90 mg and diphenylhydantoin 60 mg—peach-colored tablet

Metharbital

(Form 6)

Metharbital (Gemonil®) has been advocated by Perlstein (1950) for the treatment of childhood epilepsy and especially myoclonic forms of seizures. Peterman (1952) recommended this drug for the treatment of major convulsions. Other authors and especially Livingston (1972) have been much less favorably impressed. The drug is demethylated in the liver to barbital (Toman, 1965). Its *dosage* is similar to mephobarbital with amounts of 200 to 600 mg per day in divided dosages. Its *side effects* are scanty; drowsiness plays a major role.

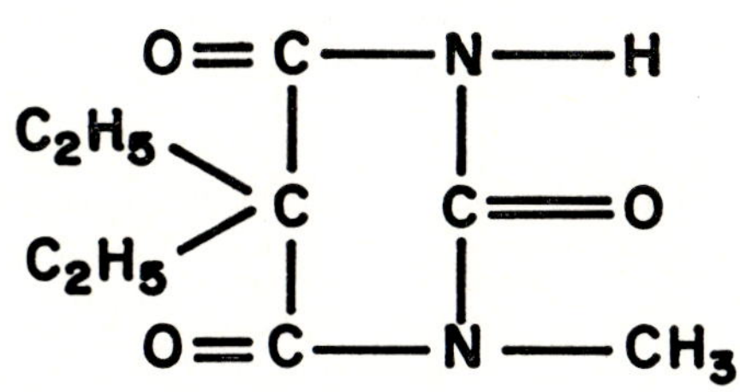

Form. 6

Supply

Gemonil Tablets—100 mg—white scored tablets

Primidone

(Form 7)

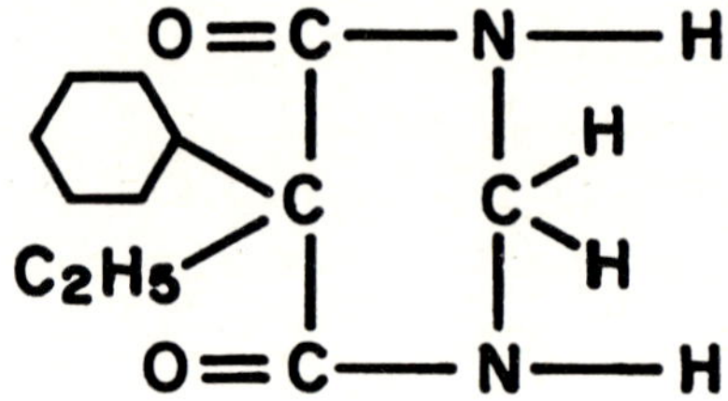

Form. 7

Primidone (Mysoline) is a desoxybarbiturate and has proved to be effective in the treatment of grand mal seizures (Handley and Stewart, 1952; Butler, 1953; Bonkalo and Arthurs, 1953; Doyle and Livingston, 1953); it has been successfully used in patients with major convulsions unresponsive to other medication. A good effect in psychomotor seizures was reported by Gibbs and Stamps (1958) and Lennox (1960).

The *absorption* rate of primidone is rather fast and in patients with long-term treatment, peak serum concentrations are reached 30 minutes after a single dose of 750 mg (Booker et al., 1970). In mice and rats, the electroconvulsive threshold is raised maximally after 3 to 6 hours (Goodman et al., 1953). The *metabolism* is somewhat complex; primidone is predominantly broken down to phenyl-ethyl-malonamide and phenobarbital, presumably as a function of hepatic enzyme activity (Gallagher and Baumel, 1972). According to Booker et al. (1970), phenobarbital cannot be detected in the serum of patients treated with primidone until at least 3 to 4 days after initiation of drug therapy. On the other hand, the primidone serum concentration is short lived with a half life of about 6 hours. About 20 percent of the primidone remains unchanged and can be found in the urine.

The average dosage for an adult is approximately 750 mg/day given in 3 single doses of 250 mg (about 10 mg/kg/day). Children receive daily amounts of 150 to 250 mg.

The therapeutic levels of *serum concentration* lie between 0.5 and 1.5 mg/100 (5-15 mcg/ml) as far as primidone itself is concerned. It becomes clear from what was said above that the serum concentration of phenobarbital as a metabolite is of great significance; these values may range from 1 to 4.5 mg/100 ml (10 to 45 mcg/ml). According to Gallagher and Baumel (1972), phenyl-ethyl-malonamide is not negligible as this metabolite of primidone treatment may act synergistically with phenobarbital; its serum concentration lies between 0.5 and 1 mg/100 ml.

Side effects of primidone are definitely more serious than those observed in the treatment with phenobarbital, mephobarbital and metharbital. *Most important is an excessive response to the very first tablet,* with lethargy or hypersomnia for up to 24 hours. This may or may not necessitate an immediate change of therapy. It is advisable for the physician to mention the possibility of such an overshooting response prior to the initiation of the treatment because a patient may resent the strong reaction to the drug or even lose his trust in his doctor. Dizziness, diplopia and ataxia may occasionally develop in the early stage of the treatment. Initial toxic effects are ascribable to primidone itself; later side effects are more likely to be due to a combined action with the metabolites. Livingston (1972) mentions gastrointestinal disturbances, sexual impotence, skin rashes and rare hemopoietic reactions.

It is obvious from the metabolic data that a combination of primidone and phenobarbital will lead to high phenobarbital serum levels which may well exceed the safe therapeutic range.

Supply

Mysoline Suspension—250 mg/5 cc (teaspoonful)—white
Mysoline tablets—50 mg—white tablet
Mysoline tablets—250 mg—white tablet

3) *Hydantoines*

(Form 8)

The hydantoines (hydantoinates) are chemically related to the barbiturates as far as the urea-component is concerned.

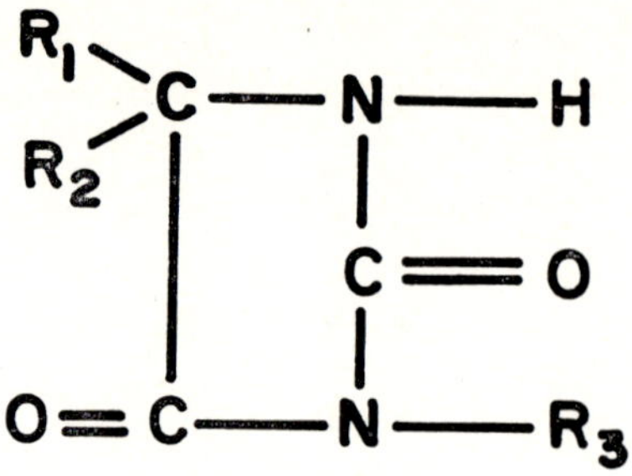

Form. 8

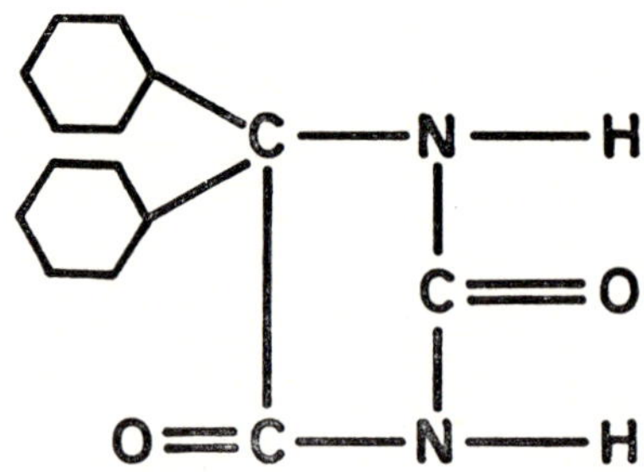

Form. 9

Diphenylhydantoin (DPH, phenytoin), marketed as Dilantin. (Form 9)

DPH was found to be the least hypnotic and most potent anticonvulsant among numerous potential antiepileptic drugs tested by Putnam and Merrit (1937) in cats subjected to electroconvulsions. Its efficacy in the treatment of epileptic patients was subsequently reported by Merrit and Putnam (1938), and over the ensuing 35 years, DPH has become one of the most commonly used anticonvulsive drugs, equalled or surpassed in use only by phenobarbital. *Its effect is directed chiefly against grand mal seizures* and, in this domain, it may be more potent than the barbiturates (when the effects of adequate and nontoxic dosages are compared). It is also valuable in the treatment of focal-cortical seizures but is much less effective against psychomotor and petit mal seizures.

The primary *neuropharmacological action* of DPH is the *stabilization of excitable membranes.* According to Morrell et al. (1958), DPH blocks repetitive firing of neurons triggered by single stimuli and it also prevents propagation of local firing. D. Woodbury (1955) demonstrated the effect of DPH on the cellular turnover of Na+ resulting in a decrease of intracellular Na+. The effect on excitable membranes (and also on subcellular structures) is widespread. It might be worthwhile to quote D. M. Woodbury and Swinyard (1972): ". . . the many sites at which DPH acts, called receptors, must be reached before its action takes place. This involves movement of DPH from the site of entrance into the body into the blood stream (absorption), distribution in the blood and extracellular fluids to the cell boundaries, passage across cell membranes into cells and across subcellular membranes into subcellular organelles. The amount of DPH that reaches the receptor and its duration of stay there depends on its rate of biotransformation and excretion from the body."

DPH is rapidly and passively absorbed across the intestinal mucosa in the non-ionized form but *absorption* is limited by its extremely slow solubility in gastrointestinal fluids. It is avidly bound to plasma proteins after entering the blood (D. M. Woodbury and Swinyard, 1972); its free form enters all tissues where it is firmly bound (at least in liver, brain and muscle). In the CNS, it has greater affinity to neuronal rather than to glial cellular structures (Yanagihara, 1972).

An important step in the *metabolism* of DPH is the *parahydroxylation* of one specific phenyl group (Butler, 1957) which is presumed to be carried out by a hepatic microsomal enzyme. According to Maynert (1960), the parahydroxylated product, 5-phenyl-5'-parahydroxy-phenylhydantoin (HPPH) lacks the pharmacological effects of DPH. After coupling with glucuronic acid or sulfate, it is excreted into the bile but mostly eliminated through the kidneys. Unmetabolized DPH is excreted in the urine in quantities of less than 5 percent whereas 60 to 70 percent of the daily intake of DPH is excreted in the urine as HPPH.

The *average dosage* customarily ranges from 4 to 8 mg/kg/

day. Thus, an adult of average weight receives usually 300 mg/day divided into 3 doses. Amounts of more than 400 mg/day are usually poorly tolerated and for this reason, a limitation of the average dosage of 4 to 6 mg/kg/day appears to be more realistic. Daily amounts of 100 to 200 mg are usually given in children. According to Wilder et al. (1972), the response to one single daily dose is equally effective as the divided administration.

The *intramuscular route* is surprisingly slower in its effect on the CNS than the oral administration (Dam and Olesen, 1966); this is due to poor water solubility. In spite of encouraging reports of a highly accelerated effect (Wallis et al., 1968), the intravenous route provides no further advantages and may lead to cardiac arrhythmias or fatal asystolia (Gellerman and Martinez, 1967; Goldschlager and Karliner, 1967; Unger and Sklaroff, 1967).

According to Svensmark et al. (1960), clinically effective *serum concentrations* are obtained within about one week; the serum levels range from 1 to 2 mg/100 ml (10-20 mcg/ml). According to Livingston (1972), there are inconsistent relationships between serum concentration, conventional dosage and seizure control whereas a good relationship exists between serum levels of DPH and signs of intoxication. Sudden withdrawal of DPH seems to have no seizure-enhancing effect. A defective parahydroxylation may lead to an enormous accumulation of DPH, signs of severe toxicity and serum levels of more than 10 mg/100 ml.

Interactions of DPH with other drugs have been recently reviewed by Kutt (1972); the often discussed phenobarbital-induced stimulation of the metabolic breakdown of DPH apparently plays no significant role in clinical treatment. An interaction with thyroid functions is important when the activity of this gland is clinically evaluated in patients taking DPH.

Side-effects of long-term use are not uncommon and rather important. Glaser (1972) has divided the manifestations of DPH toxicity into overdosage effects, probably hypersensitivity and other effects (see Table VII).

Leaving apart the acute symptomatology, the *chronic effects*

TABLE VII

DIPHENYLHYDANTOIN TOXICITY
(after Glaser, 1972)

A) *Effects of Overdosage.*
  Acute effects
    CNS (cerebello-vestibular, delirium), gastric distress
  Chronic effects
    Cerebello-vestibular syndrome
    Encephalogpathy with increased seizures, severe EEG changes, mental changes
    Peripheral neuropathy

B) *Probable hypersensitivity, "allergic" effects*
  Febrile responses with various dermatoses
  Erythema multiforme, Stevens-Johnson syndrome
  Lymphadenopathy, pseudolymphoma (? lymphoma)
  Acute systemic collagen disorder reactions (lupus erythematosus)
  Hepatitis
  Certain blood dyscrasias (neutropenia, agranulocytosis, aplastic anemia)

C) *Other effects.*
  Gum hyperplasia (effects in connective tissue)
  Megaloblastic anemia (folate deficiency)
  Endocrine effects (role in toxicity unclear)
    Adreno-cortical, pituitary
    Hirsutism in young females

on the CNS will be discussed first. The picture can be labelled as a *cerebellopontine syndrome with additional signs of diffuse toxic encephalopathy.* Ataxia, dysarthria, dizziness, vertigo and especially nystagmus are seen in association with behavioral and mental changes such as euphoria, depression, drowsiness, lethargy and general mental deterioration (Roseman, 1961). The EEG shows moderate to marked slowing; the alpha frequency gradually slows down into the theta range (below 7.5/sec) and high voltage 2 to 3/sec delta waves appear over anterior regions. These abnormally slow EEG tracings are usually remarkably free from seizure discharges but this is not always the case; return of clinical seizures and high voltage spiking has been reported by Levy and Fenichel (1965) in patients with severe DPH toxicity; one of the patients developed opisthotonic posture and even a focal (probably right parietal) syndrome developed on the top of diffuse encephalopathy (dense left hemianesthesia, mild left hemiparesis and distortion of body image). Utterback (1958) reported fatal status epilepticus grand mal in a patient with DPH toxicity; there was good neuropathological evidence of damage to Purkinje cells and granular cells in the cerebellum (this case is particularly important in view of other data stressing the role of cerebellar impairment in status epilepticus; see Chapter 7). The cerebellar pathology in patients receiving large amounts of DPH has been further substantiated by Hoffman (1958), Haberland (1962) and Dam (1970, 1972).

A reduction of the dosage will usually lead to disappearance of the neurological signs and symptoms; the toxic EEG changes require longer time for resolution. According to Buchthal et al. (1960) and Buchthal and Svensmark (1971), no severe side effects appear at serum levels below 3 mg/100 ml (30 mcg/ml) but Dam feels that nystagmus can materalize at 2 ml/100 ml, ataxia at 3 mg/100 ml and mental changes at levels about 4 mg/100 ml.

So-called "other effects" (see Table VII) are of great significance. *Gum hyperplasia* (gingival hypertrophy) is part of *the effect of DPH on connective tissue.* There is reason to presume that normal collagen catabolism is inhibited by DPH (Houck et al., 1972). This might be associated with an increase of keratinization of connective tissue and accumulation of large amounts of scleroproteins. Pituitary-adrenocortical mechanisms could also account for the effect of DPH on connective tissue (Bonnycastle and Bradley, 1960). More details on the nature and treatment of gingival hyperplasia have been given by Livingston (1972). The cosmetic and esthetic repercussions of this side-effect can become extremely severe and necessitate surgical removal of luxuriant gingiva.

Hypertrichosis or *hirsutism* are also common side effects observed in about 5 percent of patients treated with DPH (Livingston, 1972). True hirsutism implies a masculine distribution pattern while hypertrichosis simply indicates excessive growth of body hair. This disturbance is particularly embarrassing to young female patients who may even develop mustache-like hair growth. According to Livingston (1963, 1972), this is an irreversible disturbance which is unrelated to the dosage of DPH. Its detection in an early stage and subsequent change of medication will keep the hair growth in tolerable limits. One must therefore keep a watchful eye on this development, especially in girls between age 4 to 18 years.

Gastro-intestinal disturbances are usually more acute rather than chronic. Patients must be advised to take their first dosage during or after breakfast and not on empty stomach. *Dermatological effects* range from maculopapular or morbilliform rashes to purpura (thrombocytomgenic or non-thrombocytogenic) and exfoliative dermatitis. Simple rashes occur in about 10 percent of the patients (Livingston, 1972). The combination of exfoliative dermatitis and liver damage may prove to be fatal. Febrile responses have been observed and may be associated with lymphadenopathy; erythema multiforme and Stevens-Johnson syndrome are uncommon complications. Hematological changes are not very common (neutropenia, agranulocytosis, aplastic anemia), but it is worthwhile to perform blood count controls during the first months of treatment; all of these signs of hypersensitivity (rather than true toxicity) are most likely to occur during the first week after initiation of treatment.

Lupus erythematosus has been reported as a complication of DPH therapy (Rallison et al., 1961; Jacobs et al., 1963). This disease has also been ascribed to the use of other anticonvulsants (barbiturates, mephenytoin, ethosuximide, diones, carbamazepine) but the question arises as to whether the treated convulsions were nothing but the first manifestations of the connective tissue disease.

Whenever grand mal attacks occur in a diagnosed case of lupus erythematosus, phenobarbital might be preferable to DPH with its indubitable action on connective tissue.

Supply (after Livingston, 1972)

Dilantin Kapseals®—0.03 gm—hard capsule with pink band. Identification number—P-D 365

Dilantin Kapseals—0.1 gm—hard capsule with orange band. Identification number—P-D 362

Dilantin D.A. Kapseals—0.1 gm—hard special capsule formulated to delay release of contents; orange opaque band. Identification number—P-D 385

Dilantin in Oil Capsules—0.1 gm—in a vegetable oil; soluble gelatin capsule. Identification number—P-D 224

Dilantin Infatabs®—50 mg—triangular, grooved cream colored, flavored tablets. Identification number—P-D 007

Dilantin Steri-Vial®—100 mg, 250 mg—A 2.2 cc ampul of special solvent containing 40% propylene glycol and 10% alcohol in Water for Injection adjusted to pH 12 with sodium hydroxide is supplied with the 100 mg Steri-Vial; a 5.2 cc ampul of special solvent is supplied with the 250 mg Steri-Vial. The resultant solution prepared in the Steri-Vial contains Dilantin 50 mg/cc.

Dilantin—30 Suspension—30 mg/5 cc-flavored; red colored

Dilantin—125 Suspension—125 mg/5 cc-flavored; orange colored

Dilantin with Phenobarbital Kapseals—0.1 gm with phenobarbital 16 mg—hard capsule with garnet band. Identification number—P-D 375

Dilantin with Phenobarbital Kapseals—0.1 gm with phenobarbital 32 mg—hard capsule with black band. Identification number—P-D 531

Phelantin® Kayseals—Dilantin 100 mg with phenobarbital 30 mg and methamphetamine hydrochloride 2.5 mg—hard yellow capsule with transparent orange band. Identification number—P-D 394

***Mephenytoin* (*Mesantoin*®)**

(Form 10)

Mephenytoin is 5-ethyl-3-methyl-5 phenylhydantoin.

This substance was introduced by Loscalzo (1945) as an anticonvulsant with principal effect against grand mal convulsions. Its effect against other types of seizures is minimal or dubious.

The *dosage* is higher than that of DPH; Livingston (1972)

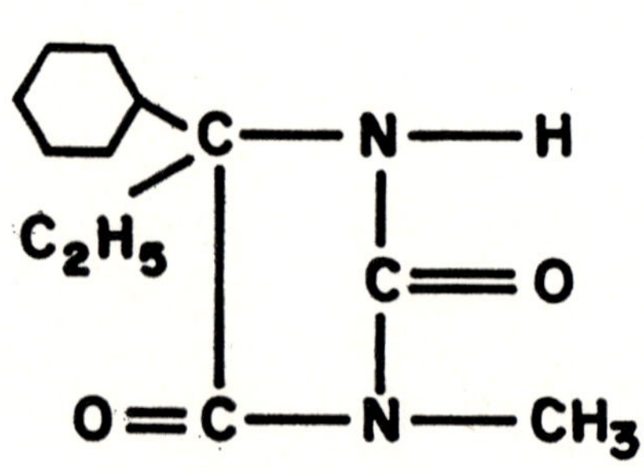

Form. 10

lists a maximum dosage of 600 mg/day for children and 1200 mg/day for adults. Neurotoxicity and gum hyperplasia are much less common in mephenytoin treatment when compared with DPH but *serious hematological changes* are a formidable drawback and fatalities have been frequently reported. Cutaneous side effects are similar to those observed with DPH therapy.

Because of the toxicity to the bone marrow, the use of this drug has become very limited; it should be used only in cases of proven unsatisfactory response to DPH and barbiturates. Its hematotoxicity may be due to its *metabolism* characterized by demethylation to 5, 5-ethylphenylhydantoin (nirvanol) which is evidently quite toxic.

For these reasons, the blood count has to be checked in regular intervals when mephenytoin is used.

Supply

Mesantoin Tablets—100 mg—pale pink color

Hydantal Tablets—a combination of Mesantoin 100 mg and phenobarbital 20 mg—glazed white tablet

***Ethotoin* (*Peganone*®)**

(Form 11)

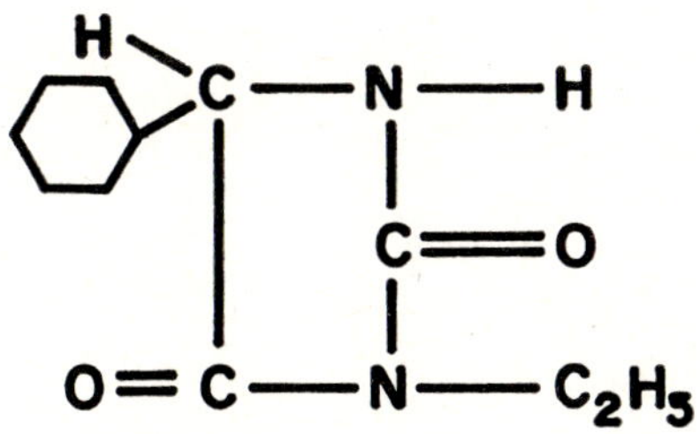

Form. 11

Ethotoin is 3-ethyl-5 phenylhydantoin

This drug was introduced by Schwade et al. (1956) and Livingston (1956) as an anticonvulsant which was found to be effective against grand mal and also, to some degree, against psychomotor seizures. Its anticonvulsive potency, however, is rather weak and, for this reason, dosages up to 4000 mg/day are required; amounts of 1500 to 2500 mg/day are average dosages for adults; children receive amounts of 500 to 1500 mg/day.

Ethotoin is a relatively safe drug; it does not give rise to gingival hyperplasia and to hypertrichosis; neurotoxic and hematological effects are uncommon (except for skin rashes) and usually not severe. According to Millichap (1972), it is probably the necessity for large doses which detracts from the practical value of the drug.

Supply

Peganone Tablets–250 mg–white, scored tablet
Peganone Tablets–500 mg–white, scored tablet

Albutoin is a further hydantoinate which has been introduced by Davis and Schwade (1959). This drug has *not been marketed thus far.* Daily dosages between 600 to 1200 mg are necessary for the treatment of major convulsions. The data of Cereghino et al. (1972) and their review of the literature are rather encouraging.

4) Acetylurea

Phenacemide (phenacetylurea, Phenurone)
(Form 12)

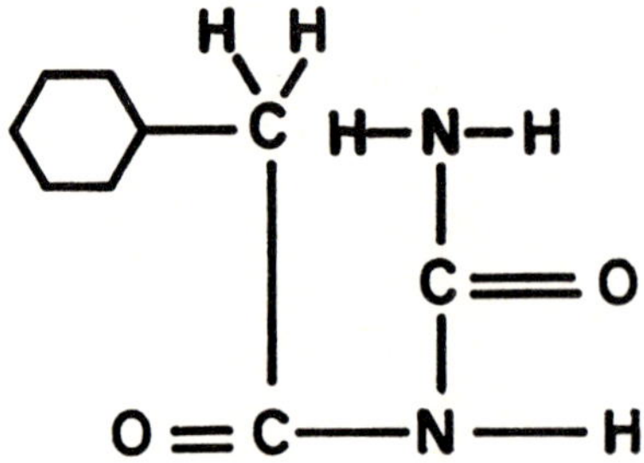

Form. 12

Phenacemide was introduced by Gibbs, Everett and Richards (1949) and was found to be particularly effective against psychomotor (temporal lobe) seizures. It is chemically characterized by an opening of the hydantoin ring structures:

Unfortunately, the toxic effects outweigh its anticonvulsive properties and the drug must be restricted to otherwise refractory cases of temporal lobe epilepsy (Forster, 1951; Livingston, 1972; Schmidt and Wilder, 1968).

The *dosage* ranges from 1000 to 6000 mg/day in adults and from 500 to 3000 mg/day in children (Livingston, 1972). *Toxic effects* are very common; fatalities have been reported from hematopoietic, hepatic and renal disturbances. Behavioral changes and acute psychosis have been observed.

Supply

Phenurone Tablets—500 mg—white tablets

5) Oxazolidinediones

The relationship of the oxazolidinediones to the other anticonvulsants is evidenced by their chemical structure. (Form 13)

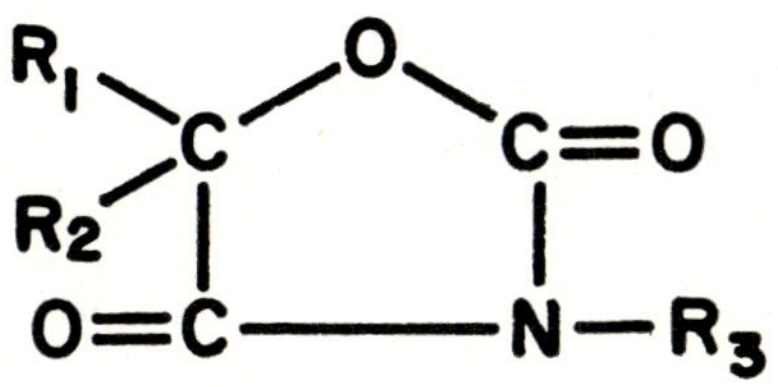

Form. 13

When we (according to Booker, 1972) consider (Form 14) the common element of the most frequently used anticonvulsants, the open ring of this joint structure may be closed as follows:

Barbiturates
(Form 15)
Hydantoins
(Form 16)

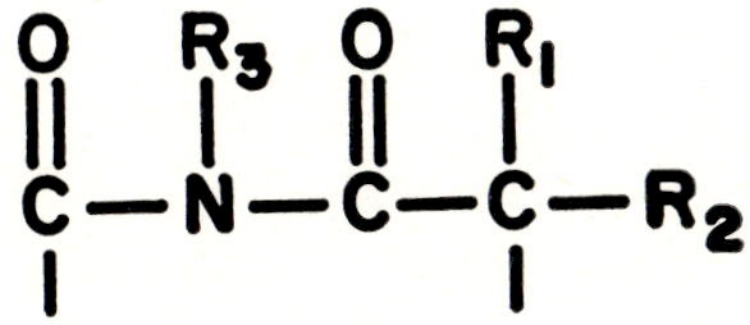

Form. 14

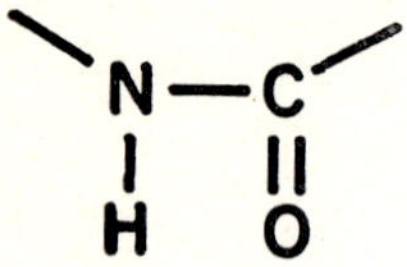

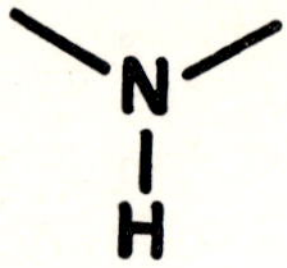

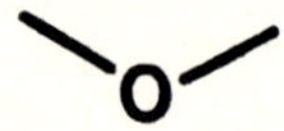

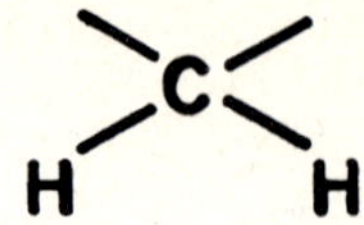

Form. 15 **Form. 16** **Form. 17** **Form. 18**

Oxazolidinediones
(Form 17)
Succinimides
(Form 18)

***Trimethadione* (*Tridione*)**
(Form 19)

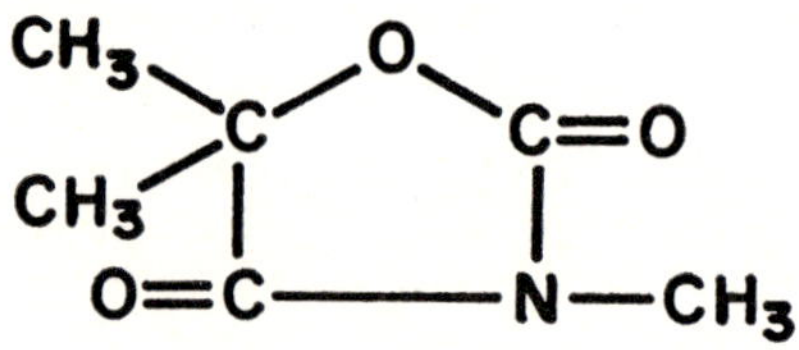

Form. 19

With 3 methyl groups in all radicals, trimethadione has the following structure:

After its introduction by Lennox (1945), this drug was generally recognized as the first anticonvulsant with *specific effect against petit mal absences.* It is obviously directed against generalized-synchronous seizure discharges and is presumed to block pentyleneterazol-induced seizures but, in clinical practice, there is no appreciable effect against grand mal attacks.

The neuronal action has been presumed to involve both inhibitory and excitatory transmission (Schmidt and Wilder, 1968); no general consensus has been reached in this respect.

According to Withrow and D. M. Woodbury (1972), trimethadione is *rapidly absorbed* in the gastrointestinal tract and quickly reaches the target organ in the course of its diffuse distribution. It is *metabolized* in the liver by means of demethylization to demethyl-oxazolidinedione which has slightly less anticonvulsive properities than trimethadione. This substance is slowly excreted in the urine.

The *dosage* ranges (according to Livingston, 1972) from 600 mg to 1800 mg/day in adults and older children and from 300 to 900 mg in children under age 6 years.

Undesirable side effects are common and sometimes serious. One of the earliest side effects after initiation of treatment is *photophobia,* which most often manifests itself as a glare experienced mainly when the patient steps out of a house into bright sun light. This disturbance probably affects the retinal level and is unrelated to the dosage; it is likely to be a hypersensitivity reaction which causes no permanent damage. Headache, diplopia, vertigo, irritability and drowsiness are less common and seen mostly when large amounts are taken. Hiccups may occur about 1 to 2 weeks after the start of treatment and usually disappear after a few days (Livingston, 1972). Dermatological reactions may occur, especially as morbilliform and urticarial rashes.

Severe renal complications have been reported; the nephrotic syndrome is in the foreground and fatalities have occurred. Most important is bone marrow toxicity leading to agranulocytosis, leukopenia, thrombocytopenia and aplastic anemia, occasionally with fatal outcome. These complications usually develop during the first year of treatment and most often during the first six months. *Blood count controls are mandatory* and should be performed in two week intervals during the first six months, later in gradually increasing intervals. Regular urinalysis is also recommended.

Supply

Tridione Capsules–300 mg–white capsule
Tridione Dulcet Tablets–150 mg–White aromatic capsule
Tridione Solution–150 mg/fl dr (3.7 ml)–aqueous, flavored, light orange color

Paramethadione (Paradione)

(Form 20)

Paramethadione was introduced by Davis and Lennox (1947) and has proved to be a very potent drug with specific effect

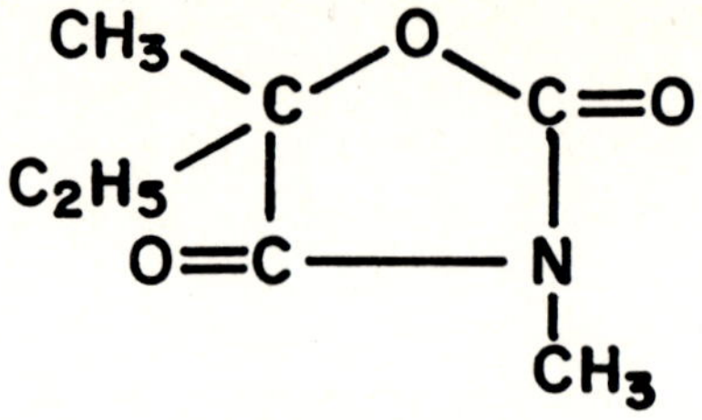

Form. 20

against *petit mal* absences. It is in most respect very similar to trimethadione but it appears to be somewhat less toxic. For this reason, Lennox (1960) considered it the treatment of choice in *petit mal* epilepsy.

Its *dosage* ranges from 600 to 1800 mg/day in older children and adults and from 300 to 900 mg/day in children below age 6 years. These are essentially the same amounts as in the treatment with trimethadione.

6) Succinimides

This group of anticonvulsants is based upon the following structure (Form 21):

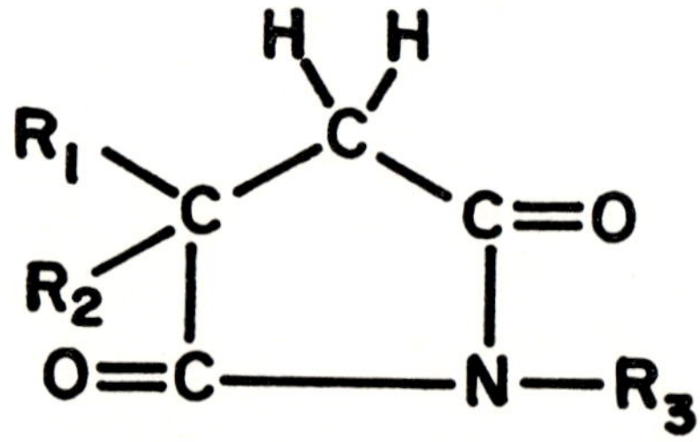

Form. 21

We will concentrate in the following on ethosuximide, the most recently introduced and most commonly used derivative; the earlier derivatives phensuximide and methsuximide will be mentioned in passing.

Phensuximide (Milontin)
(Form 22)

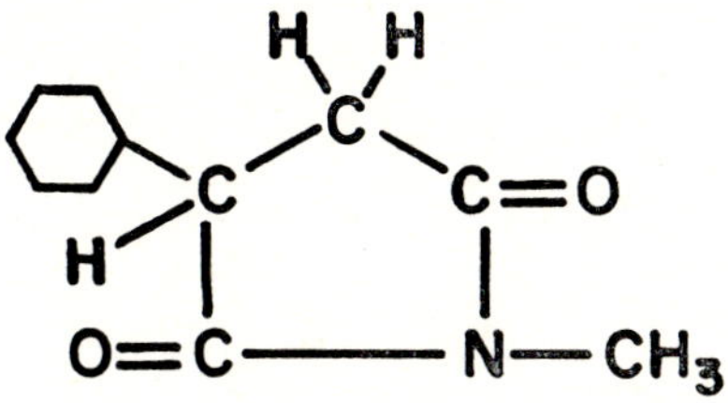

Form. 22

Phensuximide was introduced by Zimmerman (1951) and was subsequently used for the treatment of *petit mal* epilepsy but its use has been all but abandoned. It is the least effective of the succinimides presently in use. Side effects are common.

Methsuximide (Celontin)
(Form 23)

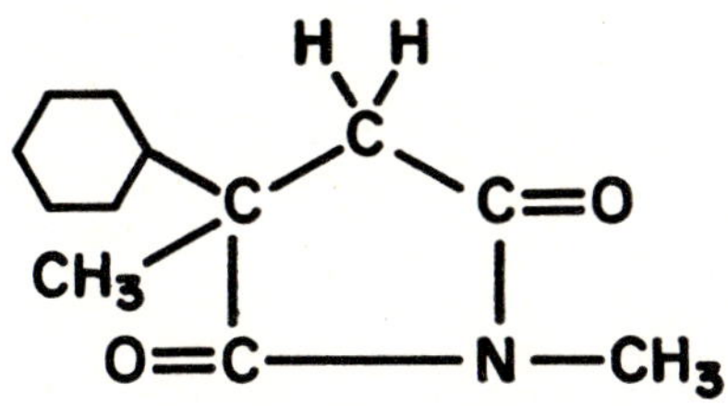

Form. 23

Methsuximide has proved to be effective against petit mal absences according to the first reports of Zimmerman (1951) and Zimmerman and Burgemeister (1954); this was confirmed by some other investigators (Vossen, 1958; Scholl et al, 1959; Trolle and Kiorboe, 1960). Some effect against psychomotor seizures has also been noted (Livingston and Pauli, 1957).

Marked drowsiness is the most commonly observed side effect and may spontaneously disappear without reduction of the dose (Livingston, 1972). Personality change, nausea, vomiting and rashes may develop; serious reactions are rare.

Supply

Celontin Kapseals (half strength)—150 mg—hard, yellow-tint capsule with brown opaque band

Celontin Kapseals—300 mg—hard, yellow-tint capsule with orange band

Ethosuximide (*Zarontin*)

(Form 24)

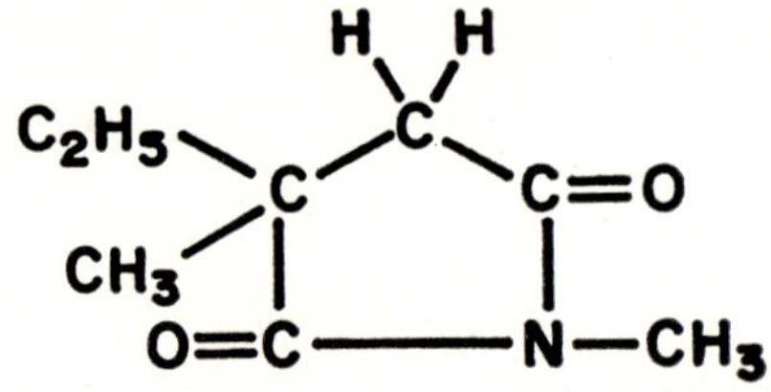

Form. 24

Ethosuximide was first presented as a new anticonvulsant with specific effect against petit mal by Zimmerman and Burgemeister (1958). Its efficacy and the moderate degree of untoward reactions were further elucidated by Vossen (1958), Sorel (1960), Lorentz de Haas and Stoel (1960), Lugaresi and Volterra (1960), Gordon (1961), Lossius (1961), Goldensohn et al. (1962), Livingston et al. (1962) and Kiorboe et al. (1964).

During the past 10 years, *ethosuximide has become the drug of choice in the treatment of petit mal absences.* Its effect against other types of seizure is probably negligible and, in order to prevent additional grand mal attacks in children with petit mal (see discussion of Common generalized epilepsy, Chapter 4), moderate amounts of phenobarbital should be added.

The neuronal action of the drug is poorly understood. Ethosuximide is rather quickly absorbed and peak concentrations in the serum are observed 1 to 3 hours after ingestion and a half-life time of 60 hours in the rhesus monkey has been reported (Dill et al., 1965; Chang et al., 1972); in man, half-life values of about 30 hours have been noted. The body distribution of the drug is diffuse the metabolic breakdown is not fully understood. About 20 percent of the ingested ethosuximide is found in the urine;

three different metabolites have been recently identified by Chang et al. (1972).

The optimum *dosage* must be determined empirically since there are no specific signs or symptoms indicative of overdosage (Livingston, 1972). The range lies between 750 to 2000 mg/day for adults, adolescents and children above age 6 and 500 to 1000 mg/day for children below this age. Because of the age determined character of petit mal, it will be seldom prescribed to adults (see Chapter 4 on common generalized epilepsy).

Therapeutic *plasma concentration levels* range from 1 to 5.5 mg/100 ml (10-55 mcg/ml) Haerer et al., 1970). *Untoward reactions* comprise nausea, hiccups, gastric distress, drowsiness, headaches and dizziness; these disturbances may necessitate permanent withdrawal. Severe bone marrow depression is very rare. Systemic lupus erythematosus has been reported by Livingston et al. (1968); this connective tissue disease has been occasionally observed during the treatment with other anticonvulsants and the primary causative effect of the drug may be debatable in such cases.

Supply

Zarontin Capsules—250 mg soluble gelatin capsule—orange color

Younger children may have difficulties swallowing these capsules and the availability of a more palatable liquid form—already used in other countries—is expected

7) Sulfonamides

Sulthiame (Ospolot) is chemically related to sulfanilamide as the following chemical structures show (Form 25, 26):

Sulfanilamide
(Form 25)
Sulthiame
(Form 26)

It was introduced in 1960 in Germany (see historical introductory remarks of this chapter) and favorable results have been reported in patients with psychomotor seizures (Engelmeier, 1960; Fenton et al., 1964); this was confirmed by Livingston et al. (1967).

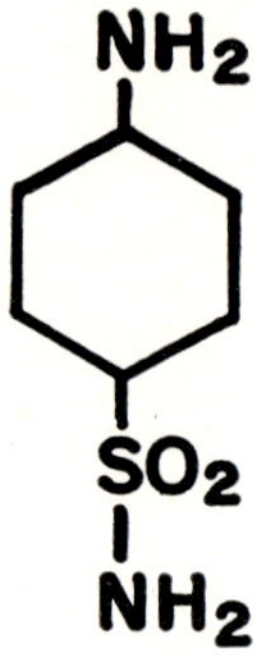

Form. 25

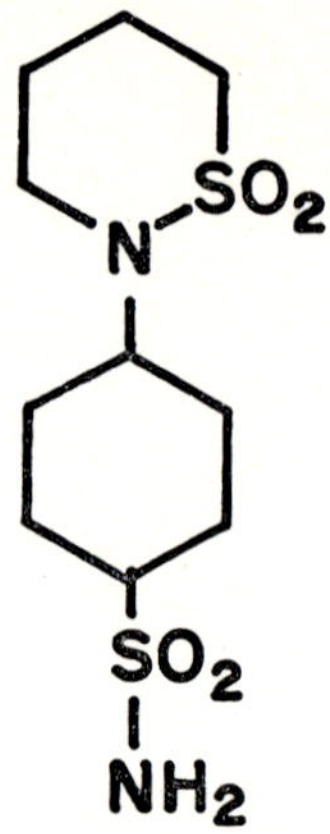

Form. 26

Sulthiame is presumed to act as a *carbonic anhydrase inhibitor* (similar to the effect acetazolamide; Millichap et al., 1955). An insufficient effect against grand mal seizures requires combination with diphenylhydatoin; increasing seizure frequency and even status epilepticus (Liske and Forster, 1963) have been reported in connection with sulthiame treatment (see Green and Kupferberg, 1972).

Among *untoward reactions,* hyperpnea and tachypnea are most common. Renal impairment has been observed but, in general, severe complications are rare. The *dosage* lies between 300 and 600 mg/day for adults. *The drug has not been marketed in the United States.*

8) Carbamazepine

Carbamazepine (Tegretol) is an imino stilbene with the structural formula (Form 27). It is chemically closely related to the widely used antidepressive drug imipramine (Tofranil®) with the structural formula (Form 28).

One of the first clinical reports on the anticonvulsive effect of carbamazepine (Jongmans, 1964) revealed good results in *grand mal and psychomotor seizures,* which was confirmed by subsequent investigations and especially by Livingston et al. (1967) who consider carbamazepine "an exceedingly effective

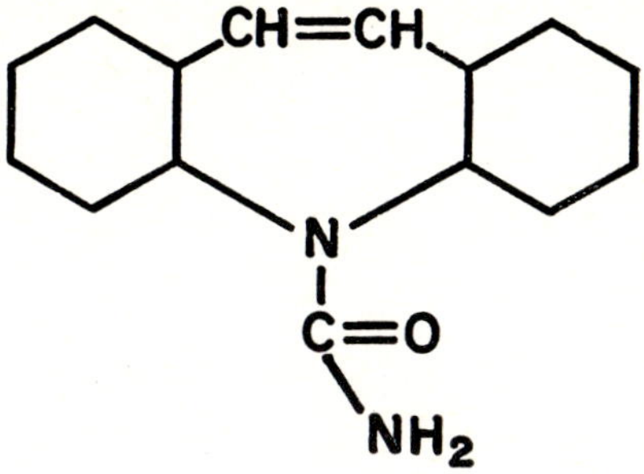

Form. 27

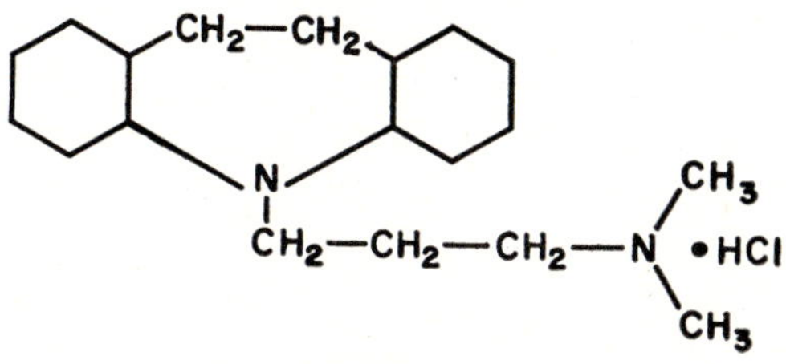

Form. 28

antiepileptic drug." *It is commercially available in the United States for the use in trigeminal neuralgia only* in spite of the general consensus that it is probably the most effective drug in the treatment of psychomotor seizures.

The *dosage* lies in the range between 400 to 800 mg/day in adults and 100 to 400 mg/day in children; considerably larger amounts (1000 to 2000 mg/day) were used in earlier clinical studies.

Untoward side effects are fairly common; diplopia was noted in 18 percent of the patients (Livingston et al., 1967); others had a "heavy feeling in the eyes," abnormal liver function tests, leucopenia or rashes. Initial drowsiness and disturbances of equilibrium gradually subsided in the further course of therapy. Many of these undesirable reactions are presumed to be dosage related and thus avoidable.

Therapeutic serum concentration levels have been found in the range of 0.1 to 0.2 mg/100 ml (1-2 mcg/ml) (Meinardi,

1972); visual disturbances occur when the level reaches 0.8 to 1.0 mg/100 ml. Very little is known about the *metabolism* of carbamazepine.

9) Bromides

Bromides and especially potassium bromide dominated the antiepileptic therapy from Locock's (1857) first report until the twenties when phenobarbital became the treatment of choice. Their effect is essentially limited to grand mal and focal seizures.

Bromides stabilize the excitable membranes and inhibit carbonic anhydrase (with subsequent intracellular accumulation of bicarbonate and hydrogen ion preventing sodium entry and thus decreasing excitability) (Tower, 1960).

Both therapeutic effect and toxicity are based upon the replacement of the Cl-ion. With *dosages* between 1000 to 3000 mg/day, a slow build-up of the Br-ion takes place in body fluids at the expense of chloride and the ion penetrates the blood-brain-barrier.

According to Livingston (1972), therapeutic serum concentration levels lie in the range of 160 to 200 mg/100 ml (20-25 mEq/1000 ml) but may be as low as 80 mg/100 ml or as high as 280 mg/100 ml. With higher serum levels, a toxic encephalopathy develops with delirium, sopor, hallucinations and coma. Gastrointestinal and dermatological (acneiform manifestations) are common. The treatment of this toxic condition requires withdrawal of bromides and administration of chloride salts and diuretics.

Livingston (1972) still recommends bromides for childhood epilepsies in amounts of 300 to 1800 mg/day; many epileptologists, however, have abandoned its use.

Supply

Three Bromides Elixir, N.F. containing 400 mg each of sodium, potassium and ammonium bromide per 5 ml (teaspoonful); to be diluted 1:4 so that 4 ml will contain 100 mg each of these three compounds.

10) Drugs with special and limited anticonvulsive action

a) Diazepam (Valium) (Form 29).

Diazepam was originally introduced as a tranquilizer; its

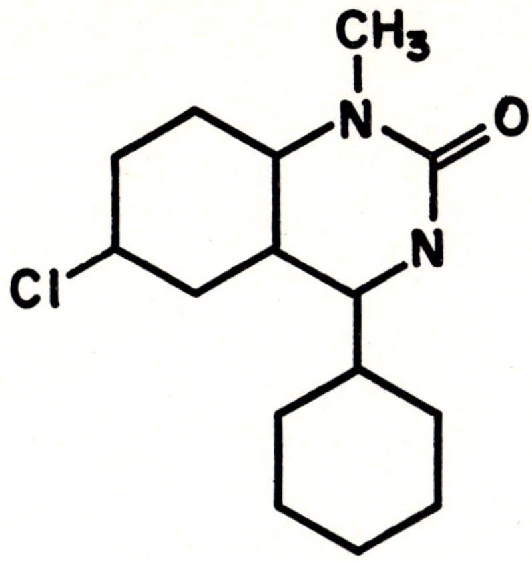

Form. 29

anticonvulsive effect was first reported by Naquet et al. (1965), Gastaut et al. (1965) and Lombroso (1966) in patients with various types of status epilepticus. These authors were impressed with the prompt response to intravenous administration.

Diazepam is a derivative of the benzodiazepines and closely related to chloriazepoxide (Librium®) with the structural formula (Form 30):

Chlordiazepoxide is well known as a "minor tranquilizer" with anxiety reducing effect but its anticonvulsive properties are clearly inferior to those of diazepam.

The practical value of diazepam is definitely associated with the treatment of status epilepticus (see Chapter 7). As a long-term oral anticonvulsant, diazepam has been tried with occasional

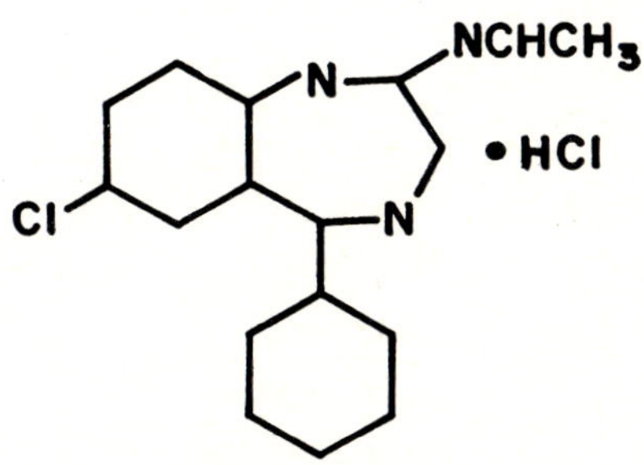

Form. 30

success in children with Lennox-Gastaut syndrome (Gastaut et al., 1966) and in other forms of epilepsy (Gross and Kaltenback, 1963; Weinberg and Harwell, 1965; Elian, 1969).

When administered intravenously in status epilepticus, its anticonvulsive action may become apparent almost immediately. The amazing rapidity of its effect was studied in 150 epileptics with spiking in the EEG (Niedermeyer, 1970 a, c) "Benign" generalized and "unstable" focal seizure discharges are suppressed for periods up to 30 minutes whereas "stable" focal spikes (such as in temporal and frontal lobe epilepsies) are much less responsive to the injected small amounts of diazepam.

The short lasting effect of i.v. diazepam in acute convulsions or status epilepticus will require repeated administration; combination with i.m. phenobarbital is particularly potent and a true synergism of both drugs is a possibility.

The serum concentration level lies around 0.02 mg/100 ml (0.2 mcg/ml) determined one hour after administration of 10 mg diazepam in adult human subjects; this amount differs little when the i.v., i.m. or oral route is chosen (De Silva et al., 1966). Maximum concentrations are followed by a decline within four hours.

Untoward reactions are not common. Respiratory depression may occur if the i.v. injection rate is faster than 1 ml/minute. Prolonged oral administration may be associated with ataxia, confusion, dysarthria, drowsiness, diplopia and various mental changes. These effects are easily avoided when the dosage is kept below the toxic range. With reduction of minor attacks, grand mal seizures may become more prominent but this view has not been substantiated.

In children with Lennox-Gastaut syndrome, diazepam i.v. may precipitate a status-like sequence of tonic seizures (Tassinari et al., 1972; Prior et al., 1972).

Supply

Valium Tablets—2 mg—scored, white
Valium Tablets—5 mg—scored, yellow
Valium Tablets—10 mg—scored, blue

Injectable Valium—2 ml ampules—5 mg/ml (not to be mixed

or diluted with other solutions or drugs, not to be added to i.v. fluids).

b) *Other benzodiazepines*

Nitrazepam (Mogadon)

This benzodiazepine was introduced for the *treatment of* infantile spasms (hypsarrhythmia) (Liske and Forster, 1963; Markham, 1964). According to Völzke et al. (1967) and Doose (1970), control of the seizures can be obtained in 50 percent of the cases. The effect becomes noticeable within 1 to 2 weeks. The optimal *dosage* lies between 0.5 to 1.0 mg/kg/day. Drowsiness is a common *side effect;* bronchial hypersecretion may also occur.

Nitrazepam has not been marked in the United States where it was withdrawn from clinical investigation by its manufacturers, Hoffmann-La Roche, Inc., in favor of clonazepam.

Clonazepam (also Ro-5-4023)

The excellent effect of this drug in the *treatment of status epilepticus* was reported by Gastaut (1970); the action was felt to be more prolonged than that of diazepam. Other authors observed favorable results in the treatment of infantile spasms (Martin, 1971) but it is still unclear whether this drug is superior to nitrazepam (Groh and Blankenhorn, 1971; Kruse, 1971).

c) *ACTH and Steroids*

The introduction of hormonal treatment with ACTH (Sorel and Dusaucy-Bauloye, 1958) was a remarkable breakthrough in the treatment of *infantile spasms* (*hypsarrhythmia*). There has been some general agreement that 50 to 70 percent of the cases can be controlled by ACTH as well as with adreno-cortical steroids. Unfortunately, relapses are common (Jeavons and Bower, 1964).

The specific anticonvulsive action of this group of hormones is completely enigmatic. One could speculate that it may be related to a normalization of neuronal activities in evoked responses since a hormonal effect on cortical evoked responses has been reported (Feldman et al., 1961).

The treatment must be started as soon as the first manifestations (jackknifing, myoclonus) are noticed. Infants with normal developmental milestones prior to the first attacks (around age 6 months) are naturally better off than babies with a history of neonatal convulsions or neurological and mental deficits (see Chapter 4).

Livingston (1972) recommends a daily i.m. injection of 25 to 30 units of repository corticotiopin (such as Acthar Gel) for 4 to 6 weeks. Further therapy is needed if this course leads to both seizure-freedom and EEG normalization. If the EEG remains abnormal, the child is placed on corticosteroids (cortisone or prednisone) for at least two months; this is also done in infants with no clinical response. Oral steroids must be tapered off after a course of a few months.

Side effects are naturally limited to the usual endocrine alteration seen in steroid treatment and generally play no major role in the above outlined treatment.

11) Adjuncts of anticonvulsive treatment

a) *Antimalarial drugs with anticonvulsive effects*

Quinacrine (Atabrine®, Atebrin®) and *chloroquine* have shown some special effects against *petit mal.*

b) *Acetazolamide* (Diamox®)

This drug is a carbonic anhydrase inhibitor and, like sulthiame, a derivative of the sulfonamides. Its diuretic effect has been found to be useful in female patients with grand mal attacks clustering around the premenstrual phase. Its truly anticonvulsive effects has been reported by Bergstrom et al. (1952), Merlis (1954) and Lombroso et al. (1956) and is chiefly directed against petit mal absences. The average dosage ranges from 500 to 1000 mg/day; its effect may wear off in the course of several months.

c) *Dextroamphetamine sulfate* (Dexedrine®)

This drug may occasionally be helpful in the suppression of petit mal absences. It is often recommended in order to counteract drowsiness caused by phenobarbital, primidone or ethosuximide but its value is debatable. It may cause insomnia; dependence and addiction are not likely to occur in epileptic patients.

d) *Folic acid.*

The work of Reynolds et al. (1966) has shown that most of the commonly used anticonvulsants (including phenobarbital, diphenylhydantoin and primidone) give rise to a disturbance of folic acid metabolism. Drug-induced folate deficiency could be the cause of mental symptoms occurring during anticonvulsive treatment.

Exciting new insights into the action and mental side-effects of anticonvulsive therapy could possibly be derived from this work.

e) *Pyridoxine*

The role of pyridoxine in convulsions due to nutritional pyridoxine deficiency and genetic dependency was mentioned in Chapter 3; pyridoxine is also useful in the treatment of convulsions occurring in isoniazid therapy of tuberculosis.

12) General principles of anticonvulsive drug therapy

a) Therapy should be initiated as soon as the evidence of epileptic seizures is well established. This is particularly important in infants with infantile spasms (hypsarrhythmia) and in children with petit mal.

b) The physician should explain to the patient or to parents or relatives the rationale of the drug treatment and the absolute necessity of a consistent intake of medication in order to maintain an optimal serum concentration.

Some patients balk at the thoughts that year or life-long medication of this type will lead to dependency or gradual chronic poisoning. The physician has to convey to the patient the basic principle that the drug will provide greater protection of his brain cells against further seizures and has to dispell all the unfounded worries about chronic toxic effects (as long as the dosage stays below toxic levels). The physician must also explain possible side effects.

This initial conversation must also cover the aspects of individual and social hygiene (see Chapter 14 and 15).

c) One type of medication is, in general, preferable to combinations of anticonvulsants. There is a notable exception from this rule; children with petit mal and the usual specific treatment with ethosuximide or diones will prophylactically require an additional dose of phenobarbital (or diphenylhydantoin) against future grand mal. In adult patients with grand mal, there is no cogent reason for "following the crowd" by prescribing both diphenylhydantoin and phenobarbital (100 mg t.i.d. respectively 32 mg t.i.d.) at the start of the treatment. A small starting dosage should be given in patients with rare seizures and increased only when the amount proves to be unsatisfactory.

The selection of the medication depends greatly on the type of seizure and partly on the type of side-effects. When avoidance of daytime-drowsiness is of utmost importance in a patient with grand mal, hydantoin is preferable to phenobarbital.

d) The proper dosage varies from patient to patient. Body weight is, of course an important factor in the determination of the optimal dosage but one must also keep in mind that, in the case of phenobarbital, a low concentration of the drug in fat tissue reduces the value of simple arithmetic.

e) One has to agree with Livingston (1970) that a divided dosage (into 3 or 4 doses per day) is preferable to one large dosage taken at bedtime even though an optimal serum concentration may be obtained with a single daily dose. Forgetfulness will lead to a marked fall of serum concentration in the latter case and this may well bring forth a return of seizures.

f) It is an essential part of the initial patient interview to point out the length of the treatment which must be conceived as a matter of years or decades. One can correctly state that complications and untoward side effects are most likely to occur during the first year or the first few months of treatment and that life-long treatment will not give rise to late and insidiously arising problems.

g) Return visits of the patient must include an investigation for possible toxic effects (CNS functions, gingiva, hematopoiesis, liver). Blood counts, liver function tests and urinalysis should be carried out prior to the initiation of potentially more toxic drugs (mephenytoin, primidone, oxazolidinediones, ethosuximide and phenacemide), then at intervals of 1 to 2 months during the first 6 months, thereafter at 3 months intervals. After several years of treatment, the intervals of laboratory examinations can be further prolonged.

h) After failure or toxicity of one drug, the change to another drug must be made gradually with an overlap period of a few weeks in which a diminishing amount of the first drug is given together with an increasing amount of the second drug.

i) The discontinuation of anticonvulsive drug therapy must be a very slow process extending over one to several years during which the drug is being tapered off. Years of credible seizure-freedom must precede the beginning of the discontinuation. The EEG should also show normalization or improvement but this is not necessarily the case. Treatment may be discontinued in the face of persisting slight to moderate paroxysmal EEG abnormalities but not in the presence of severe or even worsening changes. Keep in mind that returning seizures (following unwise discontinuation of therapy after years of seizure-freedom) may be more difficult to control than the original seizure disorder.

j) Must treatment be started at all after one seizure? In an acute brain disease (encephalitis etc.), anticonvulsive protection is advisable for a few days only. An alcohol withdrawal seizure does not require any treatment. As to febrile convulsions, see Chapter 4.

k) Treat seizures but do not treat spikes in the EEG. Spikes or sharp waves in seizure free individuals (especially children) require diagnostic attention and denote a certain cerebral disturbance but do not necessitate anti-convulsive therapy.

13) Epilogue

This chapter on anticonvulsive drug therapy might appear to be disproportionately long in comparison with the terse discussions of other epileptological topics. In spite of its length, however, this chapter does not contain a "Cook book" like precise display of the way the treatment has to be done. In reality, it consists of guidelines given after a discussion of the assets and disadvantages of each drug. A condensed view of the most commonly used anticonvulsants and their average dosage is presented in Table VIII.

TABLE VIII

AVERAGE DOSAGES OF THE MOST COMMONLY USED ANTICONVULSANTS

	Total daily dose (per kg body weight)	*Usually prescribed amounts (average body weight)*	
		Starting dosage	*Maximal advisable dosage*
Phenobarbital	1-3 mg	inf. 16 mg x 3/day	32 mg x 3/day
		child 32 mg x 2/day	48 mg x 3/day
		adult 32 mg x 3/day	65 mg x 3/day
Primidone (Mysoline®)	7-15 mg (mostly 10 mg)	inf. 25 mg x 2/day	25 mg x 6/day
		child 50 mg x 3/day	125 mg x 4/day
		adult 250 mg x 3/day	250 mg x 5/day
Diphenylhydantoin (Dilantin®)	4-8 mg	inf. 15 mg x 3/day	30 mg x 3/day
		(use not recommended in infancy)	
		child 30 mg x 3/day	50 mg x 3/day
		adult 30 mg x 3 day	50 mg x 3/day
Trimethadione (Tridione®)	10-25 mg	child 150 mg x 2/day	300 mg x 3/day
		adult 300 mg x 2/day	600 mg x 3/day
Ethosuximide (Zarontin®)	10-30 mg	child 250 mg x 2/day	250 mg x 4/day
		adults 250 mg x 3/day	500 mg x 3/day

General guidelines are preferable to the pseudoexactness of precise instructions concerning choice and amounts of drugs. There is an individual ingredient in medical treatment which corroborates the fact that the science of medicine must be linked with an element of art. With the understanding of both fundamental facets of medicine, the physician will successfully attune to the patients needs.

An important lesson to be learned in epileptology is the absolute recalcitrance of some epileptic conditions to any type of drug therapy. This refractory group may comprise 5 to 10 percent or even 15 percent (depending on how the boundaries of the epilepsies are conceived) of the total epileptic population. A small portion of the refractory group has severe focal epilepsies and may benefit from surgery (Chapter 13) but the rest will remain intractable. Therefore, needless attempts of pushing the dosage into toxic levels ought to be avoided. Severe irritability pseudo-hysteria, stuporous and psychotic episodes are a costly price to be paid for temporary seizure freedom. The wave of optimism of the late forties and early fifties(following the advent of exciting new drugs) led to the firm belief that all epilepsy could be eventually controlled by patiently finding the optimal dosage (paired with the hope that surgery would take care of the small remaining group of non-reactors).

When we keep in mind the variety of etiologies and the group of special epileptic conditions, we are today in a better position of prognosticating the course of a given seizure disorder. We can anticipate that in certain severe types of epilepsy, seizure-freedom will prove to be elusive or the "impossible dream." In such cases, we have to content ourselves to striking the balance between some seizure reduction and relative mental-physical well being. There are even patients who may be better off with no medication at all. These patients are severely brain damaged and find themselves in an institution where the seizures do not represent an additional major social problem.

Appendix: FIRST AID IN EPILEPTIC SEIZURES

When a physician witnesses a grand mal convulsion during a party, a church service or in the street, his action does not have to differ from the way he would handle a simple attack of syncopal fainting. Calm down frightened bystanders and let nature take its course; tongue biting can be avoided only in the initial stage when the mouth is wide open (with or without a moaning or sighing muffled cry) and an appropriate, preferentially padded object can be placed between the rows of teeth. More harm than good can be done with such attempts by well meaning laymen and the concern for a possible tongue bite must not be exaggerated. Protection of the head during a threatening heavy fall on a hard floor can be occasionally achieved.

The patient is apneic during the convulsion and the first stertorous inspiration indicates the return of the respiratory function; his ashen-cyanotic complexion will soon normalize. At this moment, difficulties could arise from intratracheal saliva or food particles and it is worthwhile to turn the head to the side once general flaccidity has superseded the last clonic jerks. Respiratory arrest necessitating mouth-to-mouth respiration with proper positioning of the head (neck elevated by a piece of garment, head in passive opisthotoniform retraction) is extremely rare. Acute postictal cardiovascular problems or cardiac arrest are also exceptional.

For these reasons, calling an ambulance is unnecessary in most cases; the patient's coma will soon change into a shorter or longer sleep from which he is most likely to awake in full consciousness or with some degree of confusion. Post-ictal excitation may be severe in chronic severe epileptics or in old arteriosclerotics. This is a valid reason for bringing the patient to an emergency room. Rapid succession of a second seizure is also a reason for calling an ambulance.

Psychomotor automatisms are best dealt with simple common sense; in rare instances, combative behavior or a series of such attacks could require a ride to the nearest emergency room.

The physician's calm and the way in which he tones down the embarrassing nature of the event can be a very helpful contribution to the "desensitization of the public" (see Chapter 15) and for a better understanding of the transient misfunctioning of cerebral physiology. His attitude can be a great help for the awakening patient. Epileptic laborers are best served when they are permitted to return to their work as soon as they have regained consciousness.

Chapter 13

NEUROSURGICAL TREATMENT OF THE EPILEPSIES

1) Introductory remarks

SEIZURE SURGERY IS limited to a small group of drug refractory patients but has an important place in the therapeutic armamentarium of the epilepsies. Fascinating neurophysiological insights into the functional anatomy of the human brain have been a by-product of the surgical approach.

A historical review of the surgical treatment of epilepsy would reach from the archaic ages (trephine holes of prehistoric skull presumed to be performed for the release of evil spirits in epileptics) to the modern cognizance of the epileptic focus as a removable entity; such a review cannot be included in this condensed presentation.

2) The development of neurosurgical standard procedures

Modern seizure surgery may be dated back to 1928 when Wilder Penfield, the eminent neurosurgeon-neuropathologist, joined forces with Otfrid Foerster in Breslau where this daring and brilliant neurologist neurosurgeon had ventured into the excision of traumatic epileptogenic cortical scars (Foerster and Penfield, 1930 a, b). The technical and neuroscientific refinement of the surgical approach is reflected by the work of Penfield and Gage (1933), Penfield (1936), Penfield et al. (1940), Penfield and Erickson (1941, Penfield and Steelman (141), Penfield and Flanigin (1950), Penfield and Kristiansen (1951), Penfield and

Baldwin (1952) and Penfield and Jasper (1954). This work shows Penfield's shifting emphasis from Neuropathology to Neurophysiology. Other schools contributed greatly to the development of seizure surgery (Walker et al., 1947; Walker, 1949; Walker, 1951; Walker et al., 1960; Green et al., 1951; Green, 1967; Falconer et al., 1955; Falconer, 1967; Paillas et al., 1952; Paillas, 1958; Guillaume et al., 1953; Obrador, 1953).

New impulses developed around 1950 when, on the basis of electrophysiological data and evidence of large (rather than limited) epileptogenic zones, the emphasis was placed on partial unilateral lobectomies instead of more circumscript cortical excisions. In 1947, Percival Bailey started carrying out temporal lobectomies by removing the anterior 35 to 70 mm of the lobe in patients with intractable psychomotor seizures (Bailey and Gibbs, 1951; Bailey, 1953; Bailey, 1954; Bailey, 1958), leaving intact the amygdala and the hippocampus. These areas were included in the technique used by the Montreal School (Penfield and Baldwin, 1952; Rasmussen and Jasper, 1958) and by A. Earl Walker and his associates (Walker, 1967). Other workers (Niemeyer, 1958) performed the transventricular excision of amygdala, hippocampus and hippocampic gyrus sparing the neocortical convexity of the temporal lobe. While Penfield and Baldwin (1952) and their followers remove the superior temporal gyrus along with the anterior portion of the temporal lobe, Walker leaves this structure untouched. The insula is left intact in all of these techniques.

It is interesting to read Bailey's (1958) reasons for not including amygdala and hippocampus in his technique of temporal lobectomy. All of these reasons are based on neuropathological data such as the rare involvement of these structures in trauma (according to Courville, 1958), the frequently encountered absence of sclerotic changes in amygdala and hippocampus and the rarity of psychomotor epilepsy in patients with gross lesions in this area. On the other hand, the rationale for the approach of Penfield and A. Earl Walker and their associates lies in the growing awareness of the electrophysiological role and the neurophysiological epileptogenic properties of amygdala and hippocampus which, as "low threshold areas," are likely to propagate epileptic discharges originating from temporal neocortical structures.

Because of the frequency and the severity of its involvement, the temporal lobe stands by far in the foreground of neurosurgical interest. This is somewhat different from the more widespread distribution of epileptogenic foci encountered in periods of war when lacerating brain wounds frequently affected the upper frontal, Rolandic and parieto-occipital regions. In the following, we will concentrate on temporal lobectomy as the most commonly performed procedure in the domain of seizure surgery.

3) Temporal lobectomy—Indications for this procedure and selection of cases

Clinical evidence of temporal lobe epilepsy with typical psychomotor seizures (with or without additional grand mal) must be substantiated by corresponding EEG findings which classically show anterior temporal sharp waves or spikes; nasopharyngeal or sphenoidal leads are sometimes needed for a convincing demonstration of these inter-ictal discharges. Marked bilaterality of spiking in the scalp EEG will certainly raise doubts in the mind of the neurosurgeon and his team about the validity of the indication for surgery. Several waking and sleeping records are needed for better assessment of each case. A consistent predominance of sharp wave or spike activity on one side is suggestive of the leading role of one temporal lobe in the generation of seizures but this is rather conjectural. The *intracarotid Sodium Amytal-test* (introduced by Wada, 1949, for determination of hemispheric dominance) may be used for the evaluation of the primarily involved temporal lobe (Rovit et al., 1961; Garretson et al., 1966). Less valuable is the use of intravenous pentylenetetrazol (Metrazol) (Ajmone Marsan and Ralston, 1957). The insertion of depth electrodes has become a widely accepted method aiming at a precise demonstration of deep seated epileptogenic foci.

A. Earl Walker and his co-workers have made ample use of depth electroencephalography without making this technique a mandatory prerequisite for planned seizure surgery. Depth implants and a subsequent 1 to 3 week period of daily EEG recordings (preferably recording from depth and scalp leads simultaneously) have proved to be particularly valuable in patients with equivocal lateralization of the temporal seizure discharges. Depth EEG results have often become the main reason for not performing surgery because of the marked bilaterality of deep seizure discharges. Electrical stimulation will be repeatedly carried out in all depth electrodes after a few sessions limited to recording only. The depth implant in temporal lobe epileptics preferably consists of four tresses containing 6 electrodes each with the tip lying in the amygdala or inferior temporal cortex (on either side) and in the fronto-orbital cortex (on either side). The electrodes are inserted under local anesthesia and with X-ray control.

The information obtained from depth electrodes has the advantage of greater authenticity (not being subjected to attenuating factors such as dura, skull and scalp; see Cooper et al., 1965); the disadvantages lie in the spatial limitation of the information (the set of introduced small electrodes may miss important events occurring in fairly close vicinity) and sometimes in the multitude of irrelevant details (Niedermeyer and Rocca, 1972). Complications occur in about 10 percent of the patients and usually range from minor bleedings to smoldering mild infection which latter necessitates premature removal of the electrodes; severe complications are rare.

The seizure disorder must have proved to be *unresponsive to all types of appropriate anticonvulsive medication* in subtoxic levels before a patient is considered a candidate for seizure surgery. This is a somewhat conservative philosophy and not every epileptologist will agree with it. From a strictly neurophysiological angle of view one could advocate early surgery, for instance in an older child with good evidence of temporal or frontal lobe epilepsy. The proponents of this view feel that, with increasing duration of the seizure disorder, a growing number of cerebral structures will be involved and the subserving neuronal mechanisms and pathways will become "conditioned" to epileptiform responses. On the other hand, longitudinal clinical observation has shown that many childhood seizure disorders may take a favorable course while others, such as the Lennox-Gastaut syndrome, are unlikely to be improved by surgery at any age. I feel that clinical experience must overrule neurophysiological insights (sometimes better termed speculations) in this dilemma. As to temporal lobe epilepsy, we have stressed before (Chapter 5) an element of "maturation" in this seizure disorder; interestingly, EEG findings tend to be more diffuse in childhood temporal lobe epilepsy and more clearly localized in the "mature" adult form.

4) Technique of temporal lobectomy

We will follow A. Earl Walker in this brief outline of the operation by partly using his description (1967) and the masterful illustrations of L. Schlossberg (Fig. 40 to 46).

In *preparation* for the operation, the patient is given dexamethasone in doses of 10 to 12 mg daily for 2 days before operation and for 3 days postoperatively, followed by a half dose daily until one week after the operation when the medication is stopped. Just before the patient leaves for the operating room, he is given 0.5 mg atropine and 50 mg Demerol. The operation is carried out in general anesthesia using intravenous sodium pentothal and an intratracheal tube in place. The patient is passively hyperventilated.

Scalp incision, bone flap and exposure are demonstrated in Figure 40 and 41. Electrocorticographic recordings are then carried out with a special set of sterilized wick electrodes and 2 or 3 small depth probes inserted into limbic areas (Fig. 42, see also Fig. 48). The outcome of this tracing will have not further influence on the extent of the essentially standardized procedure. The reason for performing electrocorticography is to study the distribution of seizure patterns which may be scattered beyond the Sylvian fissure and the vein of Labbé. Marked posterior temporal or fronto-Rolandic spiking may or may not suggest an unsatisfactory result; these scattered spike may later die down (as well as spikes arising from the insula)

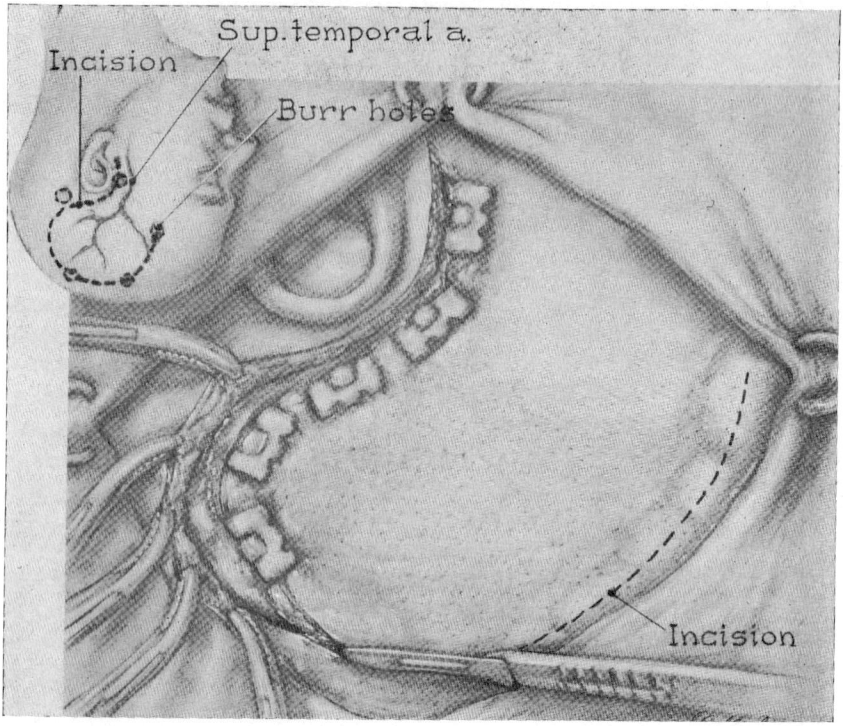

FIGURE 40. *The Scalp Incision.* This figure illustrates the question-mark incision within the hair bearing scalp which is planned so that the surgeon may turn down a scalp flag well-vascularized by the superficial temporal artery. The incision passing along the anterior margin of the pinna does not interrupt the facial branch to the frontalis muscle. Bleeding is controlled by Raney clips on the flap edge and Kolodny clamps placed on the galea aponeurotica on the outer margin of the incision. The scalp flap is then reflected anteroinferiorly. (With permission of Dr. A. Earl Walker and the Journal of Neurosurgery. The drawings of Fig. 40 through 46 were carried out by Mr. Leon Schlossberg.)

after removal of principally involved neocortical-limbic connections. Electrical stimulation is also carried out in the most active leads. The results of the stimulation are often negative; this is likely to be due to the state of general anesthesia which, however, has little attenuating effect on spontaneous cortical or limbic spiking.

The cortex appears to be normal in most cases and the

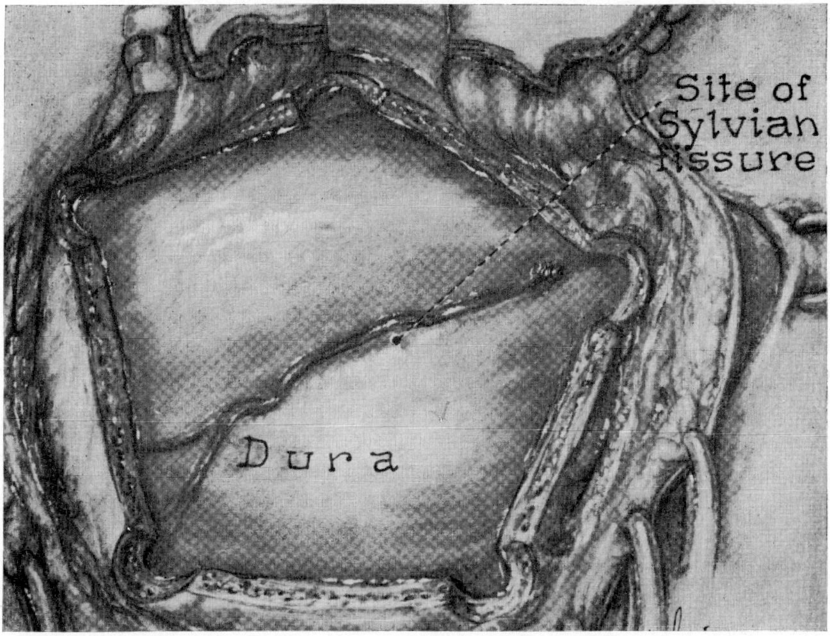

FIGURE 41. *The Bone Flap.* This figure shows four or five burr holes placed on the circumference of the proposed bone flap and usually under the temporal muscle. The anteroinferior trephination is usually just posterior to the outer canthus of the eye and within and below the anterior part of the incision (slightly lower than shown in this figure. The bone between the burr holes is cut with the Gigli saw and fractured on the inferior temporal aspect so that the flap can be reflected using the temporal muscle as a hinge. The middle meningeal vessels are coagulated as they pass onto the dura matter at the margin of the sphenoidal ridge. (With permission of Dr. A. Earl Walker and the Journal of Neurosurgery.)

removed specimen (Fig. 44) usually shows little or no gross changes; gliosis is the most common microscopic finding, while small tumors or cysts are occasional exceptions.

Postoperative complications are uncommon and usually not severe; according to Rasmussen (1970), the *mortality of seizure surgery* in general (e.g. nonneoplastic epileptogenic lesions) *is 1.0 percent.* The incidence of complications would greatly increase with additional removal of the insula (Silfvenius et al., 1964).

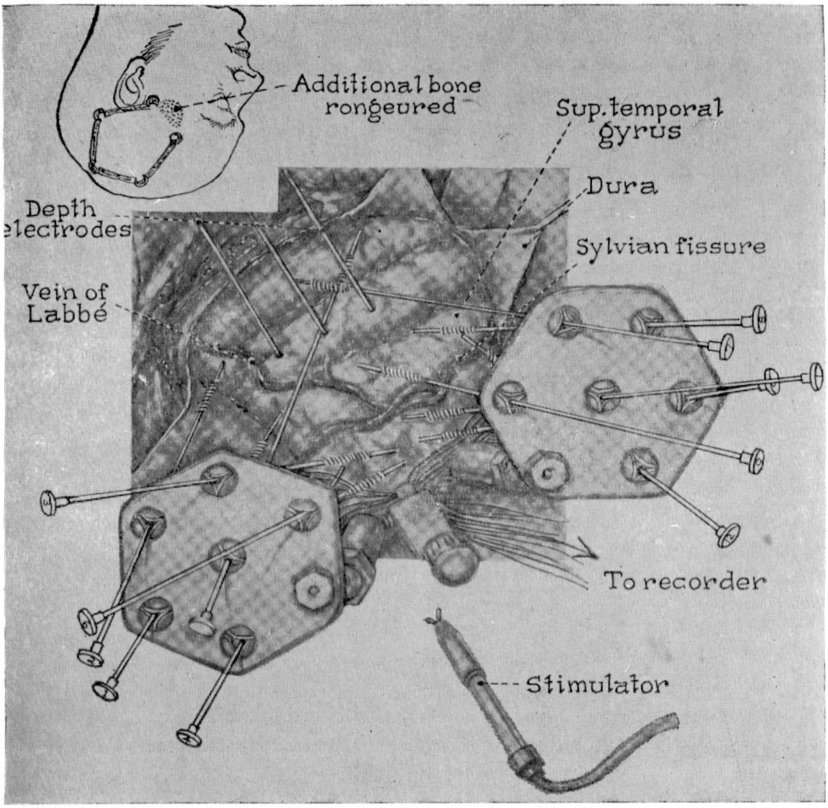

FIGURE 42. *The Exposure.* After the osteoplastic flap has been reflected, the bone is rongeured away to the base of the middle fossa and the dura mater opened as a flap so that it may be turned upwards. A radiating incision is made in the anteroinferior angle of the dura mater to expose the temporal tip. *Electrocorticography.* Three single or bipolar electrodes are then passed 3, 4, and 5 cm from the temporal pole through the second temporal convolution at right angles to its surface until they encounter resistance, usually at 4 cm. They are withdrawn 0.5 cm and left in place. An array of cortical electrodes, attached to the bone by a clamp, is then placed on the pial surface to sample at regular intervals the cortical activity. After recording the spontaneous and electrically evoked activity, the electrodes are removed. The electrocorticographic findings serve only as a guide to the extent of the ablation. If spiking is present outside the anterior temporal region, the ablation will be enlarged only if the activity is adjacent to the proposed incision. Spiking in the inferior frontal or posterior temporal regions is not considered an indication to resect those

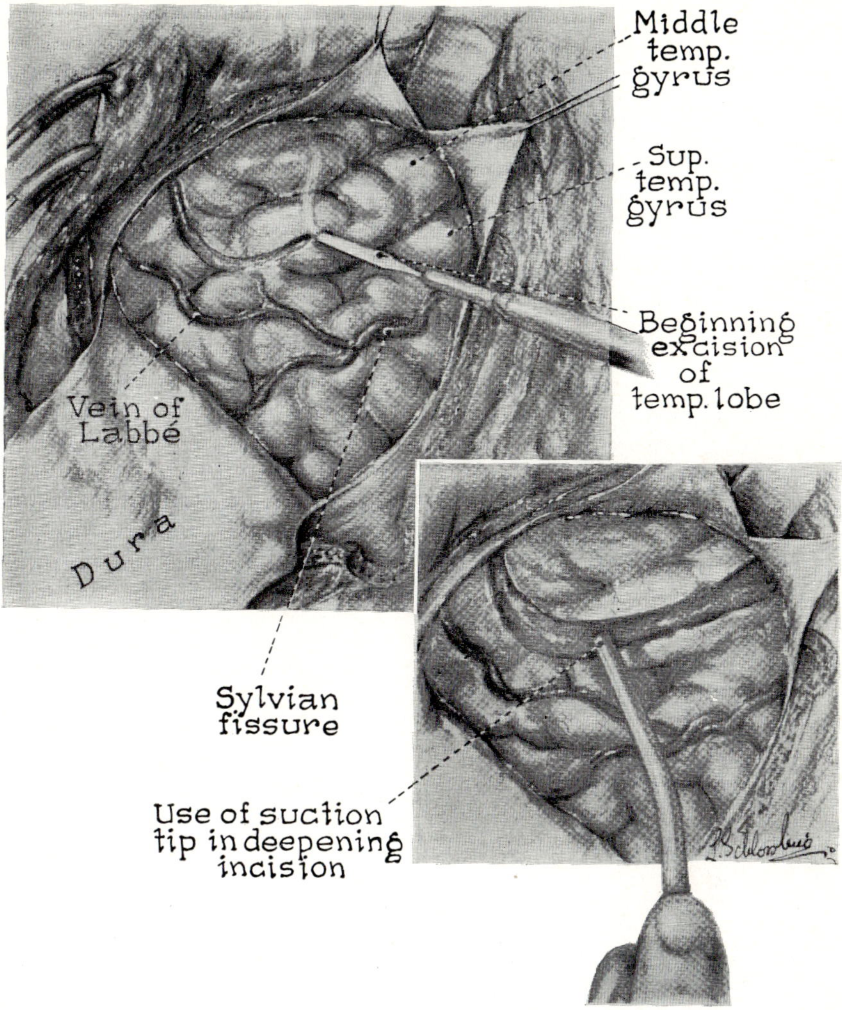

FIGURE 43. *The Ablation.* An incision is started with the electrosurgical unit along the second temporal gyrus. From the temporal tip, it is carried posteriorly 4 to 5 cm and curved inferiorly a few millimeters in front of the anastomotic vein of Labbé to the base of the temporal lobe. (With permission of Dr. A. Earl Walker and the Journal of Neurosurgery.)

---

areas. Electrical stimulation is carried out with various parameters of current and voltage and with 40 pulses/sec. The hand-held stimulating electrode (shown in this figure) is not in use any longer since the stimulating current is applied to the recording electrodes. (With permission of Dr. A. Earl Walker and the Journal of Neurosurgery.)

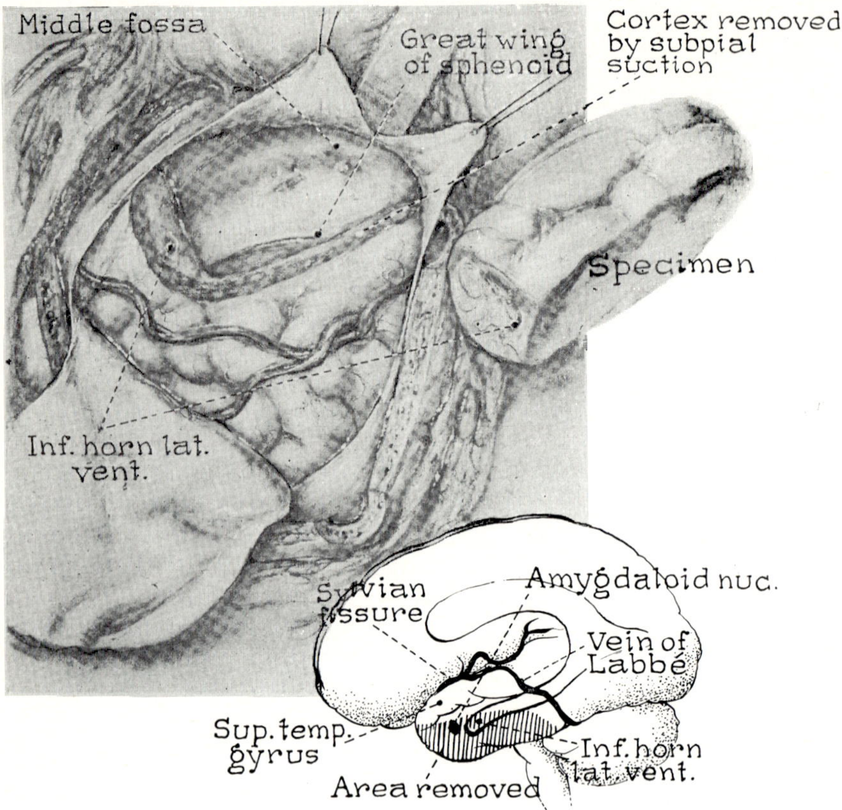

FIGURE 44. *The Ablation* (continued). After the pia arachnoid has been incised, the dissection is continued with a sucker through the white matter to the inferior horn, which is opened. The groove just dorsal to the amygdala and hippocampus is identified and the dissection carried along it to the pia on the medial surface of the temporal lobe. The latter is cauterized and cut so that the tissue may be removed in one piece. The cortex along the ventral lip of the superior temporal sulcus is sucked away subpially into the sulcus for a centimeter, or almost to the trough of the fissure, to eliminate all denervated and devascularized cortex. The amygdala and rostral part of the hippocampus is removed, so that the ablation along the floor of the middle fossa measures 5 to 6.5 cm in both right and left hemispheres. (With permission of Dr. A. Earl Walker and the Journal of Neurosurgery.)

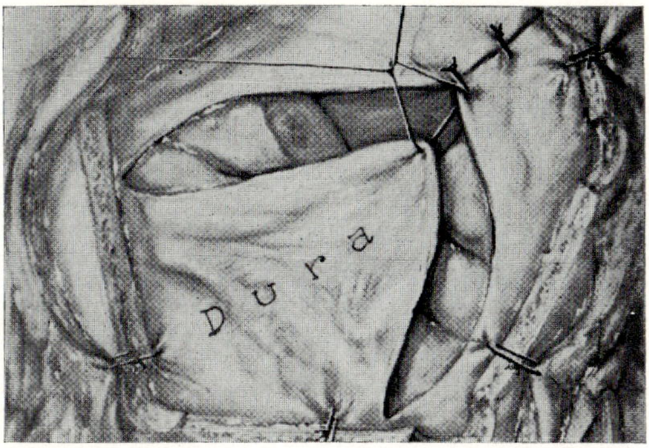

FIGURE 45. *The Dural Closure.* A control electrocorticogram is made. If spiking is present at the edge of the ablation, a further subpial sucker resection is made, but spiking at some distance from the ablation is not considered to be an indication for further resection. After a careful check for hemostasis the dura mater is closed with interrupted black silk sutures. The dura mater at the margin of the bone is held up by sutures passed to the pericranium. (With permission of Dr. A. Earl Walker and the Journal of Neurosurgery.)

Quadrantic hemianopsia may be a sequel of temporal lobectomy. Serious *memory deficits* may occur following temporal lobectomy when the opposite hippocampic area is impaired (Penfield and Milner, 1958). The Montreal School has tried to avoid this complication by the use of short memory tests under intracarotid sodium amytal (Milner et al., 1962). *Dysphasia* of the sensory type plays no role as a surgical sequel.

The *results* of temporal lobectomies may be grossly summarized as:

⅓ excellent (seizure-freedom, immediately or after a few postoperative attacks)
⅓ good or satisfactory (considerable reduction of seizures)
⅓ poor (inadequate or no reduction of seizures)

The patient will have to receive anticonvulsive medication for many years or the rest of his life in spite of seizure freedom.

These are the results of long follow-up studies (for greater detail, see Penfield and Paine, 1955; Rassmussen, 1970). In the longitudinal development, the seizure free group tends to shrink

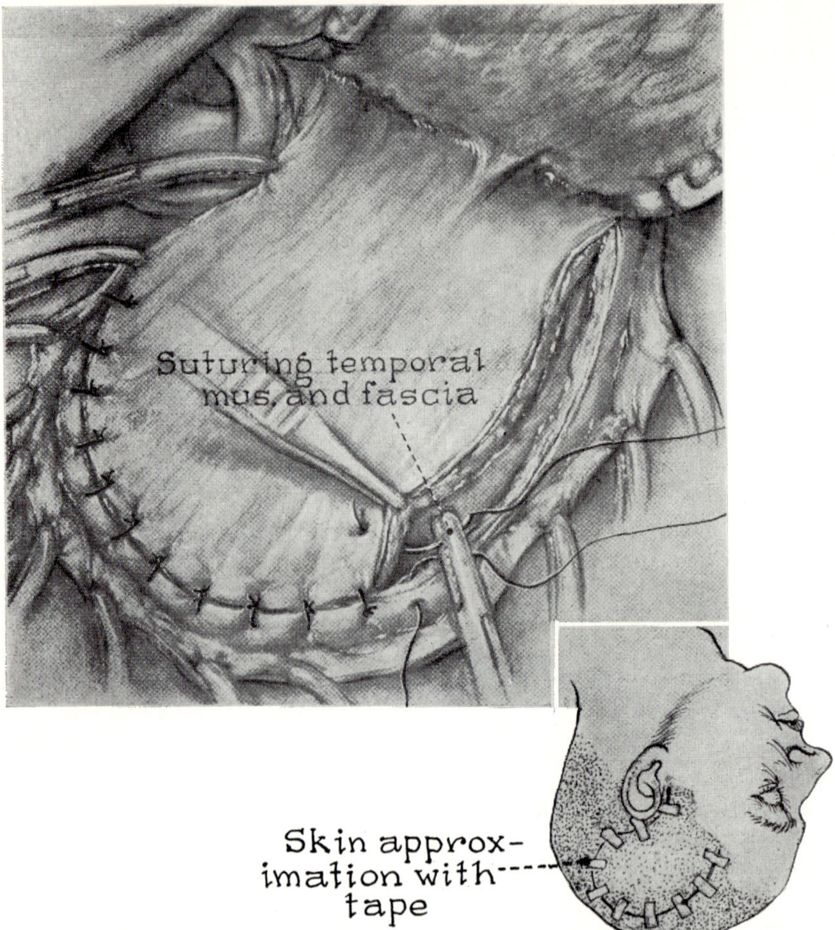

FIGURE 46. *The Bone and Scalp Closure.* The bone flap is replaced and held by one tantalum suture to the edge of the parietal bone. The temporal fascia and muscle are approximated by black silk sutures and the galea aponeurotica similarly sutured. The scalp edges are brought in apposition by plastic adhesive tapes. (With permission of Dr. A. Earl Walker and the Journal of Neurosurgery.)

in size from about 50 to 33 percent. One must also keep in mind that the patient selection is often swayed by the pressure some patients or relatives put on the neurosurgeon who may doubt the indication for surgery in some cases; the pressure may be enhanced by suicidal threats. The inclusion or omission of psychotic or psychopathic patients in the surgical material (see Chapter 5 and 11) will influence the results; frank psychosis does not respond to surgery whereas irritability, moderate aggressiveness and hyposexuality (Chapter 11) will improve together

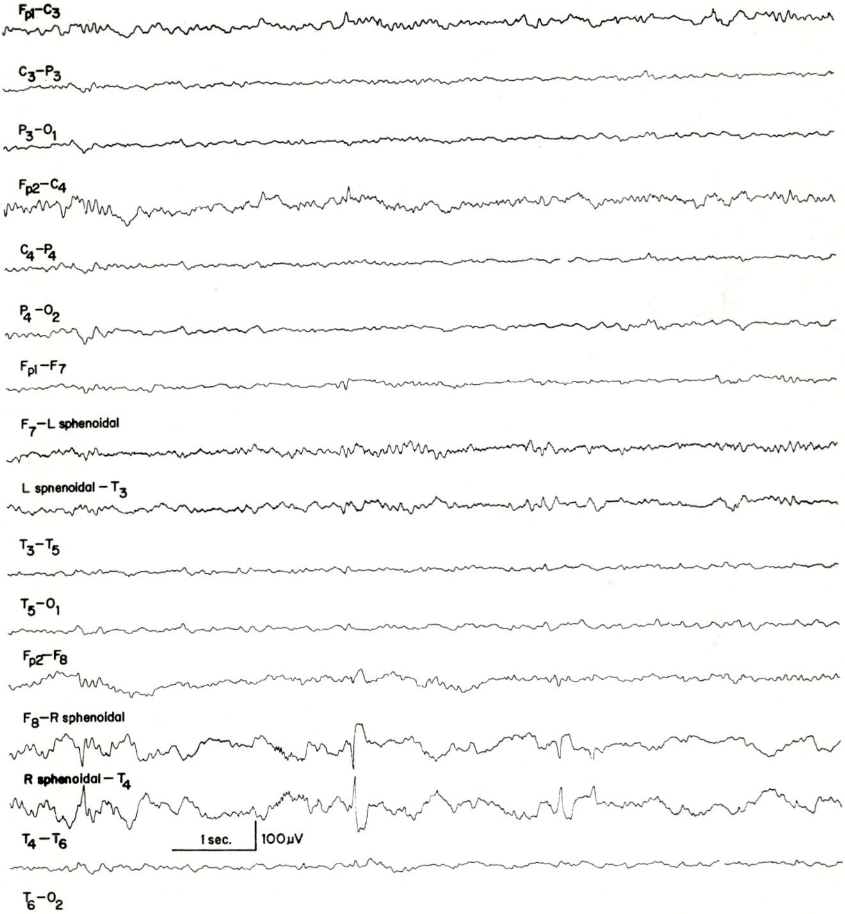

FIGURE 47. Electroencephalogram of a 23-year-old male patient with psychomotor seizures since age 10 and grand mal since age 16. Severe personality disorder (#1440800). Spikes and sharp waves are seen in the right sphenoidal electrode; this activity is barely detectable in corresponding scalp leads (F8, T4).

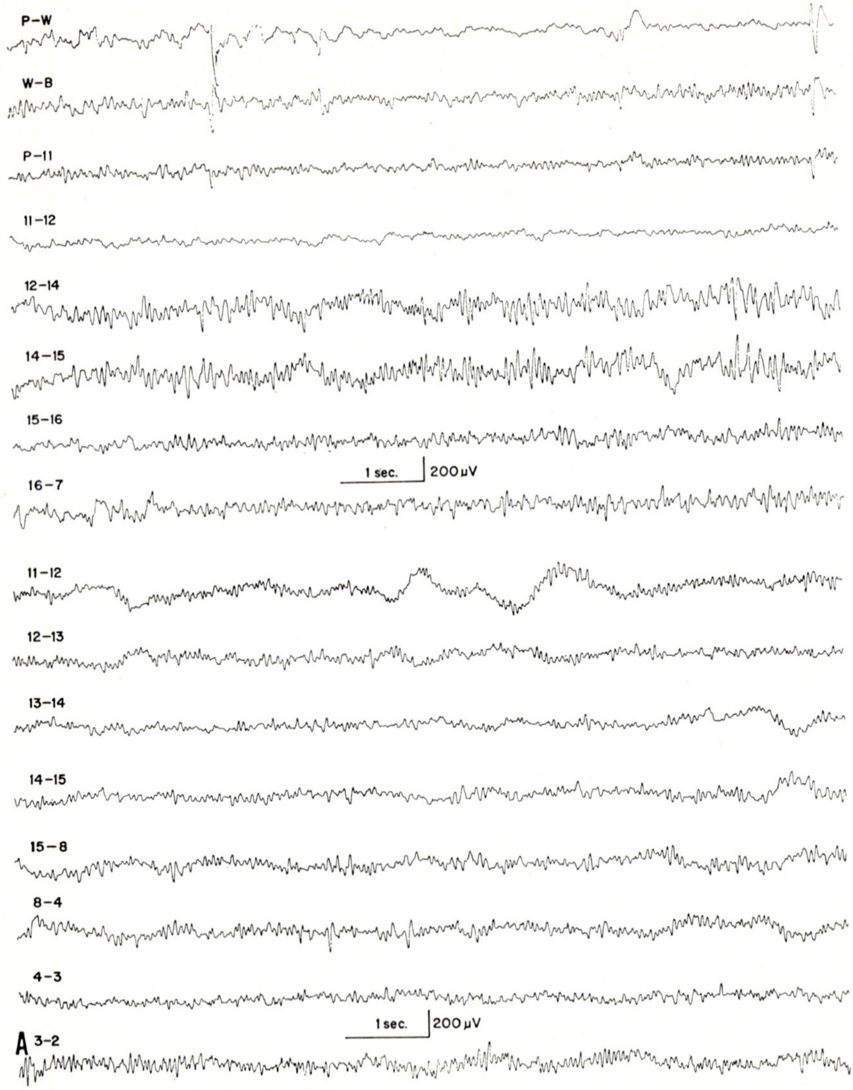

FIGURE 48. Same patient. a) Electrocorticogram during right temporal lobectomy in general anesthesia. Note marked spike activity in limbic depth leads, especially in electrode W (amygdala).

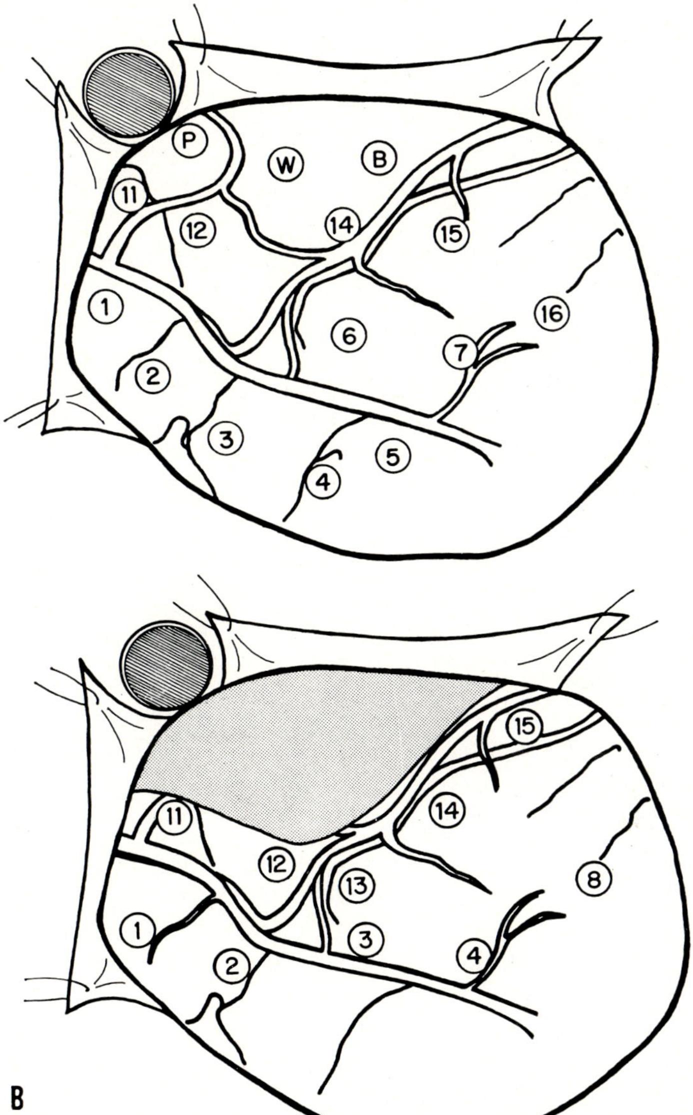

FIGURE 48. b) Localization of cortical and depth leads; extent of surgical ablation.

with good epileptological results. In most patients with excellent epileptological results, social status and professional rehabilitation parallel the improvement.

The procedure cannot be carried out on both sides; its behavioral crippling effect (Terzian, 1958) can be compared with the Klüver-Bucy syndrome in monkeys (Klüver, 1958; see also Chapter 11). Bilateral modifications of temporal lobectomy have been performed by Scoville et al (1953). These and similar attempts have aimed at behavioral changes in psychiatric rather than epileptic patients.

5) *Other major procedures*

Partial lobectomies or limited excisions of epileptogenic foci are carried out less often in areas other than the temporal lobe. This is demonstrated when one looks at the large material of the Montreal Neurological Institute from 1930 through 1965 (excluding tumors) (Rasmussen, 1970):

Temporal lobe epilepsy	551 patients
Frontal lobe epilepsy	211 patients
Parietal lobe epilepsy	87 patients

There are naturally strict surgical taboos for foci involving the major part of the precentral motor cortex or the motor speech area. Rasmussen (1963) has advocated a very extensive type of frontal lobectomy with apparently very good results.

Outside the frontal and temporal lobe, seizure surgery usually limits itself to smaller excisions (see Chapter 5 for the neurosurgical approach in a case of parietal lobe epilepsy). Cerebral commissurotomy has been used by Mann et al. (1969), in rebellious cases of epilepsy; this procedure includes both the corpus callosum and anterior commissure (presumed to be most important in the transmission of hippocampic impulses).

One wonders if micro-neurosurgical techniques will further improve the results of standard procedures by further avoidance of trauma to the tissue.

6) *Hemispherectomy*

The surgical removal of an entire hemisphere (leaving intact most of the basal ganglia) has been performed in many cases of *intractable seizure disorder associated with infantile hemiplegia* and good pneumoencephalographic evidence of *diffuse unilateral cortical sclerosis and atrophy.* This procedure was first carried out by Dandy (1933) but its use in cases of hemiplegic cerebral palsy and its technical refinement is linked chiefly with the name of Krynauw (1950).

When there is a striking difference between a severely scarred and an apparently intact other hemisphere, this operation may lead not only to seizure freedom but even to favorable slight improvement of the hemiplegic (or hemiplegic-aphasic) deficit since removal of the sclerotic tissue with its epileptogenic-irritative impact on the rest of the brain may facilitate the effectiveness of compensatory cerebral mechanisms.

Hemispherectomies are not often carried out; only a limited number of cases meet all the requirements for surgical indication and the procedure appears to be too awesome and "heroic" to the surgeon as well as to the relatives. Childhood is the best age for the operation but even young adults may respond favorably. In experienced hands, the mortality is not high.

*7) **Stereotaxic seizure surgery***

Stereotaxic production of small cerebral lesions with therapeutic effect have been extensively used in the treatment of basal ganglia diseases and especially in cases of Parkinson syndrome. Some neurosurgeons, however, have aimed with stereotaxic methods at the destruction of small epileptogenic foci or epileptogenically involved gray structures as well as fiber systems.

Stereotaxic seizure surgery evidently deals with supposedly deep seated foci and, for these reasons, petit mal absences of presumed thalamix origin (see the centrencephalic concept of common generalized epilepsy, Chapter 4) and temporal lobe (psychomotor seizures with obvious involvement of limbic masses and pathways) have been the principal object of this form of surgery. The lesions have been carried out by electrocoagulation (Spiegel and Wycis, 1952; Guiot and Brion, 1953; Riechert and Wolff, 1953), trauma such as cutting or tearing of fibers (Meyers, 1942), thermocoagulation (Leksell, 1949), chemonecrosis (Spiegel and Wycis, 1950; Narabayashi and Okuma, 1954; Cooper, 1955) and radioactive necrosis using radioactive yttrium (Campbell and Walker, 1957) or gold. More recently, Walker and his associates have inserted small metal pellets which can be heated from outside by the generation of radio frequencies.

Mullan et al. (1967), have made thalamic stereotaxic lesions for the treatment of epilepsies with generalized seizure patterns. In the case of temporal lobe epilepsy, severance of the fornix (fornicotomy) has been used by Umbach (1966). Jinnai (1966) severed the ansa lenticularis in epileptics, Diemath et al. (1966), employed cingulotomy for the treatment of intractable seizure disorders and some efforts have concentrated on amygdaloid lesions (Narabayashi and Uno, 1966). A. Earl Walker occasionally implants bilateral metal pellets into the amygdaloid nuclei; subsequent radioactive heating may be carried out more than once.

Stereotaxic lesions are certainly less damaging to the brain than major neurosurgical procedures but their effectiveness has not been convincingly demonstrated and relapses are very common. Some procedures such as amygdalotomy and cingulotomy may have additional values in the improvement of the behavioral disturbances.

Chapter 14

INDIVIDUAL HYGIENE OF THE EPILEPTIC PATIENT

1) Introductory remarks

Every comprehensive therapeutic approach to human suffering has an individual and a social facet; the former will be the topic of this chapter. The word hygiene implies that one is dealing with the patient's general health and well being rather than with the disease aspect only. The occurrence of seizures in a patient's life may result in an ever present dark cloud in the sky disturbing all his physical activities, his emotions and thoughts. It is thus needless to say that writing prescriptions for anticonvulsants and performing necessary laboratory work is not enough. The physician must be willing to shoulder the burden of giving guidelines and practical advice concerning education, professional life, recreation, activities dangerous to the patient and others, and marriage with its genetic and emotional implications. He must try to understand the life of the epileptic patient from inside. He must attempt to obtain a vivid picture of his average daily life.

Again we used the notion of "the epileptic patient" and we will have to stress over and over again in these two last chapters that epileptic seizures may occur at all levels of intelligence and that separating lines must be drawn between different levels of intellectual capabilities. Absence or presence of seizures is no crucial problem for severely mentally retarded patients; he will always remain unadjusted to the struggle for life because of his cerebral impairment. For patients capable of being gainfully employed, the occurrence of seizures is a severe blow to their livelihood and pride. While we concentrate on all aspects of epileptic seizures, we must never forget that we are dealing with patients suffering from a wide variety of cerebral insults which may be mild enough to permit intellectual top performance. Whenever we use the notion of "the epileptic," we must always be aware of the implied dangerous generalization.

2) *Nutrition (with special reference to ketogenic diet)*

Little attention is often paid to the patient's food intake. Skipping breakfast is a bad habit which could lead to hypoglycemia in the morning hours; rebound-like hypoglycemic states can result from a breakfast rich in carbohydrates but completely lacking in proteins. On the other hand, seizures in early or late morning hours are very common in patients with Common generalized epilepsy and are related mainly to the waking-sleeping cycle (Chapter 4). It would be unwise to lay excessive emphasis on the blood sugar level in such cases; we will discuss the hygienic implications of waking and sleeping in the following section.

When one prescribes medication, it is always important to point out to the patient that he must not take his tablets or capsules on empty stomach in the morning. This is a good way to find out if the patients skips breakfast. One has to insist that he takes his medicine during or shortly after his meals and that the morning dose is of great importance. Acute or chronic gastritis is likely to occur when the medication is taken on empty stomach (especially in the case of diphenylhydantoin).

There are no strict dietary rules to be given. The only well known exception is the ketogenic diet which still has a place in pediatric epileptology but is hardly useable in adults and adolescents. Other diets such as dehydration regimen (Fay, 1930) have fallen into oblivion. A recent modification of this regimen has placed particular emphasis on medium-chain-triglycerides (Huttenlocher et al., 1972).

The ketogenic diet consists of a high fat-low carbohydrate regimen leading to ketosis. It was introduced by Wilder (1921) for the treatment of childhood epilepsies. Its beneficial effect was confirmed by Keith (1947), Bridge (1949) and other workers but this treatment has never become widely accepted. Livingston has often advocated this regimen for certain forms of childhood epilepsy and his recent work (Livingston, 1972) gives a detailed account of the dietary management; this book should be consulted for the practical applications of the diet.

The ketogenic diet appears to be most effective in children with generalized seizure discharges and especially those with infantile spasms and the Lennox-Gastaut syndrome. The reduction or control of seizures is usually of temporary nature but the tranquilizing effect on the child's behavior is often quite remarkable. It is therefore worthwhile to try the ketogenic diet in children with Lennox-Gastaut syndrome who are unlikely to respond to medication.

The quality of the local nutrition department may play an important role in the effectiveness and tolerability of the regimen and this may also explain the sharp division of opinions regarding the diet's effectiveness. Parental cooperation is another very important factor. Vomiting is a common *complication* in the early stage; major complications are rare. The *duration* of the regimen may be as long as two years; thereafter, the initial 4:1 ratio of ketogenic/antiketogenic elements may be gradually reduced to 3:1, 2:1 and to normal diet.

The mechanism of the anticonvulsive effect of the diet is still obscure.

Alcoholic beverages should be avoided. There are proponents of strict abstinence while other epileptologists are somewhat more lenient in permitting restrained social drinking with a maximum of two drinks. We do not know enough about the convulsive effect of alcohol and its metabolic breakdown products; there is always a possibility that such a change of blood chemistry may be just "the straw that broke the camels back" as one of many contributory factors leading to a seizure. I feel that abstinence is a laudable goal in the treatment of seizures but one cannot be too dogmatic in this regard. As far as "alcohol epilepsy" is concerned, the role of withdrawal in patients with chronic alcoholism was pointed out in Chapter 3; this type of seizure disorder is based upon mechanisms different from the occasional seizure precipitating effect of alcohol intake in an epileptic patient.

3) Waking and sleeping

The circadian distribution of epileptic seizures with preponderant occurrence during the morning hours, during nocturnal sleep or with irregular occurence and random distribution has been studied for many years by Janz (1953, a, b, c, 1962, 1969) who established the following classification:

1) Awakening epilepsy
2) Sleep epilepsy
3) Diffuse epilepsy (random occurrence) at any time of the day

Janz has explored all possible ramifications of this subdivision; he demonstrated principal differences in the sequential distribution of sleep stages in these three groups (based on the nocturnal sleep investigations of Jovanovic, 1967). According to this work, sleep epileptics reach the stages of very deep sleep (D and E or 3 and 4) very soon after falling asleep; their seizures occur chiefly in the early phases of rapidly deepening sleep. Patients with awakening epilepsy pass through hours of very light sleep and do not reach moderately deep levels before the early morning hours. These patients spend the morning hours in a state of sleepiness in which seizures may readily occur. According to Janz, these characteristics of sleep and the circadian distribution of seizures are independent of the effect of anticonvulsants and variations of the glucose level.

There is good reason to presume that most of the patients with awakening epilepsy and some of those with sleep epilepsy belong into the group of common generalized epilepsy where deviant arousal mechanisms ("dyshormia," Niedermeyer, 1972; see Chapter 4) play a very important part. I have heard repeatedly from these patients remarks such as "I must get up slowly in the morning, I must not jump out of bed when I am sleepy etc."; we hear from these patients that they develop a strange jittery feeling, that the first myoclonic jerks develop at the breakfast table or while shaving. This is a stern warning that a major convulsion is imminent.

These premonitions of seizures are most likely to appear when the patient has had an insufficient amount of nocturnal sleep. Going out at night, watching late television shows and all excessive stresses of daily life, which alter the quantity and quality of sleep, may lead to dire consequences in the morning. In Common generalized epilepsy, the *need for regular hours of sleep and reduction of excitement-inducing factors cannot be overstressed.* It is not surprising that the upsurge of the sexual drive in adolescence facilitates grand mal seizures but probably not as a direct hormonal chain of events but by means of emotional overstimulation and consequently disturbed nocturnal sleep. There is reason to believe that sexual activities as such are not detrimental to the seizure disorder.

All this pertains to Common generalized epilepsy only. Janz (1969) is concerned about the seizure-facilitating effect of excessively long nocturnal sleep and especially of daytime naps in patients with sleep epilepsy; this investigator discusses the value of stimulants in these patients. I have no personal data to substantiate or to disprove the concept of sleep epilepsy. According to Janz (1969), patients with temporal lobe epilepsy constitute a great part of the sleep epileptics and one wonders if the above discussed changes in the limbic system with their impact on the personality (with complete lack of sexual drive and sexual response; see Chapter 5 and 11) are the cause of enhanced sleep. In all these discussions, the effects of anticonvulsants (and perhaps a different reactivity in various groups of patients) must always be taken into account.

4) Occupational activities

This segment of individual hygiene (like most of the following ones) has important interfaces with society and could also be discussed in the chapter on social hygiene. It is evident that the occasional emergence of a seizure (in an otherwise fairly well controlled seizure disorder) raises important questions concerning the suitability of the patient's occupations. All of the hazards of a seizure on the job have been frequently discussed with respect to work on high scaffolds or construction sites, in close vicinity of machinery with large moving or rotating parts and, of course, driving a motor vehicle (to be discussed later in detail). All of the *inappropriate occupations* are listed in the following (after Livingston, 1972).

Surgeon
Those which necessitate operation of a motor vehicle
Those which involve automatically controlled machinery or equipment
Policeman
Fireman
Those which necessitate altitude or ladder work
Solitary watchman or lookout
Swimming instructor or lifeguard
Nursery maid
Baby-sitter

The following list (after Livingston, 1972) comprise the *occupations considered appropriate for patients with epileptic seizure.*

Farmer
Gardener
Salesman
(not requiring auto driving)
Clerk
Mechanic
(Manually controlled equipment)
Laborer
Electrician
(repairing or bench work)
Technician
Librarian
Psychologist
Stenographer
Veterinarian
Accountant
Pharmacist
Cabinetmaker
Draftsman
Jeweler
Plumber
Forester
Florist

Photographer
Physician
(one who does not deal directly with patients)
Lawyer
(one who does not participate in court activities)
Tailor
(Manually controlled equipment)
School teacher

Successful employment of a patient with not fully controlled epileptic seizures depends to a great deal on the employer's attitude which will be discussed in the final chapter. Rehabilitation and gainful employment is basically a matter of the employee's personality and capabilities; the markedly brain-damaged epileptic will automatically have a slim chance of holding a job, whereas an epileptic with average or high intelligence must not be hampered by the fact that he may have occasional seizures (unless the attacks endanger himself or others). According to Dennerll (1970), ". . . the object of employability and employment has not been fully achieved until the individual has the attributes of a desirable employee, to counteract the adverse effect of seizure occurrence." In this light, the seizures are just one type of handicap and it is well known how well adjusted and intelligent persons can overcome handicaps by developing positive qualities which make them desirable as employees and as human beings in general.

*5) **Driving a motor vehicle***

In this modern world, the inability to drive a car has an almost "castrating" effect on an individual but driving is a social function and, in the case of a patient with a history of epileptic seizures, permission to drive a motor vehicle is strictly ruled by the state law. The well controlled epileptic can receive a temporary driver's license upon the physician's recommendation; the license may be renewed in intervals varying from state to state.

It reflects human nature when young adults with a history of unsatisfactory seizure control, suddenly report a miraculous seizure freedom. In a mood of radiant optimism they ask the doctor for a supporting letter to the department of motor vehicles in order to obtain the long desired drivers license. A 19-year-old patient of mine was asking for a medical endorsement of her application to obtain a drivers license. She insisted that she had no seizure for many years. To make matters worse, this young lady showed numerous scars and even fresh wounds from tongue bites; her EEG showed a very active focus of seizure discharges. Moreover, psychological testing revealed her intellectual functioning to be in the dull-borderline IQ range. As was the case with this unfortunate teenager, refusal to cooperate in the attempt of obtaining a driver's license usually draws a very angry response from this type of patient.

In such requests for medical approval of a drivers license, EEG improvement over previous tracings is valuable objective evidence; complete EEG normalization is even more desirable but this goal may not be reached in spite of credible seizure-freedom. The physician must take very seriously his decision to support (or not to support) the patient's application; he must find a firm position in the dilemma between his duties to the individual and Society.

The license to operate a motor vehicle necessitates the availability of automobile insurance with a sufficient amount of liability insurance. This is presently not an unsurmountable obstacle and the situation will further improve when statistical analysis can provide evidence for good driving records of such individuals. Livingston (1972) is optimistic in this regard and feels that the average driver—the so-called normal person—is more likely to assume a nonchalant attitude than the epileptic who is keenly aware of the privilege of driving a car.

6) Sports and recreation

The participation in sports and even in athletic competition should be encouraged; a prohibitive and overprotective policy is in general, out of place. There are of course, a few exceptions. Swimming must be done with some caution and, in unsatisfactorily controlled cases, it might be worthwhile to ask for the lifeguard's special attention. One of our patients almost drowned in a swimming pool. Cycling is also ill advised as seizure may lead to a severe accident. Mountaineering on exposed trails or even technical mountaineering are prohibited.

Competitive team sports with frequent body contact and the risk of traumatic impact with craniocerebral trauma are of questionable hygienic value even for a healthy person leaving aside a person with a cerebral problem. This applies mainly to American football, ice hockey and rugby. Soccer playing (European football) may be permitted but the patient has to learn to avoid cranial traumatisation by improper "heading" of the ball (which could lead to an acceleration-deceleration type trauma).

7) Marriage and having children

Our knowledge of genetic factors in epilepsies is so fragmentary that it would make no sense to look at the question of marriage primarily from a genetic-eugenic viewpoint.

What really matters is the question as to whether the patient will be able to support a family. An employable person with incomplete seizure control is likely to have no marital problems with an understanding spouse. Genetic counseling should aim to avoid marrying a partner who is likely to carry certain epileptic genes (evidenced by familial epilepsy).

The hyposexuality of a temporal lobe epileptic represents a very serious problem in marital life which is hopeless in the case of a completely impotent male. Female temporal lobe epileptics are usually unaware of their sexual defect until they get married. Their complete lack of sexual response may spell disaster for the marriage.

Sexual activities are unlikely to increase the seizure frequency unless sex interferes with a reasonably balanced amount of sleep. Enhancement of seizures by sexual abstinence is completely unproven. These old wives' tales may have some truth as far as hysterical attacks are concerned.

8) The role of emotional stress

Man has been made to endure stress and not to float gently through a life of perfect homoiostatic happiness. On the other hand, stress may reach a dangerous breaking point with pathogenetic emotional, mental and somatic consequences. Whoever listens to the history told by an epileptic patient will often hear about a return or recrudescence of seizures during periods of great emotional stress such as marital strife, separation, divorce, loss of a parent or a child. The incredible crescendo of stressful events closing in on the Prince Myshkin in Dostoievsky's great novel "The Idiot" culminates dramatically in an epileptic seizure of the hero after a long period of seizure freedom.

While the Prince Myshkin apparently suffers from temporal lobe epilepsy with fascinating experiences occurring in his psychomotor attacks (bearing the mark of Dostoievsky's own epileptic experiences), the patients who are most likely to suffer from excessive emotional stress are those with Common generalized epilepsy. A disturbed peace of mind may jeopardize the nocturnal sleep, and attacks in the morning may occur even after many years of seizure freedom.

The physician may counteract this development by the concentration of the phenobarbital intake in the evening hours in order to enforce sleep. This is a double edged sword, however, and may work to the patient's disadvantage when he finds himself in a state of a phenobarbital-induced hangover during the morning hours (with increased potential epileptogenicity). A mild daytime tranquilizer such as diazepam (Valium), chlordiazepoxide (Librium) or meprobamate (Milton®, Equanil®) may prove to be helpful. In such periods of individual crisis, the patient needs some *supportive psychotherapy* which even a physician with no psychiatric training ought to be able to deliver.

CHAPTER 15

"THE EPILEPTIC" AND SOCIETY– ASPECTS OF SOCIAL HYGIENE

1) Introductory remarks

THE CONSTANT INTERACTION between man and his environment or milieu cuts across all areas of medicine and is of great importance in a comprehensive approach to seizure disorders. The reaction of man to a fellow-man's sudden fall, coma and convulsive movements or an attack of trance-like inappropriate automatic behavior is the principal topic of this chapter. The patient with seizures cannot live in a vacuum and cannot withdraw into castles in the air; he must come to grips with a society which, in many instances, is unable to cope with his attacks. Archetypal fears beset the onlooker of a grand mal seizure and, behind the civilized facade, the spirits of bygone ages come alive.

In addition to the attitudes of society, the epileptic may suffer from society's laws. It is natural that human law has to deal with epilepsy in a protective and a restrictive sense; the resulting legal restrictions often tend to be excessive stifling and a source of constant frustration.

All this pertains chiefly to the adult patient with seizures. For the child, parental attitudes and school environment are of utmost significance.

2) The epileptic child and parental attitudes

An epileptic infant or child may stir feelings of guilt in his parents. This is a common parental response to children with cerebral palsy or mental retardation in general. It may lead to "anosognostic" denial of the child's defect, to overprotectionism and an excess of parental love at the expense of the healthy siblings. This sequence of reactions is particularly common in the most severe forms of childhood epilepsy such as the Lennox-Gastaut syndrome where seizures are always associated with mental retardation and often with neurological deficits.

It would be erroneous to construe a psychodynamic basis for the above discussed "epileptic personality" (see Chapter 11) as being a mere psychological reaction to parental attitudes. Such attempts have been made in the past and are rather unconvincing. The physician's cognizance of such parental reactions, however, is important and will give him a better comprehension of the patient's domestic milieu.

3) *School environment*

A child with seizures is likely to be taunted and jeered by his schoolmates. If he is emotionally well adjusted, he will learn to live with the unkind environment or he will start leading the life of an outcast of Society. The seriousness of this situation naturally depends on the type of seizures; frequent *petit mal* absences are better tolerated than occasional grand mal attacks or automatisms.

Teachers often do very little to alleviate the problem. Seizures are basically considered a disruption and, from this angle of view, the epileptic child is about as disruptive as the worst hyperkinetic mischief in class. Principals may share this view and the threat of expulsion often hovers over parents and child. This may occur even in well behaved and intelligent children with seizures. According to Livingston (1972), there have been recent cases of refused admission to regular public schools; the investigation revealed that the children were denied admission not because of seizures but due to mental retardation and, respectively, severe emotional problems. Such cases, however, may lead to the opinion that children with epilepsy are automatically prohibited from attending public schools.

4) *Employment*

The employer's attitude toward an employee with seizures will vary from one individual to another and there will be natural variations from periods of prosperity and labor shortage to those of depression and unemployment.

There are very encouraging examples of willingness to hire epileptics and many employers deserve praise for their attitude. The crucial problem lies in psychodynamic dimensions and seems to be a deeply entrenched fear of the uncanny seizure event which the naive person could conceive as the frightening symbol of sudden death. "I am afraid you might have a seizure in my presence" said an employer when he fired an epileptic after he had learned through the mail about his condition (Livingston, 1972). It was explicitly not the fact that the epileptic condition was concealed to the employer at the time of hiring; it was clearly and unmistakably the fear of watching a seizure.

Other employers are afraid of accident proneness, personality problems or absenteeism; they may have had some contacts with feeble-minded chronic epileptics or with chronic alcoholics with withdrawal seizures (not uncommon on Monday during working hours).

5) *The Law*

The Law reveals the general attitudes of Society toward persons with epileptic seizures. Its protective facet comes into effect when infractions of the law have been committed in a state of epileptic obnubilation of mind. The restrictive part keeps the epileptic from various privileges of the average adult citizen; the license to operate a motor vehicle is of particular importance and was discussed farther above in Chapter 14. A study of Barrow and Fabing (1966) provides ample information about various important state laws concerning the epileptic.

A part of the legal restriction deals with *eugenic marriage* and *eugenic sterilization laws.* Marriage-prohibiting laws are still in effect in three states of the United States (North Carolina, Virginia and West Virginia) while thirteen states have eugenic sterilization laws pertaining to the epileptic (Arizona, Delaware,

Indiana, Kansas, Mississippi, Montana, New Hampshire, North Carolina, Oklahoma, South Carolina, Utah, Virginia and West Virginia). These laws are based on the erroneous concept of predominantly genetic factors involved in epilepsy. According to Barrow and Fabing (1966), the eugenic sterilization laws have been virtually abandoned as far as epileptics are concerned. Many states have amended their laws with the abandonment of marriage-prohibiting paragraphs.

6) National and local organizations dealing with epilepsy; Services available for the epileptic

The *Epilepsy Foundation of America* and the *National Epilepsy League, Inc.*, are two lay epilepsy organizations on a national basis. Their goals are outlined in Livingston's study (1972). A number of regional societies and local chapters have been founded as smaller lay organizations.

Under the direction of Dr. Frank Risch, *Epi-Hab* provides the epileptic with employment, on the job training, technical instruction by qualified instructors and ultimate placement in private business and industry. It has its center at the Veterans Administration Center in Los Angeles, California, and several subcenters have been founded over the country. Its great contribution to the rehabilitation of epileptic patients can hardly be overstressed.

In addition, there are other types of vocational rehabilitation services and special epilepsy programs for children (see Livingston, 1972).

7) "Desensitization of Society" as a goal of "sociotherapy"

The work of the above mentioned foundations and chapters has aimed at the alleviation of the epileptic's lot. Medicine has concentrated on the epileptic individual's therapy but the reactions of Society can only gradually be influenced. Lectures and exhibits on the organic cerebral nature of epilepsy have tried to convey the message that seizures arise from abnormal physiology of brain cells and not from a punitive act of God.

One can summarize such work as an attempt to "desensitize" society and an action to attenuate "hypersensitivity against a fellow-man's seizures. The goal could be reached by taking the

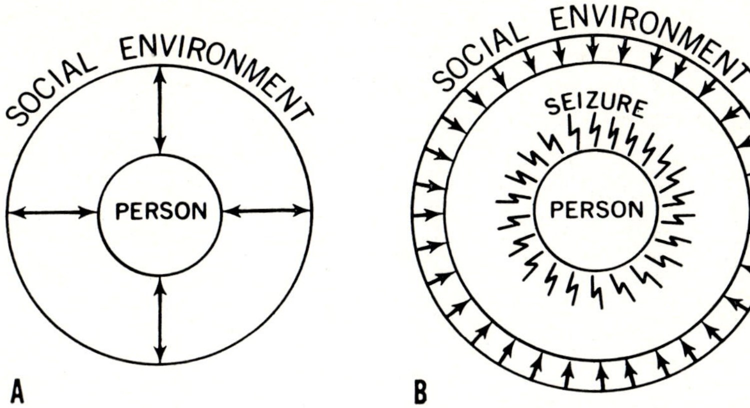

FIGURE 49. a) Normal interactions between individual and social environment. b) A seizure witnessed by other persons leads to immediate isolation of the epileptic patient. Society erects a wall which encapsulates the patient.

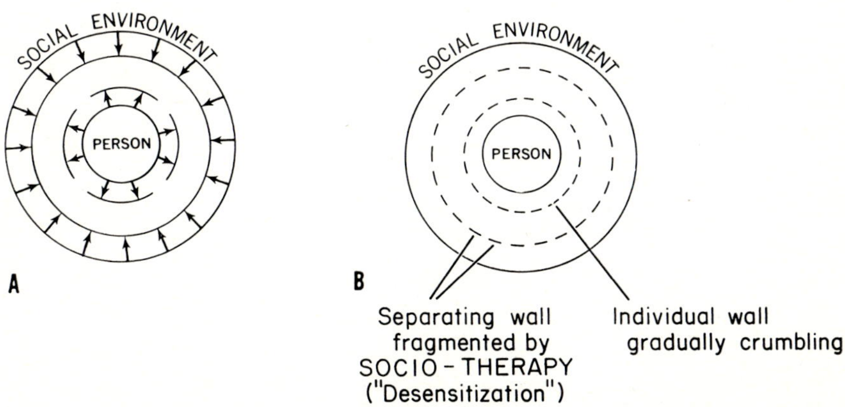

FIGURE 50. a) The socially isolated epileptic patient builds up his own wall of defense this adding further to the breakdown of interactions with Society. b) "Sociotherapy" ("desensitization of Society") gradually dismantles the separating wall. This enables the patient to break down his own walls of defense.

"spiritual sting" out of the seizure and removing the social stigma of being "struck by God" or, on a more enlightened level, of being the victim of an incurable and inherited disease. This message ought to reach parents, teachers and employers alike; it must reach society as a whole in order to tear down the wall which is constantly being erected between the epileptic individual and his environment (Fig. 49, 50). Hence, individual somatic therapy (and occasionally necessary psychotherapy) have to be supplemented with "sociotherapy" acting on society as a whole. This is painstaking work requiring years and decades of effort. Some favorable changes in public opinion have been demonstrated by Caveness, Merritt and Gallup (1969).

8) The yardstick to be used: Brain damage, not seizures as such

Rodin's (1968) thoughtful study of the prognosis of patients with epilepsy has shown that the absence or presence of intellectual deficits due to concomitant brain damage are crucial prognostic factors concerning particularly the patient's gainful employment. Behavioral deviations also play an important part in this regard.

The assessment of an epileptic individual in view of school or employment must aim at the recognition of cerebral defects and must not focus on the seizure disorder as such. This does not invalidate the fact that some occupations are not suitable for individuals with seizures.

When we place the emphasis on intellectual-behavioral performance we will have to confront the fact that, in some cases, seizures are perfectly compatible with high intelligence up to the genius level. We better dismiss the shopworn stories about Alexander the Great, Caesar and Napoleon as suffering from epileptic seizures; there is no convincing evidence for these claims that just all three of the perhaps all time greatest geniuses of statesmanship and strategy had epilepsy. I cannot see too much consolation for the average epileptic in such stories. Religious leaders and geniuses have been almost automatically listed as epileptics—(Buddha, Mohammed, St. Paul) since some investigators simply equate transcendental revelations with either psychosis or epilepsy. It might be worthwhile to concentrate on true cases of great intellectual performance in the presence of a proven epileptic disorder.

With the emphasis being laid on concomitant brain damage, there will be greater general awareness of the multitude of causes and types of cerebral pathology in patients with epileptic attacks. With this etiological and pathological pluralism in mind, people will much better understand that epileptic manifestations are nothing but abnormal reactions of the brain.

With this statement, we have returned to the very starting point of this book. In order to present a global view of the epilepsies, our journey began at the level of molecules and neurons, led to the brain and its diseases, progressed to the patient as a person and has ended with the interactions between the suffering human being and Society.

REFERENCES

Abbott, J.: The EEG in Jakob-Creutzfeldt's disease. *Electroencephalogr Clin Neurophysiol, 11*:184, 1959 (abstract).

Aicardi, J., and Chevrie, J. J.: Convulsive status epilepticus in infants and children. A study of 239 cases. *Epilepsia, 11*:187-197, 1970.

Aizawa, T.; Muramatsu, F.; Hamaguchi, K.; Tomita, M.; Kakimi, R., and Toyoda, M.: Cerebral circulation, metabolism and electrical activity during convulsion induced by megimide. *Jap Circ J, 29*:449-454, 1965.

Ajmone Marsan, C.: A newly proposed classification of epileptic seizures. Neurophysiological basis. *Epilepsia, 2*:217-228, 1961.

———, and Fuortes, M. G. F.: Electrographic study of the convulsant action of intravenously administered acetylcholine. *Electroencephalogr Clin Neurophysiol, 1*:283-290, 1949.

———, and Ralston, B. L.: *The epileptic seizure.* Springfield, Thomas, 1957.

———, and Lewis, M. R.: Pathologic findings in patients with *centrencephalic* seizure patterns. *Neurology* (Minneap), *10*:922-930, 1960.

Alajouanine, T.; Contamin, F., and Cathala, H. P.: *Le syndrome tétanie.* Paris, J. B. Baillère, 1958.

———, and Gastaut, H.: La syncinésie-sursaut et l'épilepsie-sursaut à déclenchement sensoriel ou sensitif inopiné. In T. Alajouanine (Ed.): *Bases physiologigues et aspects clinigues de l'épilepsie.* Paris, Masson, pp. 199-231, 1958.

———; Nehlil, J., and Gabersek, V.: A propos d'un cas d'épilepsie déclenchée par la lecture. *Rev neurol,* Paris, *101*:463-467, 1959.

Alzheimer, A.: Die Gruppierung der Epilepsie. *Allg Z Psychiat, 64*:418-435, 1907.

Amantea, G.: Rapporto tra eccitamenti afferenti ed epilessia sperimentale. *Boll Acad med Roma,* 1920 (quoted after Vizioli, R.).

———, and Martino, G.: Morfinizzazione ed epilessia da eccitamenti afferenti nel cane. *Boll Soc Ital Biol sper, 2*:311, 1927 (quoted after Vizioli, R.).

Ambrozy, G.: Tonusos rohamok (Tonic seizures). *Idegyok Szel, 17*:328-340, 1964.

Anderson, P.; Eccles, J. C., and Sears, T. A.: The ventrobasal complex of the thalamus: types of cells, their responses and their functional organization. *J Physiol, 174*:370-399, 1964.

Angeleri, F.; Ferro-Milone, F., and Parigi, S.: Electrical activity and reactivity of the rhinencephalic, pararhinencephalic and thalamic structures; Prolonged implanatation of electrodes in man. *Electroenceph clin Neurophysiol, 16*:100-129, 1964.

Anthony, M.; Hinterberger, H., and Lance, J. W.: Plasma serotonin in migraine and stress. *Arch Neurol, 16*:544-552, 1967.

Arseni, C., and Cristescu, A.: Epilepsy due to cerebral cysticercosis. *Epilepsia* (Amst.), *13*:253-258, 1972.

Asenjo, A.: Neurocisticercosis: generalidades. *Neurocirurgia, 19*:143-155, 1961.

Baglioni, S., and Magnini, M.: Azione di alcune sostanze chimiche sulle zone eccitabili della corteccia cerebrale del cane. *Arch Fisiol, 6*:240, 1909. Quoted after R. Vizioli.

Bailey, P.: Treatment of psychomotor states by anterior temporal lobectomy. *Res Publ Assn nerv ment Dis,* 31:341-346, 1953.

Bailey, P.: Betrachtungen über die chirurgische Behandlung der psychomotorischen Epilepsie. *Zbl Neurochir, 14*:195-206, 1954.

———: Complications of anterior temporal lobectomy. In M. Baldwin and P. Bailey (Ed.): *Temporal lobe epilepsy.* Springfield, Thomas, pp. 507-509, 1958.

———, and Gibbs, F. A.: The surgical treatment of psychomotor epilepsy. *JAMA, 145*:365-370, 1951.

Baird, R. L.; Weiss, D. L.; Ferguson, A. D.; French, J. H., and Scott, R. B.: Studies in sickle cell anemia. XXI. Clincio-pathological aspects of neurological manifestations. *Pediatrics, 34*:92-100, 1965.

Bamberger, P., and Matthes, A.: *Anfälle im Kindesalter.* Basel, Karger, 1959.

Bancaud, J.; Talairach, J.; Bonis, A.; Schaub, C.; Szikla, G.; Morel, P., and Bordas-Ferer, M.: *La stéréo-electroencéphalographie dans l'épilepsie.* Paris, Masson, 1965.

———; Talairach, J., and Bonis, A.: Physiopathogénie des épilepsies sursaut. *Rev Neurol* (Paris), *117*:441-453, 1967.

Barac, B.: Vertiginous epileptic attacks and so-called "vestibulogenic seizures." *Epilepsia, 9*:137-144, 1968.

Barolin, G. S.: Migraine and epilepsies—a relationship? *Epilepsia, 7*:53-66, 1966.

Barolin, G. S., and Scherzer, E.: Epileptische Anfälle bei Apoplektikern. *Wien Z Nervenheilk, 20*:35-47, 1963.

———; Scherzer, E., and Schnaberth, G.: Epileptische Manifestationen als Vorboten von Schlaganfällen. *Fortschr Neurol Psychiat, 39*:199-216, 1971.

Barrow, R. L., and Fabing, H. D.: *Epilepsy and the Law,* 2nd ed. New York, Hoeber Med. Div., 1966.

Batten, F. E.: Cerebral degeneration with symmetrical changes in the maculae in two members of a family. *Trans Ophth Soc, 23*:386-390, 1903.

———: Family cerebral degeneration with macular changes (so-called juvenile form of family amaurotic idiocy). *Quart J Med,* 7:444-454, 1914.

Baxter, D. W., and Bailey, A. A.: Primary reading epilepsy. *Neurology* (Minneap), *11*:437-449, 1961.

Bente, D., and Itil, T. M.: Zur Wirkung des Phenothiazinkörpers Megaphen auf das menschliche Hirnstrombild. *Arzneimittelforschg,* 4:418-423, 1954.

Berger, H.: Über das Elektrenkephalogramm des Menschen (First report). *Arch Psychiat Nervenkr,* 87:527-570, 1929.

Bergstrom, W. H.; Carzoli, R. F.; Lombroso, C.; Davidson, D. T., and Wallace, W. M.: Observations on the metabolic and clinical effects of carbonic anhydrase inhibitors in epileptics. *Amer J Dis Child,* 84:771-772, 1952.

Bickford, R. G.: Sensory precipitation of seizures. *J Mich med Soc,* 53:1018-1021, 1954.

———: The application of depth electrography in some varieties of epilepsy. *Electroenceph Clin Neurophysiol,* 8:526-527, 1956.

———: Electroencephalography. In J. A. Bastron et al. (Ed.): *Clinical examinations in Neurology.* 2nd ed. Philadelphia, Saunders, pp. 297-310, 1963.

———; Whelan, J. L.; Klass, D. W., and Corbin, K. B.: Reading epilepsy: clinical and electroencephalographic study of a new syndrome. *Trans Amer Neurol Assn,* 81:100-102, 1956.

———, and Klass, D. W.: Stimulus factors in the mechanism of television-induced seizures. *Trans Amer Neurol Assn,* 87:176-178, 1962.

———, and Klass, D. W.: Sensory precipitation and reflex mechanisms. In H. H. Jasper; A. A. Ward, Jr., and A. Pope (Ed.): *Basic mechanisms of the epilepsies.* Boston, Little and Brown, pp. 543-564, 1969.

Bielschowsky, M.: Über spätinfantile familiäre amaurotische Idiotie mit Kleinhirn-Symptomen. *Deutsch Z Nervenheilk,* 50:729, 1913.

Biltz, H.: Über die Konstitution der Einwirkungsprodukte von substituierten Harnstoffen auf Benzil und über einige neue Methoden zur Darstellung der 5, 5-Diphenylhydantoine. *Berl Dtsch Chem Ges,* 41:1379, 1908 (quoted after Glazko, 1972).

Bingel, A.: Reading epilepsy. *Neurology* (Minneap), 7:752-756, 1957.

Bingley, T.: *Mental symptoms in temporal lobe epilepsy and temporal lobe gliomas.* Copenhagen, Munksgaard, 1958.

Blom, S.: Trigeminal neuralgia: Its treatment with a new anticonvulsant drug (G-32883). *Lancet,* I:839-840, 1962.

———, and Brorson, L. O.: Central spikes or sharp waves (rolandic spikes) in children's EEG and their clinical significance. *Acta Paediat Scand,* 55:385-393, 1966.

Blumer, D.: Hypersexual episodes in temporal lobe epilepsy. *Amer J Psychiat,* 126:1099-1106, 1970.

———, and Walker, A. E.: Sexual behavior in temporal lobe epilepsy. *Arch Neurol, 16*:37-43, 1967.

Bogue, J. Y., and Carrington, H. C.: The evaluation of Mysoline®—A new anticonvulsant drug. *Br J Pharmacol, 8*:230-235, 1953.

Bonduelle, M.; Bouygues, P.; Sallou, C., and Grobuis, S.: Expérimentation clinique de l'anti-épileptique G 32. 883 (Tegretol). Resultats portant sur 100 cas observés en trois ans. *Rev Neurol* (Paris), *110*:209-214, 1964.

Bonkalo, A., and Arthurs, R. G. S.: Mysoline in treatment of epileptic and non-epileptic psychiatric patients. *Canad Med Assn J, 68*:570-574, 1953.

Bonnycastle, D. D., and Bradley, A. J.: Diphenylhydantoin and the release of adrenocorticotropic hormone in the albino rat. *Endocrinology, 66*:355-363, 1960.

Booker, H. E.; Hosokawa, K.; Burdette, R. D., and Darcey, B.: A clinical study of serum primidone levels. *Epilepsia, 11*:395-402, 1970.

Boshes, L. D., and Gibbs, F. A.: *Epilepsy Handbook.* 2nd ed. Springfield, Thomas, 1972.

Bouchet and Cazauvielh: De l'épilepsie considerée dans ces rapports avec l'aliénation mentale. *Arch Gen Med, 9*:510-542, 1825. Quoted after Peiffer.

Boudin, G.; Barbizet, J., and Labet, R.: L'association épilepsie-endocrinopathie. Epilepsie d'origine profonde avec tracé épileptique de type Petit mal et endocrinopathie d'origine diencéphalique. *Rev Neurol,* (Paris), *91*:330-346, 1954.

Bradley, K.; Easton, D. M., and Eccles, J. C.: An investigation of primary or direct inhibition. *J Physiol, 122*:474-488, 1953.

Bradshaw, P., and Parsons, M.: Hemiplegic Migraine: a clinical study. *Q J Med, 34*:65-85, 1965.

Brain, R.: Order and disorder in cerebral circulation. *Lancet, II*:857-862, 1960.

Brémer, F.: Le tétanos strychnique. et le mécanisme de la synchronization neuronique. *Arch Int Physiol, 51*:211-260, 1941.

Bridge, E. M.: *Epilepsy and Convulsive Disorders in Children.* New York, McGraw-Hill, 1949.

Brock, L. G.; Coombs, J. S., and Eccles, J. C.: The recording of potentials from motoneurones with an intracellular electrode. *J Physiol, 117*:431-460, 1952.

Bronisch, F. W., and Rauch, H. J.: Zur Pathogenese der epileptischen Anfälle bei multipler Sklerose. *Deutsch Z Nervenkr, 158*:322-344, 1947.

Broser, R.: *Die cerebralen vegetativen Anfälle.* Berlin, Springer, 1958.

Brown-Séquard, E.: D'une affection convulsive qui survient chez les animaux ayant eû une moitiée latérale de la moelle epinière coupée. *C R Soc Biol, 2*:105, 1850.

Bruens, J. H.: Psychoses in epilepsy. *Psychiat Neurol Neurochir, 74*:175-192, (1971).

Buchthal, F.; Svensmark, O., and Schiller, P. J.: Clinical and electroencephalographic correlations with serum levels of diphenylhydantoin. *Arch Neurol, 2*:624-630, 1960.

Buchthal, F., and Svensmark, O.: Serum concentrations of diphenylhydantoin (Phenytoin) and phenobarbital and their relation to therapeutic and effects. *Psychiat Neurol Neurochir, 74*:117-136, 1971.

Bumke, O.: *Lehrbuch der Geisteskrankheiten, 2nd ed.* Munich, Bergmann, 1942.

Burger, L. J.; Lopez, R. I., and Elliott, F. A.: Tonic seizures induced by movement. *Neurology* (Minneap), *22*:656-659, 1972.

Burke, J. B.: Prognostic significance of neonatal convulsions. *Arch Dis Childh, 29*:342-345, 1954.

Busse, E. W.; Barnes, R. H.; Friedmann, E. L., and Kelty, E. J.: Psychologic functioning of aged individuals with normal and abnormal electroencephalograms. I. A study of non-hospitalized community volunteers. *J nerv ment Dis, 124*:135-141, 1956.

Bush, M. T., and Sanders-Bush, E.: Chemistry and methods for determination (phenobarbital, mephobarbital and metharbital). In D. M. Woodbury; J. K. Penry, and R. P. Schmidt (Ed.): *Antiepileptic drugs.* New York, Raven Press, pp. 293-302, 1972.

Butler, T. C.: The metabolic conversion of 5, 5-diphenylhydantoin to 5-(p-hydroxyphenyl)-5-phenylhydantoin. *J Pharmacol Exp Ther, 116*:326-336, 1956.

Campbell, J. E., and Walker, A. E.: Personal communication, quoted by A. E. Walker, 1957.

Cannon, W. B.: A law of denervation. *Amer J Med Sci, 198*:737-744, 1939.

Caveness, W. F.: Ontogeny of seizures. In H. H. Jasper; A. A. Ward, Jr., and A. Pope (Ed.): *Basic mechanism of the epilepsies.* Boston, Little, Brown and Co., pp. 517-534, 1969.

———; Merritt, H. H., and Gallup, G. H.: A survey of public attitudes toward epilepsy in 1969. With an indication of trends over the past twenty years. *Epilepsia, 10*:429-440, 1969.

Cerletti, U., and Bini, L.: L'elettroshock. *Arch Gen Neurol Psichiat Psicoanal, 19*:266-270, 1938.

Chang, T.; Burkett, A. R., and Glazko, A. J.: Ethosuximide. Biotransformation. In D. M. Woodbury; J. K. Penry, and R. P. Schmidt: *Antiepileptic drugs.* New York, Raven Press, pp. 425-429, 1972.

Chatrian, G. E.: Tonic seizures. Presid. Address, Ann. Meeting Amer. Epilepsy Soc., New York, N. Y. December 2, 1971.

———; Shaw, C. M., and Leffman, H.: The significance of periodic lateralized epileptiform discharges in EEG: an electrographic, clinical and pathological study. *Electroenceph Clin Neurophysiol, 17*:177-193, 1964.

Chatrian, G. E.; Lettich, E.; Miller, L. H., and Green, J. R.: Pattern-sensitive epilepsy, Part 1 (An electrographic study of its mechanisms). *Epilepsia* *11*:125-150, 1970.

———; Lettich, E.; Miller, L. H.; Green, J. R., and Kupfer, C.: Pattern-sensitive epilepsy, Part 2. (Clinical changes, tests of responsiveness and motor output, alterations of evoked potentials and therapeutic measures.) *Epilepsia, 11*:151-162, 1970.

Chavany, J. A.; Fischgold, H.; Messimy, R., and Arfel-Capdeville, M.: Etude clinique et E.E.G. d'un cas d'épilepsia provoquée électivement par la lecture. *Rev Neurol* (Paris), *95*:381-386, 1956.

Clare, M. H., and Bishop, G. H.: Properties of dendrites; apical dendrites of the cat cortex. *Electroenceph Clin Neurophysiol, 7*:85-98, 1955.

Clementi, A.: Stricnizzazione della sfera corticale visiva ed epilessia sperimentale da stimoli luminosi. *Arch Fisiol, 27*:356-387, 1929.

Clouston, T. S.: Experiments to determine the precise effect of bromide of potassium in epilepsy. *J Ment Sci, 14*:305, 1868. Quoted after D. B. Tower, 1960.

Cooper, R.; Winter, A. L.; Crow, H. H., and Walter, W. G.: Comparison of subcortical, cortical and scalp activity using chronically indwelling electrodes in man. *Electroenceph Clin Neurophysiol, 19*:217-229, 1965.

Courjon, J. A.: Posttraumatic epilepsy in electroclinical practice. In A. E. Walker; W. F. Caveness, and M. Critchley (Ed.): *The late effects of head injury.* Springfield, Thomas, pp. 215-227, 1969.

Coursin, D. B.: Convulsive seizures in infants with pyridoxine-deficient diet. *JAMA, 154*:406-408, 1954.

Courville, C. B.: Traumatic lesions of the temporal lobe as the essential cause of psychomotor epilepsy. In M. Baldwin and P. Bailey (Ed.): *Temporal lobe epilepsy.* Springfield, Thomas, pp. 220-239, 1958.

Creutzfeldt, H. G.: Über eine eigenartige herdförmige Erkrankung des *Zentralnervensystems. Z ges Neurol Psychiat, 57*:1, 1920. Quoted after W. R. Kirschbaum, 1968.

Creutzfeldt, O. D.: Neuronal mechanisms underlying the EEG. In H. H. Jasper; A. A. Ward, Jr., and A. Pope (Ed.): *Basic mechanisms of the epilepsies.* Boston, Little, Brown and Co., pp. 397-420, 1969.

Critchley, M.: Musicogenic epilepsy. *Brain, 60*:13-27, 1937.

———: Reading epilepsy. *Epilepsia, 3*:402-405, 1962.

———; Cobb, W., and Sears, T.: On reading epilepsy. *Epilepsia, 1*:403-417, 1959/60.

Daly, D. D., and Mulder, D. W.: Gelastic epilepsy. *Neurology* (Minneap), *1*:189-192, 1957.

Dam, M.: The number of Purkinje cells after diphenylhydantoin intoxication in monkeys. *Epilepsia, 11*:313-320, 1970.

———: Diphenylhydantoin. Neurological aspects of toxicity. In D. M. Woodbury; J. K. Penry, and R. P. Schmidt (Ed.): *Antiepileptic drugs.* New York, Raven Press, pp. 227-235, 1972.

———, and Olesen, V.: Intramuscular administration of phenytoin. *Neurology* (Minneap), *16*:288-292, 1966.

Dandy, W.: Physiological studies following extirpation of the right cerebral hemispherein man. *Bull Johns Hopkins Hosp*, *53*:31-51, 1933.

Davis, J. P., and Lennox, W. G.: Comparison of Paradione and Tridione in treatment of epilepsy. *J Pediat*, *34*:273-278, 1949.

———, and Schwade, E. D.: Anticonvulsant effects of 3-allyl-5-isobutyl-2-thiohydantoin, (Box 422). *Fed Proc*, *18*:380-382, 1959.

Dawson, G. D.: Investigations on a patient subject to myoclonic seizures after sensory stimulation. *J Neurol Neurosurg Psychiatry*, *10*:141-162, 1947.

Delgado, J. M. R.: Prolonged stimulation of brain in awake monkeys. *J Neurophysiol*, *22*:458-475, 1959.

Dennerll, R. D.: Problems of rehabilitation and employability of epileptics. In E. Niedermeyer (Ed.): *Epilepsy*. Basal, Karger, pp. 326-337, 1970.

De Robertis, E.; Rodriguez de Lores Arnaiz, G., and Aberici, M.: Ultrastructural nuerochemistry. In H. H. Jasper; A. A. Ward, Jr., and A. Pope (Ed.): *Basic mechanisms of the epilepsies*. Boston, Little, Brown and Co., pp. 137-158, 1969.

DeSilva, J. A. F.; Koechlin, B. A., and Bader, G.: Blood level distribution patterns of diazepam and first major metabolite in man. *J Pharmacol*, *19*:692-702, 1966.

Diemath, H. E.; Heppner, F.; Enge, S., and Lechner, H.: Die stereotaktische vordere Cingulotomie bei therapieresistenter generalisierter Epilepsie. *Confin Neurol*, *27*:124-128, 1966.

Dill, W. A.; Peterson, L.; Chang, T., and Glazko, A. J.: Physiologic disposition of alpha-methylalpha-ethylsuccinimide (ethosuximide; Zarontin®) in animals and man. *Amer Chem Abstracts*, 149th National Meeting, Detroit, Mich., p. 30 N, 1965.

Domek, N. S.; Barlow, C. F., and Roth, L. H.: An ontogenetic study of phenobarbital-C^{14} in cat brain. *J Pharmacol Exp Ther*, *130*:285-293, 1960.

Dongier, S.: Statistical study of clinical and electroencephalographic manifestations of 536 episodes occurring in 516 epileptics between seizures. *Epilepsia*, *1*:117-142, 1959/60.

Donker, D. N. J.; Robles de Medina, E. O., and Kieft, J.: Micturition syncope. *Electroenceph Clin Neurophysiol*, *33*:328-331, 1972.

Doose, H.: Das akinetische Petit mal. *Arch Psychiat Nervenkr*, *206*:504-524, 1964.

———: Spezielle Probleme der antikonvulsiven Therapie. In E. Niedermeyer (Ed.): *Epilepsy*. Basal, Karger, pp. 246-270, 1970.

Dow, R. S.: Extrinsic regulatory mechanisms of seizure activity. *Epilepsia*, *6*:122-140, 1965.

Doyle, P. J., and Livingston, S.: Use of Mysoline in treatment of epilepsy. *J Pediat*, *43*:413-416, 1953.

Drake, W. E., and MacRae, D.: Epilepsy in multiple sclerosis. *Neurology* (Minneap), *11*:810-816, 1961.

Dreyfus-Brisac, C., and Monod, N.: Electroclinical studies of status epilepticus in the newborn. In P. Kellaway and I. Petersen (Ed.): *Neurological and electroencephalographic correlative studies in infancy.* New York, Grune and Stratton, pp. 250-272, 1964.

Durst, W., and Krump, J. E.: Elektrencephalographische und polygraphische Untersuchungen bei kreislaufbedingten Synkopen und vegetativen Anfällen. *Nervenarzt, 32*:401-405, 1961.

Dusser de Barenne, J. G., and McCulloch, W. S.: Factors for facilitation and extinction in the central nervous system. *J Neurophysiol, 2*:319-355, 1939.

Earle, K. M. M.; Baldwin, M., and Penfield, W.: Incisural sclerosis and temporal lobe seizures produced by hippocampal herniation at birth. *Arch Neurol, 69*:27-42, 1953.

Eberhart, C., and Morgan, J.: Micturition syncope. *JAMA, 174*:2076-2077, 1960.

Eccles, J. C.: *The inhibitory pathways of the central nervous system.* Springfield, Thomas, 1969.

———; Llinas, R., and Sasaki, K.: The mossy fibre granule cell relay in the cerebellum and its inhibition by Golgi cells. *Exp Brain Res, 1*:82-101, 1966.

Efron, R.: Post-epileptic paralysis: theoretical critique and report of a case. *Brain, 84*:381-394, 1691.

Elian, M.: The long-term use of valium (diazepam) in epilepsy. *Epilepsia* (Amst.), *10*:487-493, 1969.

Engel, G. L.: *Fainting.* 2nd ed. Springfield, Thomas, 1962.

———; Ferris, E. B., and Romano, J.: Focal electroencephalographic changes during scotomas of migraine. *Amer J med Sci, 209*:650-657, 1947.

Engelmeier, M. P.: Über die klinische Erprobung antiepileptischer Medikamente unter besonderer Berücksichtingung des Ospolot. *Deutsch med Wschr, 85*:2207-2211, 1960.

Erben, S.: *Diagnose der Simulation nervöser Symptome.* 3rd ed. Berlin, Urban and Schwarzenberg, 1930.

Ervin, F.; Epstein, A. W., and King, H. E.: Behavior of epileptic and nonepileptic patient with "temporal spikes." *Arch Neurol Psychiat,* paraepileptic phenomenon? *Epilepsia, 10*:417, 1969 (abstract).

Ervin, R. R.; Delgado, J.; Mark, V. H., and Sweet, W. H.: Rage: A paraepileptic phenomenon? *Epilepsia* (Amst.), *10*:417, 1969 (abstract).

Faerø, O.; Kastrup, K. W.; Lykkegard Nielsen, E.; Melchior, J. C., and Thorn, I.: Successful prophylaxis of febrile convulsions with phenobarbital. 1860. *Epilepsia, 13*:279-285, 1972.

Faeth, W. H.; Walker, A. E., and Andy, O. J.: Propagation of cortical and subcortical epileptic discharge. *Epilepsia* (Boston), *3*:37-48, 1956.

Fajans, S. S., and Thorn, G. W.: Hyperinsulinism and hypoglycemia. In T. R. Harrison et al. (Ed.): *Principles of Internal Medicine*. 5th ed. New York, McGraw-Hill, 1966, pp. 507-512.

Falconer, M. A.: Surgical treatment of temporal lobe epilepsy. *New Zeald med J, 66*:539-542, 1967.

———; Hill, D.; Meyer, A.; Mitchell, W., and Pond, D. A.: Treatment of temporal lobe epilepsy by temporal lobectomy: survey of findings and results. *Lancet, 1*:827-835, 1955.

———; Hill, D.; Meyer, A., and Wilson, J. L.: Clinical, radiological and EEG correlations with pathological changes in temporal lobe epilepsy in surgical treatment. In M. Baldwin and P. Bailey (Ed.): *Temporal lobe epilepsy*. Springfield, Thomas, 1958, pp. 396-410.

———; Driver, M. V., and Serafetinides, E. A.: Temporal lobe epilepsy due to distant lesions: Two cases relieved by operation. *Brain, 85*:521-534, 1962.

———, and Serafetinides, E. A.: A follow-up study in temporal lobe epilepsy. *J Neurol Neurosurg Psychiat, 26*:154-165, 1963.

Falret, J.: De l'état mental des épileptiques. *Arch gén Méd, 16*:661-679,

Fay, T.: The therapeutic effect of dehydration on epileptic patients. *Arch Neurol Psychiat* (Chic.), *23*:920-935, 1930.

Fegersten, L., and Roger, A.: Frontal epileptogenic Foci. *Electroenceph* Clin Neur*ophysiol, 13*:905-913, 1961.

Feindel, W., and Gloor, P.: Comparison of electrographic effects of stimulation of the amygdala and brain stem reticular formation in cats. *Electroenceph Clin Neurophysiol, 6*:389-402, 1954.

Feldman, S.; Todt, J. C., and Porter, R .W.: Effects of adrenocortical hormones on evoked potentials in the brain stem. *Neurology* (Minneap), *11*:109-115, 1961.

Fenton, G.; Serafetinides, E. A., and Pond, D. A.: The effect of sulthiame, a new anticonvulsant drug in the treatment of temporal lobe epilepsy. *Epilepsia* (Amst.), *5*:59-67, 1964.

Ferris, E. B.; Capps, R. B., and Weiss, S.: Carotid sinus syncope and its bearing on the mechanisms of unconscious state and convulsions. *Medicine* (Baltimore), *14*:377-456, 1935.

Fischer, M. H.: Elektrobiologische Auswirkungen von Krampfgiften am Zentralnervensystem. *Med Klin, 29*:15-19, 1933.

Fischer, H.: Symptomatische Epilepsie bei cerebralen Gefäszprozessen. *Arch Psychiat Nervenkr, 199*:296-310, 1959.

Fisher, C. M., and Adams, R. D.: The transient global amnesic syndrome. *Acta neurol Scand, Suppl. 9, 40*:7-82, 1964.

Flor-Henry, P.: Psychosis and Temporal lobe epilepsy. A controlled investigation. *Epilepsia, 10*:363-395, 1969.

Flügel, F.; Bente, D., and Itil, T.: Zur Stellung des Butansultamderivats Ospolot in der Behandlung zerebraler Anfallsleiden. *Deutsch med Wschr, 85*:2199-2203, 1960.

Foerster, O.: Hyperventilationsepilepsie. *Deutsch Z Nervenheilk, 83*:347-356, 1924.

———: Die Pathogenese des epileptischen Krampfanfalles. *Deutsch Z Nervenheilk, 94*:15-53, 1926.

———, and Penfield, W.: The structural basis of traumatic epilepsy and results of radical operation. *Brain, 53*:99-120, 1930.

———, and Penfield, W.: Der Narbenzug am und im Gehirn bei traumatischer Epilepsie in seiner Bedeutung für das Zustandekommen der Anfälle und für die therapeutische Bekämpfung derselben. *Z ges Neurol Psychiat, 125*:475-572, 1930.

Ford, F. R.: *Diseases of the nervous system in childhood and adolescence.* Springfield, Thomas, 1960.

Forster, F. M.: Therapy in psychomotor epilepsy. *JAMA, 145*:211-215, 1951.

———; Ptacek, L. J., and Peterson, W. G.: Auditory clicks in extinction of stroboscope-induced seizures. *Epilepsia, 6*:217-225, 1965.

Frank, K., and Fuortes, M. G. F.: Presynaptic and postsynaptic inhibition of monosynaptic reflexes. *Fed proc, 16*:39-43, 1957.

Freeman, J. M.: Neonatal seizures—diagnosis and management. *J Pediatr* (St. Louis), *77*:701-708, 1970.

Freeman, J. M., and McKhann, G. M.: Degenerative disease of the central nervous system. *Advanc Pediat, 16*:121-175, 1969.

Friedmann, M.: Über die gehäuften kleinen nicht epileptischen Absencen oder kurzen narkoleptischen Anfälle. *Deutsch Z Nervenheilk, 30*:462-492, 1906.

Gallagher, B. B., and Baumel, I. P.: Primidone. Biotransformation. In D. M. Woodbury; J. K. Penry, and R. P. Schmidt (Ed.): *Antiepileptic drugs.* New York, Raven Press, pp. 361-366, 1972.

Gänshirt, H., and Zylka, W.: Die Erholungszeit am Warmblütergehirn nach kompletter Ischämie. *Arch Psychiat Nervenkr, 189*:23-36, 1952.

Garretson, H.; Gloor, P., and Rasmussen, T.: Intracarotid Amobarbital and Netrazol test for the study of epileptform discharges in man: a note on its technique. *Electroencephalogr Clin Neurophysiol, 21*:607-610, 1966.

Gascon, G. G., and Lombroso, C. T.: Epileptic (gelastic) laughter. *Epilepsia, 12*:63-76, 1971.

Gastaut, H.: So-called "psychomotor" and "temporal" epilepsy—a critical study. *Epilepsia* (Boston), *2*:59-99, 1953.

———: Syncope and seizure. *Electroencephalogr Clin Neurophysiol, 10*:571-572, 1958.

———: A propos des symptomes cliniques rencontrés chez les épileptiques psychomoteurs dans l'intervalle de leurs crises. In T. Alajouanine (Ed.): *Bases physiologiques et aspects cliniques de l'epilepsie.* Paris, Masson, pp. 139-162, 1958.

———: A propos des décharges neuroniques developpées à distance d'une lésion épileptogène et des symptômes qui en résultent. In T. Alajouanine (Ed.): *Bases physiologiques et aspects cliniques de l'épilepsie.* Paris, Masson, pp. 163-184, 1958.

———: Un aspect méconnu des décharges neuroniques occipitales: la crise oculo-clonique ou "nystagmus épileptique." In T. Alajouanine (Ed.): *Les grandes activités du lobe occipital.* Paris, Masson, pp. 169-186, 1960.

———: A physiopathogenetic study of reflex anoxic cerebral seizures in children (syncopes, sobbing spasms, breath-holding spells). In P. Kellaway and I. Petersen (Ed.): *Clinical electroencephalography of children.* New York, Grune and Stratton, pp. 257-274, 1968.

———: Exceptional anticonvulsive properties of a new benzodiazepine (demonstrated by a screening method). In E. Niedermeyer (Ed.): *Epilepsy.* Basel, Karger, pp. 261-269, 1970.

———: Clinical and electroencephalographical classification of epileptic seizures. *Epilepsia, 11*:102-113, 1970.

———: Comments on "Petit mal variant revisited." *Epilepsia, 12*:97-99, 1971.

———; Roger, J.; Corriol, J., and Gastaut, Y.: Les forms expérimentales de l'épilepsie humaine. L'épilepsie induite par la stimulation lumineuse intermittente ou épilepsie photogénique. *Rev Neurol* (Paris), *80*:161-183, 1948.

———, and Gastaut, Y.: Correlations électroencéphalographiques et cliniques à propos de 100 cas d'épilepsie dite "psychomotrice" avec foyers sur la région temporale du scalp. *Rev Oto-neuro-ophthal, 23*:257-282, 1951.

———, and Collomb, H.: Etude du comportement sexuel chez les épileptiques psychomoteurs. *Ann méd psychol, 112*:657-696, 1954.

———, and Gastaut, Y.: Etude électroencéphalographique des syncopes. *Rev neurol* (Paris), *95*:420-421, 547-549, 1956.

———, and Roger, A.: Origine et propagation des décharges épileptiques temporales provoquées. In T. Alajouanine (Ed.): *Les grandes activités du lobe temporal.* Paris, Masson, pp. 83-134, 1955.

———; Morin, G., and Lesevre, N.: Etude du comportement des épileptiques psychomoteurs dans l'intervalle de leurs crises. *Ann méd psychol,* 1955, *I*:1-27.

———, and Gastaut, Y.: Syncopes et convulsions. A propos de la nature syncopale de certaines spasmes du sanglot et des certaines convulsions essentielles hyperthermiques ou à froid. *Rev Neurol* (Paris), *96*:158-163, 1957.

———; Naquet, R., and Fischer-Williams, M.: The pathophysiology of grand mal seizures generalized from the start. *J nerv ment Dis, 127*:21-33, 1958.

———; Regis, H.; Bostem, J., and Beaussart, M.: A propos des crises survenant au cours des spectacles télévisés et de leur mécanisme. *Presse med, 69*:1581-1583, 1961.

———; Roger, J.; Faidherbe, J.; Ouahchi, S., and Franck, G.: Non-Jacksonian hemiconvulsive seizures. One-sided generalized epilepsy. *Epilepsia, 3*:56-68, 1962.

———; Regis, H., and Bostem, F.: Attacks provoked by television and their mechanism. *Epilepsia, 3*:438-445, 1962.

———; Roger, J.; Ouahchi, S.; Timsit, M., and Broughton, R.: An electroclinical study of generalized epileptic seizures of tonic expression. *Epilepsia* (Amst.), *4*:15-44, 1963.

———; Caveness, W. F.; Landolt, H.; Lorentz de Haas, A. M.; McNaughton, F. L.; Magnus, O.; Merlis, J. K.; Pond, D. A.; Radermecker, J., and Storm van Leeuwen, W.: A proposed international classification of epileptic seizures. *Epilepsia, 5*:297-306, 1964.

———; Naquet, R.; Poiré, R., and Tassinari, C. A.: Treatment of status epilepticus with diazepam (Valium). *Epilepsia, 6*:167-182, 1965.

———, and Tassinari, C. A.: Triggering mechanisms in epilepsy. The electroclinical point of view. *Epilepsia, 7*:85-138, 1966.

———; Roger, J.; Soulayrol, R.; Tassinari, C. T.; Régis, H.; Dravet, C.; Bernard, R.; Pinsard, N., and Saint-Jean, M.: Childhood epileptic encephalopathy with diffuse slow spike-waves (otherwise known as "petit mal variant") or Lennox syndrome. *Epilepsia, 7*:139-179, 1966.

———; Rohmer, F.; Cossette, A., and Kurtz, D.: Introduction to the study of functional generalized epilepsies. In H. Gastaut; H. H. Jasper; J. Bancaud, and A. Waltregny (Ed.): *The physiopathogenesis of the epilepsies.* Springfield, Thomas, pp. 5-25, 1969.

———, and Broughton, R.: *Epileptic seizures.* Springfield, Thomas, 1972.

Gastaut, Y.: Un élément déroutant de sémeiologie électroencéphalographique: les pointes prérolandiques sans signification focale. *Rev Neurol* (Paris), *87*:488-490, 1952.

Geier, S.: A comparative Tele-EEG study of adolescent and adult epileptics. *Epilepsia, 12*:215-223, 1971.

Gellerman, G. L., and Martinez, C.: Fatal ventricular fibrillation following intravenous sodium diphenylhydantoin. *JAMA, 200*:337-338, 1967.

Gellhorn, E.: *Physiological foundations of Neurology and Psychiatry.* Minneapolis, University of Minnesota Press, 1953.

———, and Heymans, C.: Differential action of anoxia, asphyxia and carbon dioxide on normal and convulsive potentials. *J Neurophysiol, 11*:261-273, 1948.

Gibberd, F. B.: The prognosis of petit mal. *Brain, 89*:531-538, 1966.

Gibbs, C. J., Jr., and Gajdusek, D. C.: Infection as the etiology of spongiform encephalopathy (Creutzfeldt-Jakob disease). *Science, 165*:1023-1025, 1969.

Gibbs, E. L., and Gibbs, F. A.: Diagnostic and localizing value of electro-encephalographic studies in sleep. *Assn Res Nerv ment Dis, 26*:366-376, 1947.

———; Fuster, B., and Gibbs, F. A.: Peculiar low temporal localization of sleep-induced seizure discharges of psychomotor epilepsy. *Arch Neurol Psychiat, 60*:95-97, 1948.

Gibbs, F. A.: Differentiation of mid-temporal, anterior temporal and diencephalic epilepsy. In M. Baldwin, and P. Bailey (Ed.): *Temporal lobe epilepsy.* Springfield, Thomas, pp. 109-117, 1958.

———: Petit mal variant revisited. *Epilepsia* (Amst.), *12*:89-96, 1971.

———; Davis, H., and Lennox, W. G.: The electro-encephalogram in epilepsy and in conditions of impaired consciousness. *Arch Neurol Psychiat, 34*:1133-1148, 1935.

———; Lennox, W. G., and Gibbs, E. L.: The electro-encephalogram in diagnosis and in localization of epileptic seizures. *Arch Neurol Psychiat 36*:1225-1235, 1936.

———; Gibbs, D. L., and Lennox, W. G.: The influence of the blood sugar level on the wave and spike formation in petit mal epilepsy. *Arch Neurol Psychiat, 47*:1111-1116, 1939.

———; Everett, G. M., and Richards, R. K.: Phenurone in epilepsy. *Dis Nerv Syst, 10*:245-248, 1949.

———, and Gibbs, E. L.: *Atlas of electroencephalography,* 2nd ed. (Vol. 2). Cambridge (Mass.), Addison-Wesley, 1952.

———, and Stamps, F. W.: *Epilepsy Handbook.* Springfield, Thomas, 1958.

———, and Gibbs, E. L.: *Atlas of electroencephalography.* 2nd ed. (Vol. 3). Reading, Addison-Wesley, 1964.

———, and Anderson, E. M.: Treatment of hypsarrhythmia and infantile spasms with a librium analogue. *Neurology* (Minneap), *15*:1173-1176, 1965.

Glaser, G. H.: Diphenylhydantoin, Toxicity. In D. M. Woodbury; J. K. Penry, and R. P. Schmidt (Ed.): *Antiepileptic drugs.* New York, Raven Press, pp. 219-226, 1972.

Gloor, P.: Generalized cortico-reticular epilepsies. Some considerations on the pathophysiology of generalized bilaterally synchronous spike and wave discharge. *Epilepsia,* 9:249-263, 1968.

———: Neurophysiological bases of generalized seizures termed centrencephalic. In H. Gastaut; H. H. Jasper; J. Bancaud, and A. Waltregny (Ed.): *The physiopathogenesis of the epilepsies.* Springfield, Thomas, pp. 209-236, 1969.

Goldensohn, E. S.; Hardie, J., and Borea, E. D.: Ethosuximide in the treatment of epilepsy. *JAMA, 180*:840-842, 1962.

———, and Purpura, D. P.: Intracellular potentials of cortical neurons during focal epileptogenic discharges. *Science, 139*:840-842, 1963.

Goldschlager, A. W., and Karliner, J. S.: Ventricular standstill after intravenous diphenylhydantoin. *Amer Heart J, 74*:410-412, 1967.

Golla, F. L., and Winter, A. L.: Analysis of cerebral responses to flicker in patients complaining of episodic headache. *Electroenceph Clin Neurophaysiol, 11*:539-549, 1959.

Goodman, L. S.; Swinyard, E. A.; Brown, W. C.; Schiffman, D. O.; Grewal, M. S., and Bliss, E. L.: Anticonvulsant properties of 5-phenyl-5-ethylhexahydropyrimidone 4, 6-dione (Mysoline®), a new antiepileptic. *J Pharmacol Exp Ther, 108*:428-436, 1953.

Gordon, N.: The use of Ospolot in the treatment of epilepsy. *Epilepsia 5*:68-73, 1964.

Gowers, W. R.: *The borderland of epilepsy.* London, Churchill, 1907.

Graham, J. R.: *Treatment of Migraine.* Boston, Little, Brown and Co., 1955.

Green, J. D., and Shimamoto, T.: Hippocampal seizures and their propagation. *Arch Neurol, 70*:687-702, 1953.

———, and Adey, W. R.: Electrophysiological studies of hippocampal connections and excitability. *Electroenceph Clin Neurophysiol, 8*:245-262, 1956.

Green, J. R.: Temporal lobectomy with special reference to selection of epileptic patients. *J Neurosurg, 26*:584-593, 1967.

———; Duisberg, R. E. H., and McGrath, W. B.: Electrocorticography in psychomotor epilepsy. *Electroenceph Clin Neurophysiol, 3*:293-299, 1951.

Green, J. R., and Kupferberg, H. J.: Sulfonamides and derivatives. Sulthiame. In D. M. Woodbury; K. J. Penry, and R. P. Schmidt: *Antiepileptic drugs.* New York, Raven Press, pp. 477-485, 1972.

Groh, C., and Blankenhorn, V.: Weitere Mitteilungen über die klinische Wirksamkeit von Clonazepam. In R. Kruse (Ed.): *Epilepsie.* Stuttgart, Thieme, pp. 37-39, 1971.

Gross, H., and Kaltenbäck, E.: Benzodiazepine derivatives in the treatment of epilepsy. *Helv Med Acta, 30*:660-661, 1963.

Guerrero-Figueroa, R.; Barros, A.; DeBalbian Verster, H., and Heath, R. G.: Experimental "Petit mal," in kittens. *Arch Neurol, 9*:297-306, 1963.

Guillaume, J.; Mazars, G., and Mazars, Y.: Chirurgie de l'épilepsie non inhibited by patterned vision. *Arch Neurol, 13*:363-368, 1965.

Guiot, G., and Brion, S.: Traitement des mouvements anormaux par la coagulation pallidale. Technique et résultats. *Rev Neurol* (Paris), *89*:578-580, 1953.

Gumnit, R. J.; Niedermeyer, E., and Spreen, O.: Seizure activity uniquely inhibited by patterned vision. *Arch Neurol* (Chic.), *13*:363-368, 1965.

Haberland, C.: Cerebellar degeneration with clinical manifestation in chronic epileptic patients. *Psychiat Neurol* (Basel), *143*:29-44, 1962.

Haerer, A. F.; Buchanan, R. A., and Wiygul, F. M.: Ethosuximide blood levels in epileptics. *J Clin Pharmacol, 10*:370-374, 1970.

Hagen, R., and Richter, R.: Therapeutische Erfahrungen mit einem neuartigen Antiepilepticum bei Kindern und Jugendlichen. *Nervenarzt, 35*:312-314, 1964.

Halliday, A. M.: The electrophysiological study of myoclonus in man. *Brain, 86*:241-284, 1967.

Hamori, J., and Szentagothai, J.: Participation of Golgi neurone processes in the cerebellar glomeruli: An electron microscope study. *Exp Brain Res, 2*:35-48, 1966.

Handley, R., and Stewart, A. R. S.: Mysoline®: A new drug in the treatment of epilepsy. *Lancet, 1*:742-744, 1952.

Hann, J.: Petit mal Anfälle bei hypothalamisch bedingter Pubertas praecox. *Proc First Internat Congr Neurol Sci, Brussels,* 1957, Vol. 3, London, Pergamon, pp. 701-704, 1959.

———, and Franke, H.: The electroencephalogram in patients with hypersensitive carotid-sinus syndrome of cardiac type with prolonged cessation of the heart beat. *Electroencephalogr Clin Neurophysiol, 3*:50, 1953 (abstract).

Harriman, D. G. F., and Millar, J. H. D.: Progressive familial myoclonic epilepsy in three families: its clinical features and pathological basis. *Brain, 78*:325-349, 1955.

Hartman, F., and DiGaspero, H.: Epilepsie. In M. Lewandowsky (Ed.): *Handbuch der Neurologie.* Vol. 5. Berlin, Springer, pp. 832-931, 1914.

Hauptmann, A.: Luminal bei Epilepsie. *München med Wschr, 59*:1907-1918, 1912.

Haymaker, W.; Pentschew, A.; Margoles, C., and Bingham, W. G.: Occurrence of lesions in the temporal lobe in the absence of convulsive seizures. In M. Baldwin and P. Bailey (Ed.): *Temporal lobe epilepsy.* Springfield, Thomas, pp. 166-202, 1958.

Hayne, R. A.; Belinson, L., and Gibbs, F. A.: Electrical activity of subcortical areas in epilepsy. *Electroencephalogr Clin Neurophysiol, 1*:437-445, 1949.

Heath, R. G.: Common characteristics of epilepsy and schizophrenia, Clinical observations and depth electrode studies. *Amer J Psychiat, 118*:1013-1018, 1962.

Heron, J. R.: Migraine and cerebrovascular disease. *Neurology* (Minneap), *16*:1097-1104, 1966.

Herpin, T.: *Les accès incomplets d'épilepsie.* Paris, J. B. Baillière, 1867.

Hess, R.: Verlaufsuntersuchungen über Anfälle und EEG bei kindlichen Epilepsien. *Arch Psychiat Nervenkr, 197*:568-593, 1958.

———: Die epileptogenen Hirntumoren. In E. Niedermeyer (Ed.): *Epilepsy.* Basal, Karger, pp. 200-231, 1970.

Heyck, H.: *Neue Beitrage zur Klinik und Pathogenese der Migräne.* Stuttgart, Thieme, 1956.

Hill, D.: Clinical associations of electroencephalographic foci in the temporal lobe. *Arch Neurol Psychiat, 96*:379-381, 1953.

Hoefer, P. F. A.; Schlesinger, E. B., and Pennes, H. H.: Seizures in patients with brain tumors. *Res Assn Nerv ment Dis, 26*:50-58, 1947.

Hofmann, W. W.: Cerebellar lesions after parenteral Dilantin® administration. *Neurology* (Minneap), *8*:210-214, 1958.

Hooshmand, H.: Apneic seizures treated with atropine. Report of a case. *Neurology* (Minneap), *22*:1217-1221, 1972.

Hopf, H. C.; Stamatovic, A. M., and Wahren, W.: Die cerebralen Anfälle bei der multiplen Sklerose. *Z Neurol, 198*:256-279, 1970.

Houck, J. C.; Cheng, R. F., and Waters, M. D.: Diphenylhydantoin, Effects on connective tissue and wound repair. In D. M. Woodbury; J. K. Penry, and R. P. Schmidt: *Antiepileptic drugs.* New York, Raven Press, pp. 267-274, 1972.

Hughes, J. R.; Cayaffa, J. J.; Pruitt, B. A., Jr.; Boswich, J. A., Jr.; Bruck, H. M., and Borges, J.: "Post-ignitic epilepsy"-seizures following burns of the skin. Proc. Annual Meeting Amer. Epilepsy Soc., New York, N. Y., November 30, 1972.

Hunt, A. D., Jr.; Stokes, J., Jr.; McCrory, W. W., and Stroud, H.: Pyridoxine dependency: Report of a case of intractable convulsions infant controlled by pyridoxine. *Pediatrics, 13*:140-145, 1954.

Hunt, I. R.: On the occurrence of static seizures in epilepsy. *J nerv ment Dis, 56*:351-356, 1922.

Hunter, J., and Jasper, H. H.: Effects of thalamic stimulation in unaesthetized animals. *Electroencephalogr Clin Neurophysiol, 1*:305-324, 1949.

Hunter, R. A.: Status epilepticus. History, incidence and problems. *Epilepsia 1*:162-188, 1959/60.

Huttenlocher, R. R.; Wilbourn, A. J., and Signore, M. M.: Medium chain triglycerides as a therapy for intactable childhood epilepsy. *Neurology* (Minneap), *21*:1097-1103, 1972.

Ingvar, D. N.: Reproduction of the 3 per second spike and wave EEG pattern by Subcortical stimulation in cats. *Acta Physiol Scand, 33*:137-150, 1955.

———, and Lundberg, N.: Paroxysmal symptoms in intracranial hypertension. *Brain, 84*:446-459, 1961.

———, and Nyman, G. E.: Epilepsia arthmetices. A new psychological trigger mechanism in a case of epilepsy. *Neurology* (Minneap), *12*:282-287, 1962.

Isbell, H.; Altschul, S.; Kornetsky, C. H.; Eisenman, A. J.; Flanary, H. G., and Fraser, H. S.: Chronic barbiturate intoxication. An experimental study. *Arch Neurol Psychiat, 64*:1-28, 1950.

Isler, W., and Hess, R.: Verlaufsuntersuchungen über Anfälle und EEG bei fokalen Epilepsien im Kindesalter. *Arch Psychiat Nervenkr, 200*:257-266, 1960.

Itil, T. M.: Convulsive and anticonvulsive properties of neuro-psychopharmaca. In E. Niedermeyer (Ed.): *Epilepsy.* Basel, Karger, pp. 270-305, 1970.

Ito, M., and Yoshida, M.: The origin of cerebellar-induced inhibition of Deiters neurones. I. Monosynaptic initiation of the inhibitory postsynaptic potentials. *Exp Brain Res, 2*:330-349, 1966.

Jackson, J. H.: Clinical remarks on the occasional occurrence of subjective sensations of smell in patients who are liable to epileptiform seizures, or who have symptoms of mental derangement and in others. *Lancet, I*:659-660, 1866.

Jackson, J. H., and Beevor, C. E.: Case of tumour of the right temporal-sphenoidal lobe bearing on the localization of the sense of smell and on the interpretation of a particular variety of epilepsy. *Brain, 12*:346-357, 1889.

———, and Stewart, P.: Epileptic attacks with a warning of a crude sensation of smell and with the intellectual aura (dreamy state) in a patient who had symptoms pointing to gross organic disease of right temporo-sphenoidal lobe. *Brain, 22*:534-549, 1899.

Jacobs, J. C.: Systemic lupus erythematosus in childhood: Report of thirty-five cases, with discussion of seven apparently induced by anticonvulsive medication and of prognosis and treatment. *Pediatrics, 32*:257-264, 1963.

Jakob, A.: Über eigenartige Erkrankungen des Zentralnervensystems mit bemerkenswertem anatomischen Befunde (spastische Pseudosklerose, Encephalomyelopathie mit disseminierten Degenerationsherden). *Deutsch Z Nervenheilk, 70*:132, 1921 (quoted after W. R. Kirschbaum, 1968).

Janz, D.: "Aufwach"-Epilepsien. *Arch Psychiat Nervenkr, 191*:73-98, 1953.

———: "Diffuse" Epilepsien. *Deutsch Z Nervenheilk, 170*:486-513, 1953.

———: "Nacht"—oder "Schlaf"-Epilepsien. *Nervenarzt, 24*:361-367, 1953.

———: Status epilepticus und Stirnhirn. *Deutsch Z Nervenheilk, 180*: 562-594, 1690.

———: The grand mal epilepsies and the sleeping-waking cycle. *Epilepsia, 3*:69-109, 1962.

———: Differentialtypologie der idiopathischen Epilepsien. In H. Kranz (Ed.): *Psychopathologie heute*. Stuttgart, Thieme, pp. 176-194, 1962.

———: *Die Epilepsien*. Stuttgart, Thieme, 1969.

———, and Matthes, A.: Die Propulsiv Petit Mal Epilepsie. Basel, Karger, 1955.

Jasper, H. H.: Etude anatomo-physiologique des épilepsies. *Electroenceph Clin Neurophysiol, Suppl. No. 2*, pp. 99-111, 1949.

———: Functional subdivisions of the temporal region in relation to seizure patterns and subcortical connections. In M. Baldwin and P. Bailey (Ed.): *Temporal Lobe epilepsy*. Springfield, Thomas, pp. 40-57, 1958.

———: Some physiological mechanisms involved in epileptic automatisms. *Epilepsia* (Amst.), 5:1-20, 1964.

———: Mechanisms of propagation: Extracellular studies. In H. H. Jasper; A. A. Ward, Jr., and A. Pope (Ed.): *Basic mechanisms of the Epilepsies.* Boston, Little, Brown and Co., pp. 421-438, 1969.

———, and Kershman, J.: Electroencephalographic classification of the epilepsies. *Arch Neurol Psychiat* (Chic.), *45*:903-943, 1941.

———, and Droogleever-Fortuyn, J.: Experimental studies on the functional anatomy of petit mal epilepsy. *Assn Res Nerve Ment Dis, Proc, 26*:272-298, 1947.

———; Pertuiset, B., and Flanigin, H.: EEG and cortical electrograms in patients with temporal lobe seizures. *Arch Neurol Psychiat, 65*:272-290, 1951.

———, and Rasmussen, T.: Studies of clinical and electrical responses to deep temporal stimulation in man with some consideration of functional anatomy. *Assn Res Nerv Ment Dis, Proc, 36*:316-334, 1956.

Jeavons, P. M., and Bower, B. D.: *Infantile spasms. A review of the literature and a study of 112 cases.* London, Spastic cs Soc. Med. Education and Information Unit, in assoc. with W. Heinemann Med. Books, 1964.

Jennett, W. B.: *Epilepsy after blunt head injuries.* London, Heinemann, 1962.

Jinnai, D.: Clinical results and the significance of Forel-H-tomy for treatment of epilepsy. *Confin Neurol, 27*:129-136, 1966.

Jonas, A. D.: *Ictal and subictal neurosis.* Springfield, Thomas, 1965.

Jones, D. P., and Nevin, S.: Rapidly progressive cerebral degeneration (subacute vascular encephalopathy) with mental disorder, focal disturbances and myoclonic epilepsy. *J Neurol Neurosurg Psychiatry, 17*: 148-159, 1954.

Jongmans, J. W. M.: Report on the anti-epileptic action of Tegretol. *Epilepsia, 5*:74-82, 1964.

Jovanovic, U. J.: Das Schlafverhalten der Epileptiker. I. Schlafdauer, Schlaftiefe und Besonderheiten der Schlafperiodik. *Deutsch Z Nervenheilk, 190*:159-198, 1967.

Joynt, R. J., and Green, D.: Tonic seizures as a manifestation of multiple sclerosis. *Arch Neurol, 2*:293-299, 1962.

———; Green, D., and Green, R.: Musicogenic epilepsy. *JAMA, 179*: 601-504, 1962.

Jung, R.: Hirnelektrische Untersuchungen über den Elektrokrampf. Die Erregungsabläufe in corticalen und subcorticalen Hirnregionen bei Katze und Hund. *Arch Psychiat Nervenkr, 183*:206-244, 1949.

———, and Toennies, F.: Über Entstehung und Erhaltung von Krampfentladungen. Die Vorgänge im Reizort und die Krampffähigkeit des Gehirns. *Arch Psychiat Nervenkr, 185*:701-735, 1950.

Kalinowsky, L. B.: Convulsions in nonepileptic patients on withdrawal of Barbiturates, alcohol and other drugs. *Arch Neurol Psychiat, 48*:946-956, 1942.

Kalyanaraman, K.; Niedermeyer, E.; Rowe, R. ,and Wolf, K.: The electroencephalogram in congenital heart disease. *Arch Neurol, 18*:98-106, 1968.

Kandel, E. R.; Spencer, W. A., and Brinley, F. J.: Electrophysiology of hippocampal neurons. II. After-potentials and repetitive firing. *J Neurophysiol, 24*:225-242, 1961.

Keith, H. M.: Results of treatment of recurring convulsive attacks of epilepsy. *Amer J Dis Child, 74*:140-146, 1947.

Kellaway, P.: Infantile seizures: An electro-clinical study. Proc. Annual Meeting Amer. Epilepsy Soc., New York, N. Y., Dec. 2, 1971.

Kennedy, F.: Cerebral symptoms induced by angioneurotic edema. *Arch Neurol Psychiat, 15*:28-33, 1926.

———: Allergy and its effect on the central nervous system. *Arch Neurol Psychiat, 39*:1361-1372, 1938.

Kennedy, A. C.; Linton, A. L.; Luke, R. G., and Renfrew, S.: Electroencephalographic changes during hemodialysis. *Lancet*, 1963, *I*:408-411.

King, L. J.; Lowry, O. H.; Passoneau, J. V., and Venson, V.: Effects of convulsants on energy reserve in the cerebral cortex. *J Neurochem, 14*:599-611, 1967.

Kiorboe, E.; Paludan, J.; Trolle, E., and Overvad, E.: Zarontin (ethosuximide) in the treatment of petit mal and related disorders. *Epilepsia* 7:83-89, 1964.

Kirschbaum, W. R.: Zwei eigenartige Erkrankungen des Zentralnervensystems nach Art der spastischen Pseudosklerose (Jakob). *Z ges Neurol Psychiat, 92*:157, 1924. Quoted after W. R. Kirschbaum, 1968.

———: *Jakob-Creutzfeldt's disease*. New York, American Elsevier, 1968.

Klass, D. W., and Daly, D. A.: An unusual seizure induction mechanism (manugenic). *Electroencephalogr. Clin Neurophysiol, 12*:756, 1960 (abstract).

Klüver, H.: The temporal lobe syndrome. In M. Baldwin and P. Bailey (Ed.): *Temporal lobe epilepsy*. Springfield, Thomas, 1958, pp. 504-506.

Knapp, A.: *Die Geschwülste des rechten und linken Schläfenlappens*. Wiesbaden, Bergmann, 1905.

———: Die Tumoren des Schläfenlappens. *Arch Psychiat, 42*:226-240, 1918.

Kooi, K.; Guvener, A. M.; Tupper, C. J., and Bagchi, B. K.: Electroencephalographic patterns of the temporal region in normal adults. *Neurology* (Minneap), *14*:1029-1035, 1964.

———; Rajput, A. H., and DeJong, R. N.: Significance of the paroxysmal Electroencephalogram in the patient with migraine. *Proc. Sixth Int. Congr. Electroencephalogr. Clin. Neurophysiol.*, Vienna, pp. 263-266, 1965.

Koshevnikov: Eine besondere Form von Corticaler Epilepsie. *Neurol Centralbl, 14*:47-48, 1895.

Kretschmer, E.: *Medizinische Psychologie,* 11th ed. Stuttgart, Thieme, 1956.

Kristiansen, K.; Henriksen, S. F., and Ringkjob, R.: Traumatic epilepsy. Prophylaxis. In A. E. Walker; W. F. Caveness, and M. Critchley (Ed.): *The late effect of head injury.* Springfield, Thomas, 1969, pp. 261-276.

———; Kaada, B. R., and Henriksen, G. F.: Epilepsia partialis continua. *Epilepsia, 12*:263-267, 1971.

Kruse, R.: *Das myoklonisch-astatische Petit Mal.* Berlin, Springer, 1968.

———: Zusammenfassung und Diskussion der klinischen Erfahrungsberichte uber Clonazepam. In Kruse, R.: *Epilepsie.* Stuttgart, Thieme, pp. 40-46, 1971.

Krynauw, R. A.: Infantile hemiplegia treated by removing one cerebral hemisphere. *J Neurol Neurosurg Psychiatry, 13*:243-267, 1950.

Kubie, L. S.: Some implications for psychoanalysis of modern concepts of the organization of the brain. *Psychoanal Q, 22*:21-68, 1953.

Kugelberg, E., and Widén, L.: Epilepsia partialis continua. *Electroencephalogr. Clin Neurophysiol, 6*:503-506, 1954.

Kuhlo, W.: Katamnestische Untersuchungen zur Pyknolepsie. *Arch Psychiat Nervenkr, 207*:254-268, 1965.

Lafora, G. R., and Glueck, B.: Beitrag zur Histopathologie der myoklonischen Epilepsie. Z *ges Neurol Psychiat, 6*:1-14, 1911.

Lance, J. W., and Adams, R. D.: The syndrome of intention or action myoclonus as a sequel of hypoxic encephalopathy. *Brain, 86*:111-136, 1963.

Landolt, H.: Über Verstimmungen Dämmerzustande und schizophrene Zustandsbilder bei Epilepsie (Ergebnisse klinischer und elektroenzephalographischer Untersuchungen). Schweiz. *Arch Neurol Psychiat, 76*:313-321, 1955.

———: *Die Temporallappenepilepsie und ihre Psychopathologie.* Basal, Karger, 1960.

———: Die Dämmer-und Verstimmungszustande bei Epilepsie und ihre Elektrencephalographie. *Deutsch Z Nervenheilk, 185*:411-430, 1963.

Lange, J.: *Lehrbuch der Psychiatrie.* Leipzig, Thieme, 1936.

Lasater, G. M.: Reading epilepsy. *Neurology* (Minneap), *6*:492-495, 1962.

Ledermair, O., and Niedermeyer, E.: Posteklamptische Epilepsie. *Geburtsh Frauenheilk, 16*:679-685, 1956.

Leksell, L.: A stereotoxic apparatus for intracerebral surgery. *Acta chir scand, 99*:229-233, 1949.

Lennox, W. G.: The petit mal epilepsies; their treatment with Tridione. *JAMA, 129*:1069-1074, 1945.

———: *Epilepsy and related disorders,* Vol. 1. Boston, Little, Brown and Co., 1960.

Levy, L., and O'Leary, J. L.: Arrest of seizure activity. *Epilepsia, 6*:116-121, 1965.

Levy, L. L., and Fenichel, G. M.: Diphenylhydantoin activated seizures. *Neurology* (Minneap), *15*:716-722, 1965.

Lichtenstein, R. S.; Marshall, C., and Walker, A. E.: Subcortical recording in temporal lobe epilepsy. *Arch Neurol, 1*:288-302, 1959.

Lindenberg, R.: Compression of brain arteries as pathogenetic factor for tissue necrosis and their areas of predilection. *J Neuropathol Exp Neurol, 14*:223-243, 1955.

Liske, E., and Forster, F. M.: Clinical study of a new benxodiazepine as an anticonvulsant agent. *J new Drugs, 3*:241-244, 1963.

———, and Forster, F. M.: Pseudoseizures: a problem in the diagnosis and management of epileptic patients. *Neurology* (Minneap), *14*:41-49, 1964.

Livingston, S.: *The diagnosis and treatment of convulsive disorders in children.* Springfield, Thomas, 1954.

———: The use of Peganone (AC 695) in the treatment of epilepsy. *J Pediat, 49*:728-738, 1956.

———: *Living with epileptic seizures.* Springfield, Thomas, 1963.

———: *Comprehensive management of epilepsy in infancy, childhood and adolescence.* Springfield, Thomas, 1972.

———, and Pauli, L. L.: Celontin (PM-396) in the treatment of epilepsy. *Pediatrics, 19*:614-618, 1957.

———; ———, and Najmabadi, A.: Exhosuximide in the treatment of epilepsy. Preliminary report. *JAMA, 180*:822-825, 1962.

———; Torres, I.; Pauli, L. L., and Rider, R. V.: Petit mal epilepsy. Results of a prolonged follow-up study of 117 patients. *JAMA, 194*:227-232, 1965.

———; Villamater, C.; Sakata, Y., and Pauli, L. L.: Use of carbamazepine in epilepsy; results in 87 patients. *JAMA, 200*:116-120, 1967.

———; Villamater, C., and Sakata, Y.: Ospolot (sulthiame) in epilepsy: preliminary report. *Dis nerv syst, 28*:259-263, 1967.

———; Rodriguez, H.; Greene, C. A., and Pauli, L. L.: Systemic lupus erythematosus. Occurrence in association with ethosuximide therapy. *JAMA, 203*:731-732, 1968.

Locock, C.: Contribution as discussion of paper by E. H. Sieveking: Analysis of fifty-two cases of epilepsy observed by the author. *Lancet, 1*:527-528, 1857.

Lombroso, C. T.: Treatment of status epilepticus with diazepam. *Neurology* (Minneap), *17*:629-634, 1966.

———: Sylvian seizures and midtemporal spike foci in children. *Arch Neurol, 17*:52-59, 1967.

———; Davidson, D. T., Jr., and Grossi-Bianchi, M. L.: Further evaluation of acetazolamide (Diamox) in treatment of epilepsy. *JAMA, 160*:268-272, 1956.

———, and Lerman, P.: Breathholding spells (cyanotic and pallid Infantile syncope). *Pediatrics, 39*:563-581, 1967.

Lorentz de Haas, A. M., and Stoel, L. M. K.: Experiences with alpha-ethyl-alpha-methyl-succinimide in the treatment of epilepsy. *Epilepsia, 1*:501-511, 1959/60.

Lorgé, M.: Über ein neuartiges Antiepilepticum der Iminostilbenreihe (G 32883). Proc. Third Congress Internat. Coll. Neuropsychopharmacol., Munich, Sept. 1962.

Lorgé, M.: Klinische Erfahrungen mit einem neuen Antiepilepticum Tegretol® (G 32883) mit besonderer Wirkung auf die epileptische Wesensveränderung. *Schweiz med Wschr, 93*:1042-1047, 1963.

Loscalzo, A. E.: Treatment of epileptic patients with a combination of 3-methyl-5-ethyl-5-phenyl hydantoin (Masantoin) and phenobarbital (preliminary report). *J nerv ment Dis, 101*:537-544, 1945.

Lossius, H. M.: Experience with a new anti-convulsant of the succimide group, Zarontin. *Acta psychiat scand, 36 (Suppl. 150)*:200-208, 1961.

Low, N. L.; Gibbs, E. L., and Gibbs, F. A.: Electroencephalographic findings in breath holding spells. *Pediatrics, 15*:595-599, 1955.

Lowe, C. U.; Terrey, M., and MacLachlan, B. A.: Organic-Aciduria, decreased renal ammonia production, hydrophthalmos and mental retardation. *Amer J Dis Child, 83*:164, 1952.

Lugaresi, E., and Volterra, V.: Prime osservazioni su un nuovo farmaco control il "piccolo male": il PM 671 o Zarontin. *Clinica Pediatrica* (Bologna), *42*:947-956, 1960.

———; Pazzaglia, P., and Tassinari, C. A.: Differentiation of "absence status" and "temporal lobe status." *Epilepsia, 12*:77-87, 1971.

Lukash, W. M.; Sawyer, G., and Davis, J.: Micturition syncope produced by orthostasis and bladder distension. *New Engl J Med, 270*:341-344, 1964.

Lundborg, H.: *Die progressive Myoklonus-Epilepsie (Unverricht's Myoklonie)*. Upsala, Almqvist, 1903.

Lyle, C.; Monroe, J.; Flinn, D., and Lamb, L.: Micturition syncope. *New Engl J Med, 265*:982-986, 1961.

MacLean, P. D.: Some psychiatric implications of physiological studies on fronto temporal portion of limbic system (visceral brain). *Electroencephalogr Clin Neurophysiol, 4*:407-418, 1952.

———: The limbic system ("visceral brain") in relation to central gray and reticulum of the brain stem. Evidence of interdependence in emotional processes. *Psychosomat Med, 17*:355-366, 1955.

Madison, D. S., and Niedermeyer, E.: Epileptic seizures resulting from acute cerebral anoxia. *J Neurol Neurosurg Psychiat, 33*:381-386, 1970.

———, and ———: Considerations of "true" status epilepticus (grand mal). *Proc Ann Meet American EEG Soc*, Houston (Tex.), Oct. 1972.

Magnus, O.: Temporal lobe epilepsy. *Folia Psychiat Neurol Neurochir Neerland, 57*:264-297, 1954.

Malamud, N.: The epileptogenic focus in temporal lobe epilepsy from a pathological standpoint. *Arch Neurol, 14*:190-195, 1966.

Mann, L. B.; Bogen, J. E.; Vogel, P. J., and Saul, R.: Cerebral commissurotomy in man: EEG findings. *Electroencephalogr Clin Neurophysiol, 27*:660, 1969 (abstract).

Marcus, E. M.: Experimental models of petit mal epilepsy. In D. P. Purpura et al. (Ed.): *Experimental models of epilepsy—A manual for the laboratory worker.* New York, Raven Press, pp. 113-146, 1972.

———, and Watson, C. W.: Bilateral synchronous spike wave electroencephalographic patterns in the cat. Interaction of bilateral cortical foci in the intact, the bilateral cortical-callosal and a diencephalic preparation. *Arch Neurol, 14*:601-610, 1966.

———; ———, and Simon, S. A.: An experimental model of some varieties of petit mal epilepsy. Electrical-behavioral correlations of acute bilateral epileptogenic foci in cerebral cortex. *Epilepsia, 9*:233-248, 1968.

Markand, O. N., and Daly, D. D.: Pseudoperiodic lateralized paroxysmal discharges in electroencephalogram. *Neurology* (Minneap), *21*:975-981, 1971.

Markham, C. H.: The treatment of myoclonic seizures of infancy and childhood with L. A.-I. *Pediatrics, 34*:511-518, 1964.

Martin, D.: Pädiatrische Erfahrungen mit Clonazepam (Ro 5-4023). In R. Kruse (Ed.): *Epilepsia.* Sturtgart, Thieme, pp. 34-37, 1971.

Massa, T., and Niedermeyer, E.: Convulsive disorders during the first three months of life. *Epilepsia, 9*:1-19, 1968.

Matsumoto, H., and Ajmone Marsan, C.: Cortical cellular phenomena in experimental epilepsy. Ictal manifestations. *Exp Neurol, 9*:305-326, 1964.

Matthews, W. B.: Tonic seizures in disseminated sclerosis. *Brain, 81*:193-206, 1958.

———: Epilepsy and disseminated sclerosis. *Q J Med, 31*:144-155, 1962.

———, and Wright, F. K.: Hereditary primary reading epilepsy. *Neurology* (Minneap), *17*:919-921, 1967.

Maynert, E. W.: Phenobarbital, mephobarbital, matharbital. Biotransformation. In D. M. Woodbury; J. K. Penry, and R. P. Schmidt (Ed.): *Antiepileptic drugs.* New York, Raven Press, pp. 311-317, 1972.

Mazars, G.: Cingulate gyrus epileptogenic foci as an origin for generalized seizures. In H. Gestaut; H. H. Jasper; J. Bancaud, and A. Waltregny (Ed.): *The physiopathogenesis of the Epilepsies.* Springfield, Thomas, pp. 186-189, 1969.

———: Criteria for identifying cingulate epilepsies. *Epilepsia, 11*:41-47, 1970.

Mazars, Y.; Mazars, G.; Gotusso, C., and Merienne, L.: Place de l'épilepsie cingulaire dans le cadre des épilepsies focales. *Rev Neurol* (Paris), *114*:215-217, 1966.

McGeachy, T. E., and Bloomer, W. E.: The phenobarbital sensitivity syndrome. *Am J Med, 14*:600-604, 1953.

McKusick, V. A.: *Mendelian inheritance in man. Catalogs of autosomal dominant, autosomal recessive and x-linked phenotypes.* Baltimore, Johns Hopkins Press, 1966.

Meduna, L. J.: 1933, quoted after W. Sargent and E. Slater: An introduction to physical methods of treatment in Psychiatry. Edinburgh, Livingston, 1948, see p. 55. See also Meduna, L. J., and Friedman, E.: The convulsive irritative therapy of the psychoses, *JAMA, 112*:6, 1939.

Merlis, S.: Diamox: A carbonic anhydrase inhibitor; its use in epilepsy. *Neurology* (Minneap), *4*:863-868, 1954.

Merlis, J. K.: Proposal for an international classification of the epilepsies. *Epilepsia* (Amst.), *11*:114-119, 1970.

Merritt, H. H., and Putnam, T. J.: Sodium diphenyl hydantoinate in the treatment of convulsive disorders. *JAMA, 111*:1068-1073, 1938.

Metrakos, J. D., and Metrakos, K.: Genetics of convulsive disorders. Introduction to problems, methods and baselines. *Neurology* (Minneap), *10*:228-240, 1960.

———, and ———: Genetic factors in epilepsy. In E. Niedermeyer (Ed.): *Epilepsy.* Basel, Karger, pp. 71-86, 1970.

——— and ———: Genetics of convulsive disorders. II. Genetics and electroencephalographic studies in centrencephalic epilepsy. *Neurology* (Minneap), *11*:474-483, 1961.

Meyer, J. S., and Portnoy, H. D.: Post-epileptic paralysis. A clinical and experimental study. *Brain, 82*:162-185, 1959.

Meyers, R.: The modification of alternating tremors, rigidity and festination by surgery of the basal ganglia. *Res Publ Assn Nerv ment Dis, 21*:602-665, 1942.

Miller, C. A., and Long, L. M.: Anticonvulsants. I. An investigation of N-R-alpha-R_1-alpha-phenylsuccinimides. *J Am Chem Soc, 73*:4895-4898, 1951.

———, and ———: Anticonvulsants. IV. An investigation of alpha-(substituted phenyl)-succinimides. *J Am Chem Soc, 75*:6256-6258, 1953.

Millichap, J. G.: Other hydantoins. Mephenytoin, Ethotoin and Albutoin. In D. M. Woodbury; J. K. Penry, and R. P. Schmidt (Ed.): *Antiepileptic drugs.* New York, Raven Press, pp. 275-281, 1972.

———; Woodbury, D. M., and Goodman, L. S.: Mechanism of the anticonvulsant action of acetazolamide, a carbonic anhydrase inhibitor. *J Pharmacol, 115*:251-258, 1955.

———; Madsen, J. A., and Aledort, L. M.: Studies in febrile seizures. V. Clinical and electroencephalographic study in unselected patients. *Neurology* (Minneap), *10*:643-653, 1960.

———; Bickford, R. G.; Miller, R. H., and Backus, R. E.: The electroencephalogram in children with intracranial tumors and seizures. *Neurology* (Minneap), *12*:329-336, 1962.

Milner, B.; Branch, C., and Rasmussen, T.: Study of short-term memory after intracarotid injection of sodium amytal. *Trans Amer Neurol Assoc, 87*:224-226, 1962.

Minkowska, F.: Recherches généalogiques et problèmes touchant aux caractères, en particulier à celui de l'épileptoidie. *Ann Med Psychol, 81*:149-170, 1923.

Minkowski, A., and Sainte Anne-Dargassies, S.: Les convulsions du nouveau-né. *Evolut Psychiat, 1*:279-289, 1956.

Mitchell, W.; Falconer, M., and Hill, D.: Epilepsy with fetishism relieved by temporal lobectomy. *Lancet, II*:626-630, 1954.

Moniz, E.; Loff, R., and Pacheo, L.: Sur le diagnostic de la cysticercose cérébrale: à propos de deux cas. *Encéphale, 27*:42-52, 1932.

Monnier, M.: La stimulation électrique du thalamus chez l'homme. *Rev neurol* (Paris), *93*:267-277, 1955.

Moore, M. T.: Paroxysmal abdominal pain. A form of symptomatic epilepsy. *JAMA, 129*:1233-1240, 1945.

Morison, R. S., and Dempsey, E. W.: A study of thalamo-cortical relations. *Amer J Physiol, 135*:281-292, 1942.

Morrell, F.: Secondary epileptogenic lesions. *Epilepsia, 1*:538-560, 1959/60. 560, 1959/60.

———: Physiology and histochemistry of the mirror focus. In H. H. Jasper; A. A. Ward, Jr., and A. Pope (Ed.): *Basic mechanisms of the epilepsies.* Boston, Little, Brown and Co., pp. 357-370, 1969.

———; Bradley, W., and Ptashne, M.: Effects of diphenylhydantoin on peripheral nerve. *Neurology* (Minneap), *8*:140-144, 1958.

Moruzzi, G., and Magoun, H. W.: Brain stem reticular formation and activation of the EEG. *Electroencephalogr Clin Neurophysiol, 1*:455-473, 1949.

Mullan, S.; Vailati, G.; Karasick, J., and Mailis, M.: Thalamic lesions for the control of epilepsy. A study of nine cases. *Arch Neurol, 16*:277-285, 1967.

Müller, H. A.: Ein neuartiges Antiepilepticum bei chronisch anstaltsbedürftigen Epileptikern. *Nervenarzt, 34*:463-464, 1963.

Mumenthaler, M., and Altermatt, T.: Zur Klinik der tonischen Hirnstammkrämpfe. *Schweiz Arch Neurol Neurochir Psychiat, 100*:70-87, 1967.

Naquet, R., and Bostem, F.: Etude electroencéphalographique des syncopes. *Electroencephalogr Clin Neurophysiol, 16*:140-152, 1964.

———; Soulayrol, R.; Dolce, G.; Tassinari, C. A.; Broughton, R., and Lob, H.: First attempts at treatment of experimental status epilepticus in animals and spontaneous status epilepticus in man with diazepam (Valium). *Electroencephalogr Clin Neurophysiol, 18*:427, 1965 (a) (abstract).

———; Franck, G., and Vigouroux, R.: Données nouvelles sur certaines décharges paroxystiques du carrefour pariéto-temporo-occipital, rencontrées chez l'homme. *Zbl Neurochir, 25*:153-180, 1965 (b).

———; Arfel, G.; Choux, M., and Dubois, D.: Etude expérimentale de l'embolie gazeuse par voie carotidienne chez le chat. *Electroencephalogr Clin Neurophysiol, 20*:181-196, 1966.

———, and Vigouroux, R. A.: Acute cerebral anoxia and syncopal attacks. In A. Rémond (Ed.): *Handbook of Electroencephalography and clinical Neurophysiology*. Vol. 14 A, Part A, pp. 68-71. Amsterdam, Elsevier, 1972.

Narabayashi, H., and Okuma, T.: *Brain and Nerve, 6*:157-161, 1954. Quoted by Walker, A. E., 1957.

———, and Uno, M.: Long range results of stereotaxic amygdalotomy for behaviour disorders. *Confin Neurol, 27*:168-171, 1966.

Nelson, D. A., and Ray, C. D.: Respiratory arrest from seizure discharges in limbic system. *Arch Neurol, 19*:199-207, 1968.

Newnham, W.: *History of four cases of eclampsia nutans, or the "salaam"-convulsions of infancy, with suggestions as to its origin and future treatment*. Manchester, Irwin, 1849.

Niedermeyer, E.: Kasuistischer Beitrag zur Epilepsia partialis continua mit EEG-Untersuchung. *Deutsch Z Nervenheilk, 171*:482-489, 1954.

———: EEG-Untersuchungen bei suizidalem Erhängen. *Wien klin Wschr, 68*:555-556, 1956.

———: Motorische Herdepilepsie bei Thalamus-Syndrom (Kasuistische Mitteilung zur Frage der "diencephalen Jackson-Epilepsie"). *Wien klin Wschr, 69*:702-705, 1957.

———: Ein Fall von Status epilepticus, durch Tracheotomie und Sauerstoffbeatmung geheilt. Electroencephalographische und pathophysiologische Erwägungen. *Wien klin Wschr, 71*:530-533, 1959.

———: Remarques à propos de la physiopathologie de l'état de mal. *Rev Neurol* (Paris), *102*:681-684, 1960.

———: Cerebrovaculäre Altersveränderungen als Epilepsieursache. *Acta neurochir, Suppl VII*:201-206, 1961.

———: Sleep electroencephalograms in petit mal. *Arch Neurol, 12*:625-630, 1965.

———: The generalized multiple spike discharge. An electro-clinical study. *Electroencephalogr Clin Neurophysiol, 20*:133-138, 1966 (a).

———: Generalized seizure discharges and possible precipitating mechanisms. *Epilepsia* (Amst.), *7*:23-29, 1966 (b).

———: Considerations of the centrencephalic (generalized) type of epilepsy. *Delaw Med J, 38*:341-348, 1966 (c).

———: The Lennox-Gastaut syndrome: A severe type of childhood epilepsy. *Electroencephalogr Clin Neurophysiol, 24*:283, 1968 (abstract).

———: The Lennox-Gastaut syndrome: A severe type of childhood epilepsy. *Deutsch Z Nervenheilk, 195*:263-282, 1969.

———: Electroencephalographic studies on the anticonvulsive action of diazepam. *Europ Neurol, 3*:88-96, 1970 (a).

———: Common generalized epilepsy and generalized-synchronous seizure discharges. In E. Niedermeyer (Ed.): *Epilepsy*. Basal, Karger, 1970 (b), pp. 139-154.

———: Intravenous diazepam and its anticonvulsive action. *Johns Hopkins Med J, 127*:79-96, 1970 (c).

———: Spitzen über der Zentralregion und μ-Rhythmus: Gedanken zum Problem der "funktionellen" Spitzen. *Z EEG EMG, 1*:133-141, 1970 (d).

———: *The generalized epilepsies*. Springfield, Thomas, 1972.

———, and Hinchcliffe, R.: Vertigo and the electroencephalogram. *Electroencephalogr Clin Neurophysiol, 18*:78-81, 1965.

———, and Khalifeh, R.: Petit mal status. *Epilepsia, 6*:250-262, 1965.

———; McKusick, V. A.; Brunt, P., and Mahloudji, M.: The EEG in familial dysautonomia (Riley-Day syndrome). *Electroencephalogr Clin* familial dysautonomia (Riley-Day syndrome). *Electroenceph Clin Neurophysiol, 22*:473-475, 1967.

———; Laws, E. R., Jr., and Walker, A. E.: Depth EEG findings in epileptics with generalized spike-wave complexes. *Arch Neurol, 21*:51-58, 1969.

———; Walker, A. E., and Burton, C.: The slow spike-wave complex as a correlate of frontal and fronto-temporal post-traumatic epilepsy. *Europ Neurol, 3*:330-346, 1970 (a).

———; Blumer, D.; Holscher, E., and Walker, B. A.: Classical hysterical seizures facilitated by anticonvulsant toxicity. *Psychiat Clin, 3*:71-84, 1970 (b).

———, and Walker, A. E.: Mesio-frontal epilepsy. *Electroencephalogr Clin Neurophysiol, 31*:104-105, 1971 (abstract).

———; Gibbs, C. J., Jr.; Marsh, R., and Gajdusek, D. C.: EEG studies in subacute and degenerative neurological diseases experimentally produced in ferrets and chimpanzees. *Electroencephalogr Clin Neurophysiol, 33*:351-352, 1972 (abstract).

———, and Rocca, U.: The diagnostic significance of sleep electroencephalograms in temporal lobe epilepsy. *Europ Neurol, 7*:119-129, 1972.

Niemeyer, P.: The transventricular amygdala-hippocampectomy in temporal lobe epilepsy. In M. Baldwin, and P. Bailey (Ed.): *Temporal lobe epilepsy*. Springfield, Thomas, 1958, pp. 461-482.

Noell, W.: Überlebens–und Wiederbelebenszeiten des Gehirns bei Anoxie. *Arch Psychiat Nervenkr, 180*:687-712, 1948.

———, and Kornmüller, A. E.: Zur Sauerstoffmangelwirkung auf die Hirnrinde. Eine bioelektrische Untersuchung. *Pflügers Arch ges Physiol, 247*:685-712, 1944.

Obrador, S.: Personal experience in the surgical treatment of epilepsy. *J Neurosurg, 10*:52-63, 1953.

Obrist, W. D.: The electroencephalogram of normal aged adults. *Electroencephalogr Clin Neurophysiol, 6*:235-244, 1954.

Okuma, T.; Llimas, R., and Ervin, F. R.: Effect of mesencephalic reticular formation lesions on eplieptic seizure threshold. *Electroencephalogr Clin Neurophysiol, 13*:304-305, 1961.

Olds, J.: Selective effects of drives and drugs on "reward" systems of the brain. In G. E. W. Wolstenholme and C. M. O'Connor (Ed.): *Ciba Foundation Symposium on the Neurological Basis of Behaviour.* London, Churchill, pp. 124-141, 1958.

Orkand, R. K.: Neuroglial-neuronal interactions. In H. H. Jasper; A. A. Ward, Jr., and A. Pope (Ed.): *Basic mechanisms of the epilepsies.* Boston, Little, Brown and Co., pp. 737-746, 1969.

Osler, W.: The cerebral palsies of children. *Med News* (N.Y.), *53*:57, 1888.

Paal, G.: Katamnestische Untersuchungen und EEG bei Pyknolepsie. *Arch Psychiat Nervenkr, 196*:48-62, 1957.

Paillas, J. E.: Aspects cliniques de l'épilepsie temporale. Constatations faites sur une serie de 50 malades operés. In P. Bailey and M. Baldwin (Ed.): *Temporal lobe epilepsy.* Springfield, Thomas, pp. 411-439, 1958.

———; Naquet, R.; Vigouroux, R., and Vigouroux, M.: Epilepsies en foyer d'origine traumatique ou infectieuse: résultats obtenus dans 64 cas traités par interventions corticales. *Rev Neurol* (Paris), *87*:604-607,

Pakesch, E.: Untersuchungen über ein neuartiges Antiepileptikum. *Wien med Wschr, 113*:794-796, 1963.
1952.

Pampiglione, G., and Lehovsky, M.: The evolution of EEG features in Tay-Sachs' disease and amaurotic family idiocy in 24 children. In P. Kellaway and I. Petersén (Ed.): *Clinical electroencephalography in children.* New York, Grune and Stratton, pp. 287-306, 1968.

Papez, J. W.: A proposed mechanism of emotion. *Arch Neurol, 38*:725-743, 1937.

Passouant, P., and Cadilhac, J.: Physiologie normale et pathologique de l'hippocampe. In T. Alajouanine (Ed.): *Grandes activités du rhinencéphale. II Physiologie et pathologie du rhinencéphale.* Paris, Masson, pp. 145-187, 1961.

Pearce, J.: *Migraine, Clinical features, mechanisms and management.* Springfield, Thomas, 1969.

Peiffer, J.: *Morphologische Aspekte der Epilepsien.* Berlin, Springer, 1963.

Penfield, W.: Diencephalic autonomic epilepsy. *Arch Neurol, 22*:358-374, 1929.

———: Intracerebral vascular nerves. *Arch Neurol, 27*:30-34, 1932.

———: Epilepsy and surgical therapy. *Arch Neurol, 36*:449-484, 1936.

———: The cererbal cortex in man, I. The cerebral cortex and consciousness. *Arch Neurol, 40*:417-442, 1938.

———: Epileptic automatism and the centrencephalic integrating system. *Assn Res nerve ment Dis, 30*:513-528, 1952.

———: Consciousness and centrencephalic organization. *Proc. First Internat. Congr. Neurol. Sci., Brussels, 1957. Reports and dicussions, Vol. 2.* Les Editions Acta Medica Belgica, Brussels, pp. 7-18, 1957.

———, and Gage, L.: Cerebral localization of epileptic manifestations. *Arch Neurol Psychiat* (Chic.), *30*:709-727, 1933.

———; Erickson, T. C., and Tarlov, I. M.: Relation of intra-cranial tumors and symptomatic epilepsy *A.rch Neurol, 44*:300-315, 1940.

———, and Erickson, T. C.: *Epilepsy and cerebral localization.* Springfield, Thomas, 1941.

———, and Steelman, H.: The treatment of focal epilepsy with cortical excision. *Ann Surg, 126*:740-762, 1947.

———, and Flanigin, H.: Surgical therapy of temporal lobe seizures. *Arch Neurol, 64*:491-500, 1950.

———, and Kristiansen, K.: *Epileptic seizure patterns.* Springfield, Thomas, 1951.

———, and Baldwin, M.: Temporal lobe seizures and the technic of subtotal temporal lobectomy. *Ann Surg, 136*:635-634, 1952.

———, and Jasper, H. H.: *Epilepsy and the functional anatomy of the human brain.* Boston, Little, Brown and Co., 1954.

———, and Paine, K.: Results of surgical treatment of epileptic seizures. *Canad med Assn J, 73*:515-531, 1955.

———, and Milner, B.: Memory deficit produced by bilateral lesions in the hippocampal zone. *Arch Neurol, 79*:475-497, 1958.

Perez-Borja, C.; Tassinari, C. A., and Swanson, A. G.: Paroxysmal choreoathetosis and seizures induced by movements (reflex epilepsy). *Epilepsia 8*:260-270, 1967.

Perlstein, M. A.: Gemonal® (5,5 diethyl 1-methyl barbituric acid); new drug for convulsive and related disorders. *Pediatrics, 5*:448-451, 1950.

———, and Andelman, M. B.: Tridione: its use in convulsive and related disorders. *J Pediat, 29*:20-40, 1946.

———, and Gibbs, F. A.: Clinical significance of electroencephalography in cases of cerebral paralysis. *Arch Neurol Psychiatry, 62*:682-685, 1949.

———; Gibbs, E. L., and Gibbs, F. A.: The electroencephalogram in infantile cerebral palsy. *Amer J Phys Med, 34*:477-496, 1955.

Peterman, M. G.: Treatment of convulsions in childhood. *Amer J Dis Child, 84*:409-415, 1952.

Petersén, I.; Sorbye, R.; Gelin, L. E.; Johansson, and Avellan, L.: EEG and burns. *Electroencephalogr clin Neurophysiol, 17*:210, 1964) (abstract).

Petsche, H.: Epileptischer Anfall und kortikale Neuronenpopulation. *Wien Z Nervenkeilk, 24*:46-55, 1968.

Pfleger, L.: Beobachtungen über Schrumpfung und Sklerose des Ammonshorns bei Epilepsie. *Allg Z Psychiat, 36*:359-380, 1880.

Phillips, C. G.: Intracellular records from Betz cells in the cat. *Q J Exp Physiol, 41*:58-69, 1956.

Plum, F.; Posner, J. B., and Troy, B.: Cerebral metabolic and circulatory responses to induced convulsions in animals. *Arch Neurol, 18*:1-13, 1968.

Poblete, R.; Ruben, R. J., and Walker, A. E.: Propagation of afterdischarge between temporal lobes. *J Neurophysiol, 22*:538-553, 1959.

Poiré, E.: Hypoglycemic epilepsy: Clinical, electrographic and biological study during induced hypoglycemia in man. In H. Gastaut; H. H. Jasper; J. Bancaud, and A. Waltregny (Ed.): *The physiopathogenesis of the epilepsies.* Springfield, Thomas, pp. 75-110, 1969.

Pollen, D. A.: Intracellular studies of cortical neurons during thalamic induced wave and spike. *Electroencephalogr Clin Neurophysiol, 17*:398-404, 1964.

———; Peret, P., and Reid, K. H.: Experimental bilateral wave and spike from thalamic stimulation in relation to level of arousal. *Electroencephalogr Clin Neurophysiol, 15*:1017-1028, 1963.

Pond, D. A.: The E.E.G. in Paediatrics. In J. D. N. Hill and G. Parr (Ed.): *Electroencephalography.* New York, Macmillan, pp. 207-231, 1963.

Pope, A.: Perspectives in Neuropathology. In H. H. Jasper; A. A. Ward, Jr., and A. Pope (Ed.): *Basic mechanisms of the epilepsies.* Boston, Little, Brown and Co., pp. 773-781, 1969.

Portnoy, B. A., and Herion, J. C.: Neurological manifestations of sickle cell disease. With a review of the literature and emphasis on the prevalence of hemiplegia. *Ann Int Med, 76*:643-652, 1972.

Pradhan, S. N., and Ajmone Marsan, C.: Chlorambucil toxicity and EEG "centrencephalic" patterns. *Epilepsia, 4*:1-14, 1963.

Prichard, J. S.: The character and significance of epileptic seizures in infancy. In P. Kellaway and I. Petersén (Ed.): *Neurological and electroencephalographic correlative studies in infancy.* New York, Grune and Stratton, pp. 273-285, 1964.

Prill, A.; Quellhorst, E., and Scheler, F.: Epilepsy: Clinical and electroencephalographic findings in patients with renal insufficiency. In H. Gastaut; H. H. Jaspe,; J. Bancaud, and A. Waltregny (Ed.): *The physiopathogenesis of the epilepsies.* Springfield, Thomas, pp. 60-68, 1969.

Prince, D. A.: Modification of focal cortical epileptiform discharge by afferent influences. *Epilepsia, 7*:181-201, 1966.

———: Cortical cellular activities during cyclically occurring interictal epileptiform discharges. *Electroencephalogr Clin Neurophysiol, 31*:469-484, 1971.

———, and Wilder, B. J.: Control mechanisms in cortical epileptogenic foci. *Arch Neurol, 16*:194-202, 1967.

Prior, P. F.; Maclaine, G. N.; Scott, D. F., and Laurance, B. M.: Tonic status epilepticus prepitated by intravenous diazepam in a child with petit mal status. *Epilepsia, 13*:467-472, 1972.

Purpura, D. P.: Relationship of seizures susceptibility to morphologic and physiologic properties of normal and abnormal immature cortex. In P. Kellaway and I. Petersén (Ed.): *Neurological and electroencephalographic correlative studies in infancy.* New York, Grune and Stratton, pp. 117-154, 1964.

———, and Grundfest, H.: Nature of dendritic potentials and synaptic mechanisms in cerebral cortex of cat. *Neurophysiol, 19*:573-595, 1956.

Rabe, F.: *Die Kombination hysterischer und epileptischer Anfälle.* Berlin, Springer, 1970.

Raffauf, H.-J.: Die Behandlung zerebraler Anfallsleiden mit Ospolot. *Deutsch med Wschr, 85*:2203-2207, 1960.

Rallison, M. L.; Carlisle, J. W.; Lee, R. E., Jr.; Vernier, R. L., and Good, R. A.: Lupus erythematosus and Stevens-Johnson syndrome. *Amer J Dis Child, 101*:725-738, 1961.

Randow, R.; Sonnichsen, N., and Schulz, H.: Epilepsie als Frühsymptom des Lupus erythematodes. *Derm Wschr, 151*:1283-1289, 1965.

Rasmussen, T.: Surgical therapy of frontal lobe epilepsy. *Epilepsia 4*:181-198, 1963.

———: The neurosurgical treatment of focal epilepsy. In E. Niedermeyer (Ed.): *Epilepsy.* Basal, Karger, pp. 306-325, 1970.

———, and Jasper, H. H.: Temporal lobe epilepsy: Indication for operation and surgical technique. In P. Bailey and M. Baldwin (Ed.): *Temporal lobe epilepsy.* Springfield, Thomas, pp. 440-460, 1958.

Reilly, R. H.; Killiam, K. F.; Jenney, E. H.; Marshall, W. H.; Tausig, T.; Apter, N .S., and Pfeiffer, C.: Convulsant effects of isoniazid. *JAMA, 152*:1317-1321, 1953.

Renshaw, B.: Influence of discharge of motorneurones upon excitation of neighboring motorneurones. *J Neurophysiol, 4*:167-183, 1941.

Ribstein, M., and Walter, M.: Convulsions du prémier mois. *Rev Neurol* (Paris), *99*:91-99, 1958.

Richards, R. K., and Everett, G. M.: Tridione®; A new anticonvulsant drug. *J Lab Clin Med, 31*:1330-1336, 1946.

Riechert, T., and Wolff, M.: Über ein neues Zielgerät zur intrakraniellen elektrischen Ableitung und Ausschaltung. *Arch Psychiat Nervenkr, 186*:225-230, 1951.

Rodin, E. A.: *The prognosis of patients with epilepsy.* Springfield, Thomas, 1968.

———: Grand mal seizures and visual evoked responses. In E. Niedermeyer (Ed.): *Epilepsy.* Basel, Karger, pp. 105-119, 1970.

———: Psychomotor epilepsy and aggression. Proc. Annual Meeting Amer. Epilepsy Soc., New York, N. Y., Nov. 30, 1972.

———; DeJong, R. N.; Waggoner, R. W., and Bagchi, B. K.: Relationship between certain forms of psychomotor epilepsy and "schizophrenia." *Arch Neurol Psychiat, 77*:449-463, 1957.

———; Gonzales, S.; Caldwell, D., and Laginess, D.: Photic evoked responses during induced epileptic seizures. *Epilepsia* (Amst.), 7:202-214, 1966.

———; Onuma, T.; Wasson, S.; Porzak, J., and Rodin, M.: Neurophysiological mechanisms involved in grand mal seizures induced by Metrazol and Megimide. *Electroencephalogr Clin Neurophysiol, 30*:62-72, 1971.

Rose, A. L., and Lombroso, C. T.: Neonatal seizure states. A study of clinical, pathological and electroencephalographic features in 137 full-term babies with a long-term follow-up. *Pediatrics, 45*:404-425, 1970.

Roseman, E.: Dilantin toxicity. A clinical and electroencephalographic study. *Neurology* (Minneap), *11*:912-921, 1961.

Rosen, H., and Walker, A. E.: Hypnotic studies of patients with convulsions. *Curr Psychiat Ther, 3*:138-149, 1963.

Rosenbaum, H. E.: Familial hemiplegic migraine. *Neurology* (Minneap), *10*:164-170, 1960.

Rossi, G. F.; Walter, R. D., and Crandall, P. H.: Generalized spike and wave discharge and non-specific thalamic nuclei. *Arch Neurol, 19*:174-183, 1968.

Rovit, R.; Gloor, P., and Rasmussen, T.: Intracarotid amobarbital in epilepsy. *Arch Neurol, 5*:606-625, 1961.

Rowbotham, S. F.: *Acute injuries of the head.* Edinburgh, Livingstone, 1964.

Ruttner, F.: Über den Elektrokrampf. Neurologische Beobachtungen. *Deutsch Z Nervenheilk, 157*:169-192, 1944.

Sager, O.; Chivu, V.; Moiseanu, M., and Bazilesco, S.: Le complexe "Pointeonde" obtenu chez les animaux decortiqués bilatéralement pendant l'accès convulsif metrazolique. *Proc First Internat Congr Neurol Sci, Brussels, Vol. 3, 1957.* London, Pergamon, pp. 111-120, 1959.

Samt, P.: Epileptische Irreseinformen. *Arch Psychiat Nervenheilk, 6*:110-216, 1876.

Sauer, H.: Über gehäufte kleine Anfälle bei Kindern (Pyknolepsie). *Mschr Psychiat Neurol, 40*:276-300, 1916.

Schadé, J. P.: On the contribution of neuroglia to the function of the cerebral cortex. In P. and I. Petersen (Ed.): *Neurological and electroencephalographic correlative studies in infancy.* New York, Grune and Stratton, pp. 37-51, 1964.

Scherman, R., and Abraham, K.: "Centrencephalic" electroencephalographic patterns in precocious puberty. *Electroencephalogr Clin Neurophysiol, 15*:559-567, 1963.

Schmidt, R. P.: Sequelae of febrile convulsions. *Med Clin N Amer, 42*:389-397, 1958.

———, and Wilder, B. J.: *Epilepsy*. Philadelphia, Davis, 1968.

Scholl, M. L.; Abbott, J. A., and Schwab, R. S.: Celontin—a new anticonvulsant. *Epilepsia, 1*:105-109, 1959/60.

Scholz, W.: *Die Krampfschädigungen des Gehirns*. Berlin, Springer, 1951.

Schröder, M.: Die Lokalisation der Ammonshornschädigung im arteriellen Grenzgebiet. *Inaug Diss Med Fac Unviers.* Munich (34 p.), 1962.

Schumacher, G. A., and Wolff, H. G.: Experimental studies on headache. *Arch Neurol Psychiat, 45*:199-214, 1941.

Schuman, S. H., and Miller, L. J.: Febrile convulsions in families. *Clin Pediat, 5*:604-608, 1966.

Schwade, E. D.; Richards, R. K., and Everett, G. M.: Peganone®, a new anticonvulsant drug. *Dis Nerv Syst, 17*:155-158, 1956.

Scollo-Lavizzari, G., and Hess, R.: Sensory precipitation of epileptic seizures. *Epilepsia, 8*:157-161, 1967.

Scott, D. F.; Groethuysen, U. C., and Bickford, R. G.: Lambda responses in the human electrencephalogram. *Neurology* (Minneap), *17*:770-781, 1967.

———; Moffett, A., and Swash, M.: Observations on the relation of migraine and epilepsy. An electroencephalographic, psychological and clinical study using oral tyramine. *Epilepsia, 13*:365-375, 1972.

Scott, J. S., and Masland, R. L.: Occurrence of "continuous symptoms" in epilepsy patients. *Neurology* (Minneap.), *3*:297-301, 1953.

Scoville, W. B.; Dunsmore, R. H.; Liberson, W. T.; Henry, C. E., and Pepe, A.: Observations on medial temporal lobotomy and uncotomy in the treatment of psychotic states. Preliminary review of 19 operative cases compared with 60 frontal lobotomy and undercutting cases. *Assn Res Nerv ment Dis Publ, 31*:347-369, 1953.

Serafetinides, E. A.: Psychiatric aspects of temporal lobe epilepsy. In E. Niedermeyer (Ed.): *Epilepsy*. Basel, Karger, pp. 155-169, 1970.

———, and Falconer, M. A.: The effects of temporal lobectomy in epileptic patients with psychosis. *J ment Sci, 108*:584-593, 1962.

———, and Falconer, M. A.: Speech disturbances in temporal lobe seizures. *Brain, 86*:333-346, 1963.

Servit, Z.: Phylogenetic development of susceptibility to and symptomatology of epileptic seizures. *Epilepsia, 1*:95, 1959/60.

———: Focal epileptic activity and its spread in the brain of lower vertebrates. A comparative electrophysiological study. *Epilepsia, 11*:227-240, 1970.

Shanzer, S.; April, R., and Atkin, A.: Seizures induced by eye deviation. *Arch Neurol, 13*:621-626, 1965.

Sherrington, C. S.: Decrebrate rigidity and reflex coordination of movements. *J Physiol* (Lond.), *22*:319-332, 1898.

Silfvenius, H.; Gloor, P., and Rasmussen, T.: Evaluation of insular ablation in surgical treatment of temporal lobe epilepsy. *Epilepsia, 5*:307-320, 1964.

Small, J. G.; Milstein, V., and Stevens, J. R.: Are psychomtor epileptics different? *Arch Neurol, 7*:187-194, 1962.

Sommer, W.: Erkrankungen des Ammonshornes als ätiologisches Moment der Epilepsie. *Arch Psychiat Nervenkrankh, 10*:631-675, 1880.

Sorel, L.: Action antiépileptique expérimentale et clinique du Zarontin. *Acta Neurol Belg, 60*:551-559, 1960.

———: L'épilepsie myokinétique grave de la prémière enfance avec pointeonde lente (Petit mal variant) et son tratement. *Rev Neurol* (Paris), *110*:215-223, 1964.

———, and Dusaucy-Bauloye, A.: A propos de 21 cas d'hypsarrhythmie de Gibbs; son traitement spectaculaire par l'ACTH. *Rev neurol* (Paris), *99*:136-138, 1958.

Speranski, A. D.: *A basis for the theory of medicine*. New York, International Publishers, 1935.

Spiegel, E. A., and Wycis, H. T.: Pallidothalamotomy in chorea. *Arch Neurol Psychiat, 64*:295-296, 1950.

———, and ———: *Stereoencephalotomy*. New York, Grune and Stratton, 1952.

Spielman, M. A.: Some analgesic agents derived from oxazolidine-2, 4-dione. *J Am Chem Soc, 66*:1244-1245, 1944.

Spielmeyer, W.: Über eine besondere Form von familiärer amaurotischer Idiotie. *Neurol Centralbl, 25*:51-55, 1906.

———: Die Pathogenese des epileptischen Krampfes. Histopathologischer Teil. *Z ges Neurol Psychiat, 109*:501-520, 1927.

———: Funktionelle Kreislaufstörungen und Epilepsie. *Z ges Neurol Psychiat, 148*:285-298, 1933.

Starzl, T. E.; Niemer, W. T.; Dell, M., and Forgrave, P. R.: Cortical and subcortical electrical activity in experimental seizures induced by Metrazol. *J Neuropath exp Neurol, 12*:262-276, 1953.

Stauder, K. H.: Epilepsie und Schläfenlappen. *Arch Psychiat Nervenkrankh, 104*:181-212, 1935.

———: *Konstitution und Wesensveränderung der Epileptiker*. Leipzig, Thieme, 1938.

Stefanis, C., and Japer, H. H.: Recurrent collateral inhibition in pyramidal tract neurons. *J Neurophysiol, 27*:855-877, 1964.

Steinmetz, E. F., and Vroom, F. Q.: Transient global amnesia. *Neurology* (Minneap.), *22*:1193-1200, 1972.

Stevens, H.: Reading epilepsy. *New Engl Med, 257*:165-170, 1957.

———: Allergy and epilepsy. *Epilepsia, 6*:205-216, 1965.

———: Paroxysmal choreoathetosis: A form of reflex epilepsy induced by movements. *Trans Amer Neurol Assn, 90*:92-93, 1965.

Stevens, J. R.; Kodama, H.; Lonsbury, B., and Mills, L.: Ultradian characteristics of spontaneous seizure discharges recorded by radio telemetry in man. *Electroencephalogr Clin Neurophysiol, 31*:313-325, 1971.

Stewart, L. F., and Dreifuss, F. E.: "Centrencephalic" seizure discharges in focal hemispheric lesions. *Arch Neurol, 17*:60-68, 1967.

Strauss, H.: Paroxysmal blindness. *Electroenceph Clin Neurophysiol, 15*:921, 1963. (Abstract).

Strömgren, E.: Om den ixothyme Psyke. *Hospitalstid, 79*:637-648, 1936.

Svennerholm, L.: The distribution of lipids in the human nervous system. *J Neurochem, 11*:839-853, 1964.

Svensmark, O.; Schiller, P. J., and Buchthal, F.: 5,5-Diphenylhydantoin (Dilantin®) Blood levels after oral or intravenous doses in man. *Acta Pharmacol Toxicol* (Koh.), *16*:331-346.

———, and Buchthal, F.: Diphenylhydantoin and phenobarbital. Serum levels in children. *Amer J Dis Child, 108*:62-67, 1964.

Takahashi, T.; Niedermeyer, E., and Knott, J. R.: The EEG in older and younger adult groups with convulsive disorder. *Epilepsia* (Amst.), *6*:24-32, 1965.

Talairach, J.; Hecaen, H.; David, M.; Monnier, M., and Ajuriaguerra, J.: Recherches sur la coagulation thérapeutique des structures sous-corticales chez l'homme. *Rev neurol* (Paris), *81*:4-24, 1949.

Tasaki, I.; Polley, E. H., and Orrego, F.: Action potentials from individual elements in cat geniculate and striate cortex. *J Neurophysiol, 17*:454-474, 1954.

Tassinari, C. A.; Dravet, C.; Roger, J.; Cano, J. P., and Gastaut, H.: Tonic status epilepticus precipitated by intravenous benzodiazepine in five patients with Lennox-Gastaut syndrome. *Epilepsia, 13*:421-435, 1972.

Temkin, O.: *The falling sickness.* 2nd ed. Baltimore, Johns Hopkins Press, 1971.

Terzian, H.: Abservations on the clinical symptomatology of bilateral partial or total removal of the temporal lobe in man. In P. Bailey and M. Baldwin (Ed.): *Temporal lobe epilepsy.* Springfield, Thomas, pp. 510-529, 1958.

Tharp, B. R.: Orbital frontal seizures. An unique electroencephalographic and clinical syndrome. *Epilepsia, 13*:627-642, 1972.

Titeca, J.: L'épilepsie musicogénique. Revue générale à propos d'un cas personnel suivi pendant quatorze ans. *Acta neurol Belg, 65*:598-648, 1965.

Toman, J. E. P.: Drugs effective in convulsive disorders. In L. S. Goodman and A. Giman (Ed.): *The pharmacological basis of therapeutics.* 3rd ed. New York, Macmillan, pp. 215-236, 1965.

Tower, D. B.: *Neurochemistry of epilepsy.* Springfield, Thomas, 1960.

———: Arrest of seizure activity. Biochemical aspects and pharmacology. *Epilepsie* (Amst.), *6*:141-155, 1965.

Trachtenberg, M. C., and Pollen, D. A.: Neuroglia: Biophysical properties and physiologic function. *Science, 167*:1248-1252, 1970.

Trolle, E., and Kiorboe, E.: Treatment of petit mal epilepsy with the new succinimides: PM 680 and Celontin. *Epilepsia, 1*:587-591, 1959/60.

Trouillas, P., and Courjon, J.: Epilepsy with multiple sclerosis. *Epilepsia* (Amst.), *13*:325-333, 1972.

Tükel, K., and Jasper, H. H.: The electroencephalogram in parasagittal lesions. *Electroencephalogr Clin Neurophysiol, 4*:481-494, 1952.

Tyler, H. R., and Clark, D. B.: Incidence of neurological complications in congenital heart disease. *Arch Neurol, 77*:17-22, 1957.

———, and ———: Loss of consciousness and convulsions with congenital heart disease. *Arch Neurol, 79*:506-510, 1958.

Udvarhelyi, G. B., and Walker, A. E.: Dissemination of acute focal seizures in the monkey. I. From cortical foci. *Arch Neurol, 12*:333-356, 1965.

Umbach, W.: *Elektrophysiologische und vegetative Phänomene bei stereotaktischen Operationen*. Berlin, Springer, 1966.

Unger, A. H., and Sklaroff, H. J.: Fatalities following intravenous use of sodium diphenylhydantoin for cardiac arrhythmias. Report of two cases. *JAMA, 200*:335-336, 1967.

Unverricht, H.: *Die Myoclonie*. Leipzig, Deuticke, 1891.

Utterback, R. A.: Parenchymatous cerebellar degeneration complicating diphyenylhydantoin (Dilantin®) therapy. *Arch Neurol, 80*:180-181, 1958.

Vahlquist, B., and Nylander, I.: Cyclic vomiting with recurring EEG changes and severe course. *Acta Paediat Sued, 43/Suppl. 100*:608-623, 1954.

Van Buren, J. H.: The abdominal aura. A study of abdominal sensations occurring in epilepsy and produced by depth stimulation. *Electroencephalogr Clin Neurophysiol, 15*:1-19, 1963.

Van Reeth, P. C.; Dierkens, J., and Luminet, D.: L'hypersexualité dans l'épilepsie et les tuumeurs du lobe temporal. *Acta neurol Belg, 2*:194-218, 1958.

Veith, G.: Die Residualepilepsie vom Standpunkt des Pathologen. *Nervenarzt, 30*:552-554, 1959.

Victor, M.: The role of alcohol in the production of seizures. In E. Niedermeyer (Ed.): *Epilepsy*. Basel, Karger, pp. 185-199, 1970.

———, and Brausch, J.: The role of abstinence in the genesis of alcohol epilepsy. *Epilepsia, 8*:1-20, 1967.

Vizioli, R.: A clinical and EEG survey on infantile and childhood epilepsy. *Epilepsia, 3*:1-13, 1962 (a).

———: The Italian contribution to the problem of reflex epilepsy. *Epilepsia, 3*:229-235, 1962 (b).

Vogt, C., and Vogt, O.: *Sitz und Wesen der Krankheiten im Lichte der topistischen Hirnforschung und des Variierens der Tiere*. Leipzig, Barth, 1937.

Vogt, H.: Über familiäre amaurotische Idiotie und verwandte Krankheitsbilder. *Mschr Psychiat Neurol, 18*:161, 1905. Quoted after G. Pampiglione and M. Lehovsky, 1968.

Völzke, E.; Doose, H., and Stephen, E.: The treatment of infantile spasms and hypsarhythmia with Mogadan. *Epilepsia, 8*:64-70, 1967.

Vossen, R.: Über die antikonvulsive Wirkung von Succinimiden. *Deutsch med Wschr, 83*:1227-1230, 1958.

Wada, J.: (A new method for the determination of the side of cerebral speech dominance—a preliminary report on the intracarotid injection of sodium amytal in man—in Japanese). *Med. Biol.* (*Tokyo*) (*Igaku to Seibutsaki*), *14*:221-222, 1949.

———, and Rasmussen, T.: Intracarotid injection of sodium amytal for the Cateratination of cerebral speech dominance: experimental and clinical observation. *J Neurosurg, 17*:266-282, 1960.

Waldinger, C., and Berg, R. B.: Signs of pyridoxine dependency manifest at birth in siblings. *Pediatrics, 32*:161-168, 1968.

Walker, A. E.: *Post-traumatic epilepsy*. Springfield, Thomas, 1949.

———: Electrocorticography in epilepsy. An appraisal. *Electroenceph Clin Neurophysiol, 2*:30-37, 1949.

———: Treatment of cortical epilepsy by cortical excision. *J Pediat, 38*:285-298, 1951.

———: Temporal lobectomy. *J Neurosurg, 6*:641-649, 1967.

———: The propagation of epileptic discharge. In E. Niedermeyer (Ed.): *Epilepsy*. Basel, Karger, 1970, pp. 13-28.

———; Marshall, C., and Beresford, E. N.: Electrocorticographic characteristics of the cerebrum in post-traumatic epilepsy. *Res Assn Nerv ment Dis Publ, 26*:502-512, 1947.

———; Lichtenstein, R. S., and Marshall, C.: A cortical analysis of electrocorticography in temporal lobe epilepsy. *Arch Neurol, 2*:172-182, 1960.

———, and Jablon, S.: *A Follow-up Study of Head Wounds in World War II*. Washington, D.C., V. A. Medical Monograph, Government Printing Office, 1961.

———, and Marshall, C.: The contribution of depth recording to clinical medicine. *Electroencephalogr Clin Neurophysiol, 16*:88-99, 1964.

———, and Udvarhelyi, S. B.: Dissemination of acute focal seizures in monkeys. II From subcortical foci. *Arch Neurol, 12*:357-380, 1965.

———, and Morello, G.: Experimental petit mal. *Trans Amer Neurol Assn*, pp. 57-61, 1967.

———, and Erculei, F.: Post-traumatic epilepsy 15 years later. *Epilepsia, 11*:17-26, 1970.

Wallis, W.; Kutt, H., and McDowell, F.: Intravenous diphenylhydantoin in treatment of acute repetitive seizures. *Neurology* (Minneap.), *18*: 513-525, 1968.

Walter, W. G.; Dovey, V. J., and Shipton, H.: Analysis of electrical responses of the human cortex to photic stimulation. *Nature, 158*:540-541, 1946.

Ward, A. A., Jr.: Decerebrate rigidity. *J Neurophysiol, 10*:89-103, 1947.

———: The epileptic neuron. *Epilepsia, 2*:7080, 1961.

Weber, R.: Musikogene Epilepsie. *Nervenarzt, 27*:337-340, 1956.

Weil, A. A.: EEG findings in a certain type of poychosomatic headache: dysrhythmic migraine. *Electroencephalogr Clni Neurophysiol, 4*:181-186, 1952.

Weinberg, W. A., and Harwell, U. L.: Diazepam (Valium) is myoclonic seizures. *Amer J Dis Child, 109*:123-127, 1965.

Weinmann, H.: Behandlung von Blitz-Nick-Salaam-Krämpfen mit Mogadan "Roche." *Munch med Wschr, 108*:727-730, 1966.

Weir, B.: Spikes-Wave from stimulation of the reticular core. *Arch Neurol, 11*:209-218, 1964.

———, and Sie, P .G.: Extracellular unit activity in cat during the spike-wave complex. *Epilepsia, 7*:30-43, 1966.

Weiss, J.; Capps, R. B.; Ferris, E. B., and Munro, D.: Syncope and convulsions due to a hyperactive carotid sinus reflex. *Arch Int Med, 38*:407-415, 1936.

Westmoreland, B. F., and Klass, D. W.: Studies of "small spikes" with depth electrography. *Epilepsia, 13*:346-347, 1972 (abstract).

Westrum, L. E.; White, L. E., Jr., and Ward, A. A., Jr.: Morphology of the experimental epileptic focus. *J Neurosurg, 21*:1033-1046, 1964.

White, J. C.: Epileptic nystagmus. *Epilepsia, 12*:157-164, 1971.

Whitty, C. W. M.: Familial hemiplegic migraine. *J Neurol Neurosurg Bychiat, 16*:172-177, 1953.

Wikler, A., and Essig, C. F.: Withdrawal seizures following chronic intoxication with barbiturates and other sedative drugs. In E. Niedermeyer (Ed.): *Epilepsy*. Basel, Karger, pp. 170-184, 1970.

Wilder, B. J.; Streiff, R. R., adn Hammer, R. H.: Diphenylhydantoin. Absorption, distribution and excretion: Clinical studies. In D. M. Woodbury, J. K. Penry and R. P. Schmidt: (Ed.): *Antiepileptic drugs.* New York, Raven Press, pp. 137-148, 1972.

Wilder, R. M.: The effect of Ketonuria on the course of epilepsy. *Mayo Clinic Bull, 2*:307, 1921.

Williams, D.: A study of thalamic and cortical rhythms in "petit mal." *.Brain, 76*:50-67, 1953.

———: The structure of emotions reflected in epileptic experiences. *Brain, 79*:29-67, 1956.

Withrow, C. D., and Woodbury, D. M.: Trimethadione and other oxazolidinediones. Absorption, distribution and excretion. In D. M. Woodbury; J. K. Penry, and R. P. Schmidt (Ed.): *Antiepileptic drugs.* New York, Raven press, pp. 389-394, 1972.

Wolff, H. G.: *Headache and other head pain.* New York, Oxford University Press, 1948.

Woodbury, D. M.: Effect of diphenylhydantoin on electrolytes and radiosdodium turnover in brain and other tissues of normal, hyponatremic and postictal rats. *J Pharmacol Exp Ther, 115*:74-95, 1955.

———: Mechanisms of action of anticonvulsants. In H. H. Jasper; A. A. Ward, Jr., and A. Pope (Ed.): *Basic mechanisms of the epilepsies.* Boston, Little, Brown and Co., pp. 647-681, 1969.

———, and Swinyard, E. A.: Diphenylthydantoin. Absorption, distribution and excretion. In D. M. Woodbury; J. K. Penry, and R. P. Schmidt (Ed.): *Antiepileptic drugs.* New York, Raven Press, pp. 113-126, 1972.

Woodbury, J. W.: Biophysics of nerve membrane. In H. H. Jasper; A. A. Ward, Jr., and A. Pope (Ed.): *Basic mechanisms of the epilepsies.* Boston, Little, Brown and Co., pp. 41-75, 1969.

Wulff, M. H.: The barbiturate withdrawal syndrome. A clinical and electroencephalographic study. *Electroenceph Clin Neurophysiol, Suppl., 14*: 173, 1959.

Yanagihara, T.: Distribution of diphenylhydantoin in the neuronal and glial fractions. In D. M. Woodbury; J. K. Penry, and R. P. Schmidt (Ed.): *Antiepileptic drugs.* New York, Raven Press, pp. 125-126, 1972.

Zellweger, H.: Die Krämpfe im Kindesalter. Basel, Schwabe, 1948.

Zimmerman, F. T.: Use of methylphenylsuccinimide in treatment of petit mal epilepsy. *Arch Neurol Pschiat* (Chic.), *66*:156-162, 1951.

Zimmerman, F. T., and Burgemeister, B. B.: Use of N-Methyl-alpha, alphamethylphenyl-succinimide in treatment of petit mal epilepsy. *Arch Neurol Psychiat* (Chic.), *72*:720-725, 1954.

Zimmerman, F. T., and Burgemeister, B. B.: A new drug for petit mal epilepsy. *Neurology* (Minneap.), *8*:769-775, 1958.

Zlotlow, M.: Primary reading epilepsy. *NY St J Med, 64*:2472-2474, 1964.

ADDITIONAL REFERENCES

Bickerstaff, E. R.: Basilar migraine. *Lancet, I*:15-17, 1961.

Courville, C. B.: Traumatic lesions of the temporal lobe as the essential cause psychomotor epilepsy. In Baldwin, M. and Bailey, P. (Eds.): *Temporal Lobe Epilepsy.* Springfield, Thomas, 1958, pp. 220-239.

Cossa, P. and Martin, P.: L'automatisme psychomoteur des epilepsies. *Rev Neurol, 84*:317-327, 1951.

Jouvet, M.: Mechanisms of the states of sleep. *Res Publ Assoc Res Nerv Ment Dis, 45*:86-126, 1967.

Koella, W. P.; Smythies, J. R.; Bull, D. M., and Levy, C. K.: Physiological fractionation of the effect of serotonin on evoked potentials. *Am J Physiol, 198*:205-212, 1960.

Kutt, H.: Diphenylhydantoin. Interactions with other drugs in man. In Woodbury, D. M., Penry, J. K. and Schmidt, R. P. (Eds.): *Antiepileptic Drugs.* New York, Raven Press, 1972, pp. 169-180.

Levy, L. L. and Fenichel, G. M.: Diphenylhydantoin activated seizures. *Neurology* (Minneap.), *15*:716-722, 1965.

Meinardi, H.: Carbamazepine. In Woodbury, D. M., Penry, J. K. and Schmidt, R. P. (Eds.): *Antiepileptic Drugs.* New York, Raven Press, 1972, pp. 487-496.

Passouant P., and Cadilhac, J.: Décharges épileptiques et sommeil. In Niedermeyer, E. (Ed.): *Epilepsy.* Basel, Karger, 1970, pp. 87-104.

Pujol, J. F.: The role of the nonoaminergic neurons in the sleep-waking cycle. In Chase, H. (Ed.): *The Sleeping Brain.* Perspectives in the Brain Sciences, Vol. pp. 147-150. Los Angeles, Brain Information Service/Brain Research Institute, U.C.L.A., 1972.

Reynolds, E. H., Chanarin, I., Milner, G. and Matthews, D. M.: Anticonvulsant therapy, folic acid and vitamin B-12 metabolism and mental symptoms. *Epilepsia* (Amst.), 7:261-270, 1966.

Rothballer, A. B.: The effect of phenylephrine, methamphetamine, cocaine and serotonin upon the adrenaline-sensitive component of the reticular activating system. *Electroenceph Clin Neurophysiol,* 9:409-417, 1957.

Schlichther, W., Bristow, M. E., Schultz, S. and Henderson, A. L.: Seizures occurring during intensive chlorpromazine therapy. *Canad Med Assn J,* *74*:364-366, 1956.

Tchicaloff, M., and Pennetti, F.: Résultats thérapeutiques d'un nouvel antiépileptique, le Tegretol. *Schweiz Med Wschr,* 93:1664-1666, 1963.

Wilson, S. K.: The epilepsies. In Bumke, O. and Foerster, O. (Eds.): *Handbuch der Neurologie,* Vol. 17. Berlin, Springer.

NAME INDEX

C

D

E

F

G

H

M

N

T

U

V

W

Y

Z

SUBJECT INDEX

B

C

D

E

F

G

H

I

J

K

L

N

O

P

U

V

W

Z